THE CHILD WITH CANCER

For Baillière Tindall

Senior Commissioning Editor: Inta Ozols
Project Development Manager: Karen Gilmour
Project Manager: Jane Shanks
Design Direction: George Ajayi

THE CHILD WITH CANCER:
Family-Centred Care in Practice

Edited by

Helen Langton RGN RSCN RCNT RNT BA(Hons)

Head of Child School, Faculty of Health and Social Care,
University of the West of England, Bristol

Foreword by

Anne Casey RSCN MSc

Editor, Lecturer and Adviser, Royal College of Nursing, UK

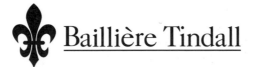 Baillière Tindall

Edinburgh • London • New York • Philadelphia • St Louis • Sydney • Toronto

BAILLIÈRE TINDALL
An imprint of Harcourt Publishers Limited

© Harcourt Publishers Limited 2000

 is a registered trademark of Harcourt Publishers Limited

The right of Helen Langton to be identified as editor of this work has been asserted by her in accordance with the Copyright, Designs and Patents Act 1988

First published 2000

0 7020 2300 0

British Library Cataloguing in Publication Data
A catalogue record for this book is available from the British Library

Library of Congress Cataloging in Publication Data
A catalog record for this book is available from the Library of Congress

Note
Medical knowledge is constantly changing. As new information becomes available, changes in treatment, procedures, equipment and the use of drugs become necessary. The editors, contributors and the publishers have, as far as it is possible, taken care to ensure that the information given in this text is accurate and up-to-date. However, readers are strongly advised to confirm that the information, especially with regard to drug usage, complies with the latest legislation and standards of practice.

Printed in China
NPCC/01

The publisher's policy is to use **paper manufactured from sustainable forests**

Contents

Experience of life as a potential cause of uncertainty about
 bone marrow transplantation
Information giving pre- bone marrow transplantation
Legal and ethical issues affecting families consenting to bone
 marrow transplantation and nurses involved in the
 families' preparation
Family and health care provider relationships and information
 giving in preparation for bone marrow transplantation
Bone marrow donation
The future of bone marrow transplantation
The hospitalised period
The post-discharge period
The interface between curative and palliative care for
 children undergoing bone marrow transplantation
Staffing issues
Conclusion

Introduction
Who are the survivors?
Issues affecting the successful normalisation process of the
 cancer experience

Contributors

Jane Bishop MSc BSc(Hons) BA(Hons) RGN RSCN CCN Community Children's Nurse, Child Health Services, London NHS Trust, North Hampshire Hospital, Basingstoke, Hampshire

Moira Bradwell RGN RSCN (ENB 870/998)
Paediatric Macmillan Nurse, Birmingham Children's Hospital NHS Trust, Birmingham

Susan Bulley RGN RSCN Dip ANC (ENB 240)
Paediatric Outreach Specialist Nurse, CLIC Domiciliary Nurse, Outreach Office 3, Derriford Hospital, Plymouth

Anita Jane Cox (nee Hall) RGN RSCN Dip (ANC) Paed Onc BSc(Hons)
Clinical Nurse Specialist Paediatric Oncology, Royal London Hospital, London

Sally Curnick RGN RSCN NDN PWT Dip Hum Psy
CLIC Domiciliary Nurse, Bristol Royal Hospital for Sick Children, Bristol

Rosemary Harding BSc(Hons) RSCN RGN RCNT DipN(Lond) Cert Ed(FE) (ENG 237/240/998)
Senior Lecturer (Child School), Faculty of Health and Social Care, University of the West of England, Bristol

Anne Harris RSCN RGN QSW
Sargent Team Leader, Bristol Children's Hospital, Bristol

Jeanette Hawkins RGN RSCN DipN (ENB 240/998)
Oncology/Haematology Day Care Manager, Oncology/Haematology Day Care, Birmingham Children's Hospital NHS Trust, Birmingham

Sarah Kirk RGN RSCN (ENB 240)
Senior Nurse, Ward 15, Birmingham Children's Hospital, Birmingham

Helen Langton RGN RSCN RCNT RNT BA(Hons)
Head of Child School, Faculty of Health and Social Care, University of the West of England, Bristol

Tracey Lawrance BSc(Hons) RGN RSCN Oncology Cert Bone Marrow
Transplantation Cert
Bone Marrow Transplant Co-ordination Sister, Birmingham
Children's Hospital NHS Trust, Birmingham

Alison Slade RGN RSCN (ENB 240)
Senior Staff Nurse, Haematology/Oncology, Great Ormond
Street Hospital for Children, London

Mervyn Townley RGN RMN Post-Reg Diploma (Children's Nursing) DipN
Dip Ned MA
Senior Lecturer, Child School, Faculty of Health and Social Care,
University of the West of England, Bristol

Stuart Welton RMN
Senior Nurse, The Riverside Adolescent Unit, Blackberry Hill
Hospital, Bristol

Kath Wilkinson-Carr RGN RN(Child) CM DMS FACTC
Sister, Paediatric Head Injury Unit, Royal National Hospital for
Rheumatic Diseases, Bath

Foreword

For each family the diagnosis of cancer or leukaemia in a child is the worst thing that has ever happened to them. Living through treatment, adapting to life after treatment or coping with life after a child's death are the most challenging tasks they will ever face. I worked in paediatric oncology in the late '70s and early '80s when the promise and the problems of aggressive therapies were just beginning. During that time, I learnt about partnership nursing from the children, their families, from experienced nurses and other professionals who faced these challenges together. This book reflects the years of progress that have been made since then, both in this specialty and in the wider world of child health care: family centred philosophies and partnerships in care are the reality now, not just the way that a few skilled professionals worked 20 years ago.

Partnership with children and families is not an easy option. It requires skill, experience, diplomacy and a huge store of personal strength, especially in oncology where the decisions to be faced and the treatments to endure are so difficult. The explicit and implicit exploration in successive chapters of the concept of partnership and what it means in practice, provide new insights for the reader. It is good to see a recognition of the effect on nurses of working in this specialty: you cannot have an effective partnership if the nurses themselves are not supported adequately to become the friends and carers of the child and family.

Partnerships with fellow professionals and between agencies such as health, social services and education are also complex. The importance of co-ordination and communication are beautifully illustrated in the chapters on discharge planning and care in the community.

One of the striking things about the book is that the contributors are almost all clinical nurses, writing with the knowledge and confidence of expert practitioners. This is the way that nurses in the real world help children and families to steer a course through the trauma of diagnosis, through treatment and survivorship or death. Case studies illustrate and emphasise the key principles of care and reflective prompts encourage the reader to relate these principles to his or her own practice.

Although it is possible to list the likely effects on the child and family of cancer and treatment – from first learning the diagnosis through to late effects in survivors – it is the lived experience of each individual child and family which is at the heart of paediatric oncology nursing. This focus, not on the general facts and figures, but on identifying meaning and impact in each case, is what makes this book exceptional. You can have confidence that while reading the book the challenges of the future will be met with the same commitment and dedication and the same goal of seeking to reduce the negative impact that cancer has on the lives of the whole family.

Anne Casey

Introduction

The developments in diagnosis and treatment of the child with cancer have increased steadily over the past few decades. While the incidence has increased, the mortality rate has decreased, with childhood cancer being the third most common cause of death in the UK after accidents and congenital abnormalities. This ability to reduce the mortality rate has allowed practitioners to begin to explore the other aspects that a diagnosis has on the child and family – the psychosocial impact of disease and the quality-of-life issues experienced from diagnosis, through treatment, to either survivorship or death.

Within generalist children's nursing there has also been a shift of emphasis from a medical model of care to one of partnership in care, with the child as the central focus and the parents and nurse as partners in caring for the child through negotiation and empowerment. This has allowed the potential for a change in control from the nurse to the child and family. It has also encouraged nurses to explore the effect on the family of a child's illness.

This book seeks to combine these two concepts of care by addressing the psychosocial needs of the child with cancer through a partnership approach to caring.

Chapter 1 explores the concept of partnership in care and sets the scene for the ensuing discussion. Partnership is explored from the philosophical perspective, and then this is interpreted from the child's view, the parents' view and the nurses' view. All three are seen as important if a relationship is to develop based on partnership and trust.

Chapter 2 takes this further and develops the aspect of negotiation, empowerment and locus of control when attempting to practise from a partnership philosophy. Much of the literature suggests that this is difficult to achieve and difficulties are highlighted within this chapter.

Chapter 3 moves away from the philosophical debate and concentrates on the impact of diagnosis and treatment on the child and family. This comprehensive chapter offers good insight into the disruption of fit experienced by children and their families while learning about a diagnosis and beginning to adapt to treatment.

Chapter 4 follows this by looking specifically at the impact of treatment upon the child, and demonstrates an in-depth review of the literature with reference to specific therapies, for example chemotherapy, and how these affect the child and his/her life. While some aspects of treatment are explored, this is not from a physiological point of view, but rather a look at concepts such as altered body image and psychological distress caused by the disease and treatment.

In Chapter 5, having looked at the impact of treatment on the child, the focus is shifted to the family. While separating the family from the child is difficult, it is important to acknowledge the identity of the family as a unit, but with individuals within it who have needs of their own as a result of living with a child with cancer. Stigma is explored and cultural issues are raised, giving rise to the need for further studies in this area.

Chapter 6 seeks to address the impact of treatment on the nursing staff. The cost of caring and working in partnership with families is often not acknowledged, and therefore this is an important chapter. Multidisciplinary team working is explored and the concept of shared care is discussed. A study by the author is presented which, while local, may help others to identify with and address the issues raised. In an age of a declining workforce, the pressures on children's oncology nurses are ever increasing. It is important that the stress of working in this area is acknowledged and that managers are proactive in developing strategies to reduce the potential of burnout.

In Chapter 7, this theme of coping strategies is taken further, with a comprehensive overview of key strategies and how staff can support children and family throughout the cancer experience. It is important to look at both the range of strategies and the way in which stages of development impact onto coping, as well as other variables such as cultural background and socioeconomic status. This chapter gives good insight into literature and strategies that nurses may adopt to enhance coping and is also useful when looking at coping from the nurses' perspective.

Chapter 8 focuses primarily on bone marrow transplantation (BMT). Aspects covered in previous chapters are applied specifically to the child and family within the BMT Unit. New treatments are referred to, giving the chapter a contemporary focus. The relationship between BMT and the paediatric intensive care unit (PITU) is well addressed; this is an area that often causes great anxiety to staff, families and the child and it is good to see how a successful partnership in care between the two specialities can be achieved.

Chapter 9 offers an excellent description of the need for the development of discharge planning. A framework for discharge planning is offered based on an extensive review of the literature. Discharges planning is often given a low priority, and the chapter raises it to the fore as a concept which should be present from the start of admission, rather than an afterthought.

The logical flow of the text insists that Chapter 10 looks at care in the community following discharge. This is a vital chapter in the light of the move to ambulatory and community care in the treatment of children with cancer. The authors feel strongly about the need to integrate children back into their local communities and give recommendations based on experience as to how this could be achieved, for example through school visits and involvement of the primary health care team. Specialist roles such as the paediatric oncology community outreach nurse and social workers are explored in an effort to demonstrate how seamless care is to be provided to families. While many models of community children's nursing are in operation, this chapter seeks to share examples of good practice in order to help future practitioners develop their thinking regarding care for children with cancer in the community.

Chapter 11 looks at the resolution of the cancer experience through the concepts of survivorship and rehabilitation. This is a full and extensive chapter that uses a wide range of literature to explore the ways in which a child and family work towards building their cancer experience into their life story and moving on. Practical examples are given which give nurses ideas about how they may be involved in helping a child and family move along this continuum.

The difficulty with any book of this nature is the decision of where to place the chapter which looks at the dying child. The logical flow suggests a final chapter, but this leads the reader to associate death and dying as a last port of call with an air of inevitability around it. The final chapter does deal with the care of the dying child. However, the concept of normality and the maintenance of the family unit are discussed within the partnership framework. Options of care setting such as acute, home and hospice are addressed and the role of the paediatric community nurse is discussed. While death is seen as 'the end' in terms of the cancer experience, this is not so for the family and this is discussed in detail with issues such as the ongoing role of the nurses' involvement highlighted.

As a result of the above discussion, it was felt inappropriate to end the book with this chapter. There is, therefore, a concluding chapter that pulls together the themes of the book and looks at the challenges the children's oncology nurses of the future face in the realm of psychosocial care for this client group. While prevention, early detection and treatment are continuing to be

advanced in the treatment of the child with cancer, the foresee-
able future does not hold hope for an eradication of disease. It is,
therefore, important that the impact of cancer upon the child and
family continues to be acknowledged, and practice is developed
to minimise the psychosocial impact of cancer. A partnership
between nurses, the family and child is seen as one way to work
towards achieving this.

Interspersed throughout the text are a number of helpful
Activity, Reflection, Case study and Discussion boxes:

 Activities relate to the practicalities of family-centred care;

 Reflection points request the reader to consider chapter
themes as reflected in their work;

 Case studies serve as precise illustrations of the general
situations discussed within the chapters;

 Discussion points consider the broader aspects of family-
centred care philosophy.

Partnership in care

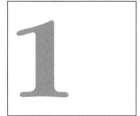

JANE BISHOP

In memory of Luke Margery and with thanks to his family

Key points
- What is partnership?
- Working with others
- Linking the parts
- Who is partnership with?
- Child and family
- GP and other members of the primary health care team
- Hospital multidisciplinary team
- Multi-agency
- Own nursing team
- Why have partnership?
- Practical aspects of care
- Support
- Resource
- Companionship
- Where does partnership take place?
- Home
- Hospital
- School
- Play
- Wherever the child is
- When does partnership occur?
- Availability
- Flexibility
- Long term
- How does partnership take place?
- Negotiation
- Dynamic
- Enabling
- Care in partnership
- Trust
- Compassion, diplomacy, respect
- Compromise
- Recognising separateness
- Consideration

Introduction

Partnership is a term which is widely used in paediatric nursing and promoted as an ideal basis for the care of sick children in hospital or at home. In this chapter the idea of partnership will be examined in terms of:

- What is partnership and who are the partners?
- Why have partnership and where does it take place?
- When and how does partnership occur?

Partnership as a framework for caring for children with cancer and their families will be considered in relation to these questions.

The concept of partnership has been adopted eagerly by children's nurses and appears in most statements of philosophy. One example is the Royal College of Nursing's 'Paediatric Nursing: a philosophy of care' (Royal College of Nursing, 1996), which includes a section entitled 'Partnership with the family' (Box 1.1).

Box 1.1   RCN paediatric philosophy of care: partnership with the family (reproduced from Royal College of Nursing, 1996)

All Royal College of Nursing policies relating to the care of children who are ill or have a disability are based on the principles and commitments set out in this guidance document.

THE NEEDS OF THE CHILD AS AN INDIVIDUAL

In working towards the provision of appropriate facilities for sick children, nurses should:

- recognise each child as a unique, developing individual whose best interests must be paramount
- listen to children, attempt to understand their perspectives, opinions and feelings and acknowledge their right to privacy
- consider the physical, psychological, social, cultural and spiritual needs of children and their families
- respect the right of children, according to their age and understanding, to appropriate information and informed participation in decisions about their care.

PARTNERSHIP WITH THE FAMILY

Nurses should:

- recognise that good health care is shared with families – who should be closely involved in their child's care at all times unless, exceptionally, this is not in the best interests of the child
- promote the active participation of children and their families in care and, by providing teaching and support, assist them to be partners in care
- promote the right of children to have a parent accompany them during hospitalisation and treatment.

FACILITIES FOR SICK CHILDREN AND THEIR FAMILIES

The Royal College of Nursing:

- asserts the right of all children in all settings to be nursed by appropriately educated and skilled staff and believes that staffing levels and skill mix must reflect the special needs of children who are ill or disabled and their families
- continually works to identify trends which may threaten the health and well being of children
- endorses the development of comprehensive, integrated child health services
- promotes the provision of hospital accommodation and facilities appropriate to the needs of children and young people and separate from those provided for adults
- advocates the reduction of hospital admissions and inpatient stay by promoting family participation in care, ambulatory services, day services and paediatric community nursing services.

The RCN encourages nurses to pursue these objectives within their own sphere of practice and to promote the educational opportunities necessary to advance the art and science of paediatric nursing.

The Royal College of Nursing has given its support to:

- The United Nations Convention on the Rights of the Child (1989)
- The Resolution of the European Parliament on a Charter for Children in Hospital (1986)
- Action for Sick Children (formerly National Association for the Welfare of Children in Hospital) *10 Targets for the 1990s* (1991)
- The principles of the Children Act (1989)
- The Department of Health guidance document *Welfare of Children and Young People in Hospital* (1991) and similar guidance issued for Northern Ireland, Wales and Scotland
- The recommendations of the Audit Commission Report *Children First: A Study of Hospital Services* (1993)
- The recommendations of the Allitt Inquiry (1994).
- The NHS Patients' Charter – Services for Children and Young People (1996).

Parents' groups and organisations lobbying for improved facilities and care for children, such as the Association for Children with Life-Threatening Conditions (ACT*), also use the term 'partner' or 'partnership'. An example of this is clause two of the ACT Charter

---

*ACT is a national voluntary organisation, created by and for individual professionals and professional bodies, national and local voluntary organisations, children's hospices, parent support groups and parents. It exists as a reference point for the exchange of information for anyone involved in the care of children with any life-threatening or terminal condition and their families, including children with cancer. The ACT strongly upholds the notion of partnership with parents and children.

(ACT, 1994), which states: 'Parents should be acknowledged as the primary carers and shall be centrally involved as partners in all care and decisions involving their child' (Box 1.2).

Despite wide usage of the term however, there has been limited explanation of what is meant by 'partnership' or of how partnership is implemented or realised by either nurses or sick children and their families. The term is often used interchangeably with ideas such as 'parental participation' and 'family-centred care'. The 'partnership model' has been adopted as a distinct model by

---

Box 1.2   ACT Charter for children with life-threatening illness (reproduced with permission from the copyright holders Act Bristol)

1. Every child shall be treated with dignity and respect and shall be afforded privacy whatever the child's physical or intellectual ability.
2. Parents shall be acknowledged as the primary carers and shall be centrally involved as partners in all care and decisions involving their child.
3. Every child shall be given the opportunity to participate in decisions affecting his or her care, according to age and understanding.
4. Every family shall be given the opportunity of a consultation with a paediatric specialist who has particular knowledge of the child's condition.
5. Information shall be provided for the parents, and for the child and the siblings according to age and understanding. The needs of other relatives shall also be addressed.
6. An honest and open approach shall be the basis of all communication which shall be sensitive and appropriate to age and understanding.
7. The family shall remain the centre of caring whenever possible. All other care shall be provided by paediatric trained staff in a child-centred environment.
8. Every child shall have access to education. Efforts shall be made to enable the child to engage in other childhood activities.
9. Every family shall be entitled to a named key worker who will enable the family to build up and maintain an appropriate support system.
10. Every family shall have access to flexible respite care in their own home and in a home-from-home setting for the whole family, with appropriate paediatric nursing and medical support.
11. Every family shall have access to paediatric nursing support in the home when required.
12. Every family shall have access to expert, sensitive advice in procuring practical aids and financial support.
13. Every family shall have access to domestic help at times of stress at home.
14. Bereavement support shall be available for as long as required.

ACT, 1994

paediatric nursing with minimal explanation of what partnership is in practice.

In this chapter it is hoped to offer a deeper exploration of the notion of partnership in nursing children with cancer and their families. This will include within the scenario an exploration of who the partners are in such a relationship, and how the roles of the partners are identified, clarified and negotiated. The function of partnership in children's nursing and the dynamics of the constantly changing relationships within the partnership model are also discussed. In addition, the concept of partnership as a framework for caring with respect to nursing the child with cancer and the family is emphasised.

Historical background to partnership in nursing

Political and organisational changes within the health service in the last decade have influenced changes in the management and organisation of nursing and resulted in the emergence of 'the new nursing' (Salvage, 1990). This incorporated an ideology of 'partnership' which implies a therapeutic nurse–patient relationship based on respect, trust and equality of worth. The Patient's Charter (Department of Health, 1996), for example, encouraged patients to exercise their right to information about treatment options, to be involved in decision making but also to accept responsibility for the choices they make regarding treatment. Such attempts to empower patients or to raise awareness in consumers of health care services of their rights and expectations and concomitant responsibilities in the care of their own health, has necessitated re-examination by nurses of their role in patient care.

In paediatric nursing this shift occurred earlier and in a different way. The emergence of psychological theories relating to child care, in particular Bowlby's (1965) ideas on maternal deprivation and the work of Robertson (1970) on the effects of hospitalisation on children and separation anxiety, were influential in this process. The Platt Report on the 'Welfare of Children in Hospital' (Platt Report, 1959) drew on these theories and emphasised the need to consider children's emotional and psychological well being in hospital. In the 1960s parents themselves formed the National Association for the Welfare of Children in Hospital (NAWCH), now named Action for Sick Children (ASC), and have lobbied persistently and to a large extent effectively, to improve access and facilities for parents of sick children. Hawthorn's (1974) research clearly demonstrated that parents actually had a role to play in the care of their ill child over and above that of simply

Figure 1.1 Casey's partnership model of paediatric nursing (reproduced with permission from Casey 1988)

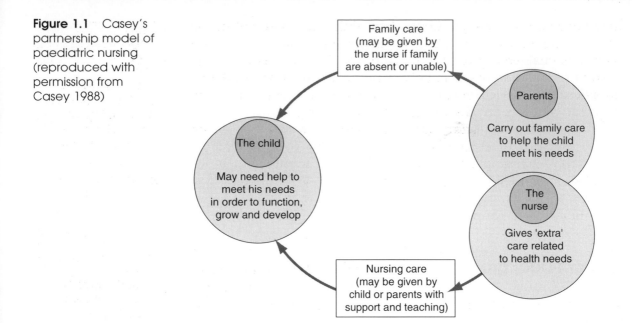

being present with the child, but did not elaborate on how this might be achieved universally.

Casey (1988) explains that her partnership model (Figure 1.1) was derived from children's nursing practice at the time and stated simply that: 'the paediatric nurse complements parental care by doing those things for the child, or his parents, to meet the child's needs' and that the process of nursing is carried out in partnership with the child and his or her family.

Farrell (1992), who worked in the paediatric intensive care unit of the children's hospital where this nursing model was implemented, expands a little on our understanding of partnership. He states that: 'partnership nursing aims to establish a relationship of equality between the professional carers and parents'. Farrell concludes: 'the success of the model depends on paediatric nurses being able to identify clearly what their role is, and how they should function when faced with particular health care problems'.

Casey's (1988) model originally views partnership as simply the level of care carried out by children's nurses and family carers depending on the child's needs. For example when a child is first diagnosed with cancer and commences a chemotherapy regimen via a central line, the paediatric nurses undertake most of the work relating to the care of the line. As the parents or carers begin to adjust to the initial shock of the diagnosis and learn more about the condition and treatment and feel more confident about their child's care, some of the tasks relating to the care of the child's central line may be taken on by the parents. Later on, the parents may become completely independent in the management of the line. At other times, for example when the child is acutely ill again with a neutropenic fever requiring hospitalisation, parents may wish to hand some of the child's physical care back to paediatric nursing staff. This shifting and transferring of care requires careful negotiation which will be discussed in Chapter 2.

As more and more acute care of children, including those with cancer, is taken out of the hospital setting with the development of skilled, experienced Community Children's Nursing teams, so the idea of 'partnership' has changed. Gould (1996), a community children's nurse, presents a slightly different perspective of the concept of partnership. She points out that caring for a sick child with cancer involves many different partnerships on different levels and not simply that between child, family and nurse: '... in community work, additional partnerships are forged and maintained to ensure that the child and family receive appropriate levels of support and assistance to achieve optimum well-being' (Figure 1.2).

The concept of partnership

The notion of partnership is clearly important to paediatric nurses. The word 'partnership' appears regularly in the majority of journal articles describing the care of sick children, and the involvement of parents or children themselves in the management of their illness is upheld as desirable.

Further questions inevitably arise as to the nature of partnership in children's cancer nursing:

■ What is the role of the children's nurse in a partnership scenario?
■ How can or should partnership be practised when caring for children and families?
■ How do children's nurses explain about partnership to parents?

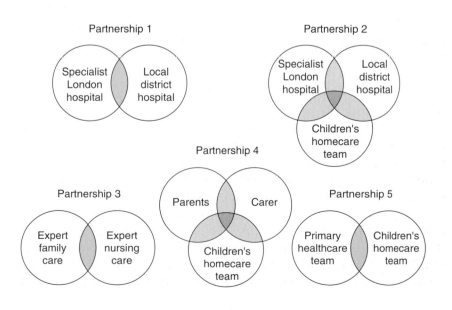

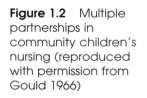

Figure 1.2 Multiple partnerships in community children's nursing (reproduced with permission from Gould 1966)

The general understanding of the term partnership describes a contractual relationship between two or more people (*Webster's New Collegiate Dictionary*, 1965). Implicit in this definition is that a working arrangement has been negotiated between the participants, each of whom has a contribution to make to the process. Palmer (1993) notes that purely in terms of sharing the work in caring for a sick child, the relationship between nurses and parents is different today from that of 20 years ago: 'this change has resulted in a decrease in active physical care by many nursing staff towards their patients, and an increase in the educative role of preparing, teaching, assessing, and supporting parents to nurse their own child'.

Foley (1993), Director of Paediatric Nursing at the Sloan Kettering Cancer Centre, New York also describes partnership in terms of the distribution of tasks and functions: 'For the family with cancer, effective communication is related to offering and receiving emotional support, and to fulfilling role responsibilities'. Partnership here is seen as a means to an end and as a strategy to be exploited to enable parents to fulfil their responsibilities in order to attain clinical goals: 'the goal of parental partnership is aspired to in most settings, although achievement is uneven'.

Partnership is seen as a way of gaining cooperation, albeit for the benefit of the child and family. 'Parents may not perceive that they are partners in the quest for clinical cure. Conversely they may or may not consider health team members as parties in achieving positive emotional outcomes for the family' (Foley, 1993). Partnership in this light has little to do with the relationship itself, and is simply used as a mechanism for achieving an outcome.

Darbyshire (1993), in a critical review of the available literature on partnership with parents in children's nursing, observes likewise: 'the literature of parental involvement was notable for its basis in an instrumental and technological understanding of parents as being essentially of functional value'. Darbyshire (1993) concentrates his research instead on the lived experience of parents caring for their sick child in hospital and that of nurses dealing with resident parents. Furthermore, he notes that 'the "cardinal principle" of paediatric nursing i.e. parental participation has been viewed largely as philosophically and professionally unproblematic.' He is diplomatically pointing out that paediatric nurses have not questioned nor tried to understand the concept of partnership.

In nearly all of the literature on children's nursing that mentions partnership, no mention is made of the social or psychological functions of partnership as part of a human relationship. Morse (1991), a nurse educationist in the USA, in a research study into negotiating commitment and involvement in the nurse–patient relationship, focuses her enquiry on the development of a relationship as a process from the perspective of both nurses and patients.

Darbyshire (1994), a British children's nurse tutor, comments briefly on similar such research and cautions against rigorous attachment to processes with stages, as a means of implementing the notion of partnership. Central to Morse's (1991) thesis is her concern that there is insufficient emphasis on the process of building relationships in the teaching of communication skills. The sample for her research included participants from paediatrics and palliative care, among other clinical areas. From her data she identifies four levels within a mutual relationship, or partnership, and suggests that both nurses and patients (or parents) use various strategies for maintaining control within the relationship by inhibiting or facilitating involvement. Morse (1991) also suggests that the strategies employed by patients (or parents) to sustain this partnership have more to do with whether the nurse meets their criteria as a person, than as a competent technician. Included among these criteria are personal qualities such as trustworthiness, reliability and gentleness. Morse (1991) describes these as internal factors which influence a relationship and observes that external factors such as the organisation of care, for example primary nursing, will also affect the way in which a partnership develops. She acknowledges the fragility and reciprocal nature of such relationships and in so doing introduces a more human element to the idea of partnership.

Palmer (1993), an experienced British paediatric oncology nurse, observes: 'the success of parental involvement is dependent on both parents' and staffs' attitudes, enthusiasm and willingness to work together'. This statement perhaps pinpoints the problem in any notion of partnership – that of clarifying and negotiating roles. And this particular statement highlights the difficulties of power and control in a partnership. Palmer (1993), in the very phrasing of the idea, suggests that it is paediatric nurses who need to involve parents, rather than parents retaining their rightful authority and engaging the help of health professionals in the care of their child. The Department of Health's 'Patient's Charter: services for children and young people' (1996) supports this approach by setting out standards in terms of parents' rights and expectations for the care of a sick child.

Palmer (1993) offers the view that: 'an alteration in the parent's role consequently alters the role of the paediatric nurse'. It is the realisation of this and the threat to their own position that may account for the enthusiasm with which paediatric nurses have embraced the idea of partnership. By promoting the ideology of partnership in paediatric nursing, it could be argued that children's nurses have been able to retain and protect their professional role.

Evaluation of 'care-by-parent' units showed that there was resistance by some nursing staff, but that this resistance was explained variously by them as fears about accountability in a hospital situation, and inappropriateness of the ward geography (Palmer, 1993). By empowering parents to care for their sick child some nurses felt that they were undermining their own position as professional carers. Malin and Teasdale (1991) support this by arguing that: 'there is a tension between the concepts of caring and empowerment' and that in caring *for* patients 'the power base of the relationship between nurse and patient is not equal'.

Moving from the acute care setting to the child's home, the shifting of power within the partnership relationship becomes more obvious as community children's nurses transfer care and support of families into a different arena. Cribb, Bignold and Ball (1994) note that specialist paediatric oncology nurses: 'work with an empowerment model of care which serves to shift the locus of definition, and the meeting of needs, towards families'. These authors are exploring the idea of holistic nursing as practised by specialist paediatric oncology nurses.

From their interviews with specialist paediatric oncology nurses, Cribb *et al.* (1994) observe that in the home: 'they rely on the same alloy of clinical and mediating skills (as they use in hospital), they have to strike the same balance between encouraging independence and creating dependence, and they have to recognise the expertise and "power" of parents'. Partnership is important, but peripheral, to the main focus of the study reported by Cribb *et al.*, but if a part is considered to be an integral element, or one of the portions into which something is divided and which together constitutes the whole (*Webster's New Collegiate Dictionary*, 1965), then partnership is in a sense a way of attempting to maintain the whole. Cribb *et al.* (1994) see this 'linking of the parts' variously as: boundary crossing, diplomacy, mediation, collaboration and translation.

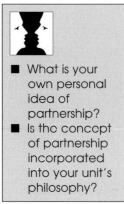

- What is your own personal idea of partnership?
- Is the concept of partnership incorporated into your unit's philosophy?

Partnership in practice

Paediatric nurses have different views as to what form parental involvement in their child's care in hospital should take. This was borne out by a study by Webb, Hull and Madeley (1985), which found that staff and parents appeared to be unaware of each other's expectations, understanding and willingness to participate actively in the care of the sick child. Campbell (1993), a children's nurse tutor, 8 years later notes that: 'the unstated and unexamined acceptance of family-centred care in practice might lead to different interpretations by nurses'.

Difficulties in clarifying roles may occur and situations can arise where one partner thinks the other is giving the practical care, for example, dressing the child's central line site. Gould (1996) points out that making clear-cut distinctions between family care and nursing care even with practical tasks is not easy. Application of the paediatric partnership model is not simple and requires skill and sensitivity: 'for example, the care in relation to the central line would require expert nursing input at least initially, but the very existence of the line may impede performance of normal family care, such as bathing'. The 'family-centred care' approach has also been used interchangeably, but mistakenly so, with the idea of partnership and has led to further confusion. Brunner and Suddarth (1991, p. 60) stated that: 'the goal of family-centred care is to maintain or strengthen the roles and ties of the family with a hospitalised child in order to promote normality of the family unit'.

While this is an admirable aim and one to which paediatric nurses should aspire, it could be said that some nurses view so-called family-centred care as a way of enhancing the idea of partnership in children's nursing, and even as a useful strategy for maintaining and protecting their own role in the care of sick children without being entirely clear as to what either term means.

Banoub-Badour and Laryea (1992) prefer to use the term 'culture brokering' when discussing ways of working with parents. Speaking particularly about assessing cancer pain in very young children, they describe the role of nurses working in partnership with parents as: 'acting as a culture broker to bridge the gap between child, parents and the health care team'. They use the anthropological term culture brokering to mean interpreting the child's needs via the parents and nurse. Culture brokering is a translation of messages, institutions and belief systems from one group to another. Banoub-Badour and Laryea (1992) suggest that parental beliefs inform the child's pain perception, expression and response, and that: 'each encounter between the child, family and nurse constitutes a cultural encounter where the incongruencies of views about the causation, meaning and treatment of cancer pain in the child are likely to occur'. They therefore see partnership, or culture brokering, as crucial in order to validate what the nurse and parents perceive the young child's pain to be.

The following case study aims to highlight some of the above points relating to partnership in practice.

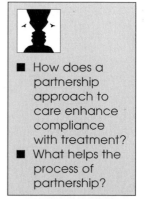

■ How does a partnership approach to care enhance compliance with treatment?
■ What helps the process of partnership?

Case study 1.1

Luke was a 15 year old who was diagnosed as having non-Hodgkin's lymphoma 21 months ago. His treatment was uneventful and followed the usual pattern of transferring briefly from the children's unit of the district general hospital in the town where he lived, to the regional paediatric oncology unit 30 miles away.

The first partnerships were therefore set up in the first few days of what would be a relationship lasting for several years: that between Luke and his family and the local consultant paediatrician who would be managing most of his care, advised by the regional centre; and that between the specialist unit and the local district unit.

Having had his diagnosis confirmed by biopsy of the mediastinal mass which caused his presenting symptoms of a rasping cough, shortness of breath and facial swelling, Luke had a central line inserted and started on the induction phase of a 100-week programme of cytotoxic chemotherapy following national guidelines. After a few days he was transferred back to his local hospital for continuation of the induction phase, then a few days at home followed by the first intensification block of chemotherapy. This intensive stage of treatment went hand in hand with meeting numerous health professionals who would be involved in Luke's care.

One of the first people whom Luke and his family met was a community children's nurse based at the children's unit of the local district general hospital. She visited at home one Saturday afternoon, shortly after Luke had completed his induction chemotherapy, and met the whole family: Luke, his identical twin brother, his 18-year-old sister, his mother and stepfather, and his 2-month-old baby half-sister. This was the first opportunity for both sides in what would constitute the main 'partnership' throughout Luke's treatment to meet each other and to find out about each other as individuals. This is a crucial step in laying the foundations for a long-term working relationship.

The community children's nurse was able to find out how each member of this cohesive family felt about Luke's illness and how having a member of the family who was ill and needing a good deal of extra care and attention affected them as individuals. Luke's mother was a practising theatre nurse and stated from the outset what she wanted from the partnership and that as her field of nursing was so different from children's or oncology nursing she requested that staff treated her 'like any other mother'. This meeting also deliberately offered an unhurried opportunity for Luke and his family to clarify some of the information they had been given in the privacy and familiarity of their own home.

Further visits at a later stage were used to continue to build the partnership from both sides while starting the process of enabling Luke and his family to take on some of the care themselves. This is a tentative, sensitive process of finding out when carers feel ready to take on additional responsibilities in the care of their child at the same time as having themselves to adjust to the idea of having a child with a potentially life-threatening illness, in addition to the usual day-to-day family care which in this situation included that of a small baby. As time went on Luke decided to manage the care of his central line himself and was meticuluous about his personal hygiene and mouth care, while his mother remained responsible for giving his daily medication.

Another partnership that was set up in the early stages of Luke's illness was with his school which formed a major part of his life. A meeting was held with Luke's and his parent's permission between the headteacher, Luke's year head, the school nurse and the community children's nurse. This was an example of linking together some of the parts of Luke's life, the purpose being to ensure that key school staff had factual information about his illness, some understanding of what his treatment involved and what effect it might have on him. For example, permission was given by the headteacher for Luke to wear a cap or hat at all times indoors and outside as he was very conscious of his hair loss. In an effort to disrupt his lessons as little as possible, the school nurse made her medical room available for half an hour once a week during break times for Luke to come and meet the community children's nurse and to have his blood taken for his weekly blood count, and his central line and general condition to be checked. Luke was given the responsibility of attending punctually which he did without fail, and the community children's nurse brought all the equipment needed with her. This was the agreed partnership and it worked well.

Luke's blood results would then be discussed back at the district general hospital with the local lead consultant paediatrician for oncology at the weekly multidisciplinary meeting, and Luke's doses of oral cytotoxic chemotherapy adjusted for the next week. Later in the day the community children's nurse would then telephone the family to inform them of the decisions.

Luke's mother's balanced approach towards developing her children extended to the management of Luke's illness, and this almost equal partnership in care between mother and teenage son gave Luke appropriate opportunity to develop his independence within the continuing security of a stable family. He was encouraged to continue his paper round, and to particpate in all school activities including work experience, and later to make a smooth transition to college with some of his friends from school. While allowing him these freedoms, his mother had many adjustments to make herself both with Luke's illness and with the new baby. In order to be more available to Luke in case he was unwell, or 'just wanted to know she was around', she altered her shift patterns. This accommodating approach is one of the hallmarks of a successful partnership: flexibility and negotiation as to the degree of parental involvement in care between child, parent and nursing/medical staff and other key people such as the school personnel.

Recognition that the boundaries between the partners are changing constantly and dynamically as one circumstance impacts on another, enabled this partnership to work well. For example, Luke's increased dependence on his mother and the nursing staff during admission to the children's unit with acute illness and neutropenic fever, compared with his easy transition to independence when relatively well again.

Regrettably, Luke suffered a relapse of his condition while on active treatment a few months before the end of his original 100-week programme. He developed a cough which his mother recognised instantly as the same cough present on initial diagnosis. The results of immediate investigations were given to Luke and his parents together, by the consultant paediatrician with the community children's nurse most closely involved present. By this time, after 18 months of partnership with the same team throughout, Luke felt secure enough to be able to express openly there and then his disappointment, anger and frustration at this setback. He also trusted the team sufficiently to be able to ask many questions about the continuing treatment and the bone marrow transplant he now faced.

Partnership as a framework for caring

By promoting partnership in paediatrics, children's nurses are indeed sharing knowledge and skills enabling parents to care *for* an ill child, but when the balance of power and control changes within the relationship and parents or other 'partners' take on the physical tasks relating to the child's needs, the nurse's role in caring *about* the child and family continues to be of as equal importance as before. This is particularly the case when caring for a child with cancer or other life-threatening illness. The impact on the family, which will be dealt with in Chapter 5, is enormous and the nursing role, especially in the community setting, is equally one of being available for support and ensuring a smooth transition for the child and family between episodes of care in the acute setting and home and school, as it is about taking blood samples and checking the child's central line.

Cribb *et al.* (1994) comment on the 'indeterminacy' of health care work: 'the commitment of the specialist paediatric oncology nursing services to families is open-ended. It is not defined by specific tasks, nor is it clearly circumscribed by kind of task, or by episodes or events, including the death of a child.' Callery and Smith (1991), in a study of role negotiation between nurses and parents of hospitalised children, note that: 'there is no consensus amongst children's nurses about what form participation should take and how far that participation should extend'. The same authors observe that in the 1970s when free access to children's wards began to be encouraged, the position of parents resident with a sick child was similar to that of actually being a patient themselves. The parents experienced loss of freedom and autonomy with respect to how they carried out their usual parenting role and care of their child, and in addition were themselves stressed by the context of their situation and the anxiety of having an ill child.

Gibson (1995), in a recent Canadian study, examines the process of empowerment of mothers of chronically ill children. This included children with cancer where most often nurses, parents and child are establishing a relationship that will last for up to 2 years, or sometimes more. A distinct process emerged from the data: there was frustration in the early stages where parents relied on health professionals to make sound decisions for them and their child. At this stage parents saw themselves as recipients of care and not active participants. Through a cyclical process of critical reflection and experience in caring for their chronically ill child, parents achieved what Gibson (1995) calls 'participatory competence'. Parents become experts in their child's care and condition, and gained a total knowledge of their child which nurses who have intermittent contact can never hope to have about the child.

Cain *et al.* (1995) suggest that the degree of collaboration between, for example, children's nurses and parents, may depend on a perceived difference of status between health professional and lay person based on knowledge and experience. Nevertheless most children's nurses readily acknowledge that parents, particularly in the case of children with a well-established diagnosis of a chronic, long-term or life-threatening illness, are extremely knowledgeable and experienced in the care of their child. Gibson (1995) adds that parents valued a: 'partnership where there was mutual respect and open communication between the health care professionals and the mothers as well as the commitment to a common goal'.

Gibson (1995) also notes the relational aspect of partnership in the process of empowerment: 'mothers perceived that health care professionals were receptive and responsive'. Both the positives and negatives within such a partnership acted as catalysts to empowerment. From her research Gibson (1995) conceptualises empowerment as: 'a social process of recognising, promoting and enhancing people's abilities to meet their own needs, solve their own problems and mobilise the necessary resources in order to feel in control of their own lives'.

Nevertheless, even when parents had gained a sense of control within the situation and had adjusted to living with a chronically ill child, partnership with others was still important. This underlines the idea of partnership as something ongoing and dynamic.

Griffin's (1983) analysis of caring as having distinct but complementary elements, that is, active and affective components, could be said to be intrinsic to the concept of partnership as a human relationship and corresponds to some extent to Morse's (1991) understanding of partnership discussed earlier, as a mutual relationship between two or more people involving care and concern.

Cribb *et al.* (1994) note that: 'although specialist paediatric onco-logy nurses cannot pretend to deal with every sort of concern that families have, they can *attend* to every concern and maintain the infrastructure of care, that is, by being available, by sitting with, being with, and listening to family members'. This is partner-ship in terms of caring but is an aspect which has not yet been sufficiently addressed nor fully acknowledged by paediatric nurses. For example, partnership in human terms such as com-panionship with parents caring for a child who is dying, 'a being alongside the suffering, impotent as they are impotent, mute as they are mute, sharing their darkness' (Cassidy, 1988, p. 115), may be a notion with which some children's nurses can identify, but which they may not have articulated.

Parents in Gibson's (1995) study described a period of simply 'holding on' in coming to terms with the diagnosis of a chronic and potentially life-threatening illness in their child. This aspect of partnership, that simply of pastoral care, has been neglected, or unacknowledged, in paediatric nursing. Campbell (1986, p. 15) describes this holding on for another person as steadfastness within a relationship: 'Pastoral care is grounded in mutuality, not in expertise; it is possible because we share a common humanity'. Roach (1991, p. 9) disputes this idea of shared humanity, saying that: 'nursing is no more no less than the professionalisation of the human capacity to care through the acquisition and applica-tion of the knowledge, attitudes and skills appropriate to nursing's prescribed roles'.

It must be remembered that partnership in nursing children with cancer and their families is very often not so much about competence as about: 'the mediation of steadfastness ... not the offering of advice at an intellectual level, nor the eliciting of insight at an emotional level' (Campbell, 1986. p. 16). In this sense partnership is not a process to be learned, nor a technique to be practised, but what Cassidy (1988, p. 38) describes with eloquent simplicity as: 'an endless circular dance of loving'.

Conclusion

Partnership is fluid and dynamic, and role boundaries between parents, nurse and child change constantly over a prolonged period of time such as the course of a 2-year cancer treatment protocol. Rather than professionalising caring as Roach suggests, nursing needs to go beyond its self-imposed professional role and draw on the wisdom and experience of others in order to understand partnership more fully. As a starting point, Darbyshire (1993) suggested: 'If paediatric nursing is to continue to advocate

and develop a philosophy of care based on mutuality and partnership with parents, then nursing needs a deeper understanding
of the nature of parental experiences and how these relate to their
own nursing practice'.

Likewise Bowden (1997, p. 112), in an illuminating chapter
on caring and nursing, emphasises the centrality of the client's
experience to the nurse–patient relationship: 'Nursing care is a
particular way of entering the world of another person ...'. Writing
about the ethical dimension of nursing practice Bowden (1997,
p. 112) reiterates that 'the patient's perspective adds crucial insight
to understanding'. This viewpoint, which perhaps necessitates
close personal identification within the partnership relationship,
raises questions about the extent to which paediatric nurses
should become involved with a child and family on an emotional
level. Cribb *et al.* (1994) state that 'the philosophy of specialist
oncology paediatric nursing rests upon the necessity of partnership'. They acknowledge that this entails several roles and relationships and that 'these roles may pull in different directions.
Achieving some balance is a matter of personal and professional
judgement'. Indeed, if children's nurses recognise and affirm the
human aspect of partnership, then the emotional elements must
also be considered.

Cribb *et al.* (1994) comment 'for professionals, the emotional
labour includes the self-conscious management of emotional distance'. Bowden (1997), in direct contrast, suggests that distinctions
between detachment and engagement, or impersonal and personal
care, are artificial in nursing. Instead, Bowden supports the work
of Benner and Wrubel (1989), who demonstrate through their
examples of the 'expert' practitioner that as nursing is essentially about interpersonal relations, emotional connections provide
greater insight into the patient's world: 'Emotions give access to
the kind of global understanding and attunement to the complexity of the patient's world that is the hallmark of expert nursing
care' (Bowden, 1997, p. 108).

Bowden cites Gadow (1980, p. 111), who maintains that nursing
involvement is unique and distinctive in that it allows for the
integration of knowledge and feelings leading to 'a more reflective, directed intensity of involvement'. Bowden (1997) views this
blending of the 'instrumental' and 'expressive' roles of the nurse
as offering 'emotionally engaged attention and responsiveness' to
the individual situation of that child and family. As such this gives
credence to the idea of partnership as participation in, and understanding of, the emotionally charged and complex situations
in which children's nurses find themselves when caring for a child
with cancer. Bowden (1997) observes that the limitations of this
type of partnership approach are not so much the uncertainties

that may arise relating to involvement with or detachment from a child and family, as tensions resulting from organisational and managerial constraints.

There is also a paradox in partnership. The strength of partnership in human terms lies in the atmosphere of trust, commitment, humility and respect of each partner for the others. And in the context of working with families with a sick child, as in any partnership, one needs to uphold the individuality of the partners and foster independence by nurturing and not stifling or overshadowing, nor insisting on conformity to one's own viewpoint. Gibran (1926, p. 12) when writing of partnership in marriage advised: 'but let there be space in your togetherness. Love one another, but make not a bond of love … And stand together yet not too near together.' Separateness within a partnership must be recognised and respected. Nevertheless, for the child with cancer and the family, if practised with thought and sensitivity, partnership as a reciprocal, reflective and dynamic process can offer support to both patient and practitioner.

References

ACT (Association for Children with Life-Threatening or Terminal Conditions and Their Families) (1994) *The ACT Charter for Children with Life-threatening Conditions and their Families.* Bristol: ACT.

Banoub-Badour, S. & Laryea, M. (1992) Culture-brokering: the essence of nursing care for preschool children suffering from cancer related pain. *Canadian Oncology Nursing Journal,* 2(4), 132–136.

Benner, P. & Wrubel, J. (1989) *The Primacy of Caring: stress and coping in health and illness.* Menlo Park, CA: Addison-Wesley.

Bowden, P. (1997) *Caring: gender-sensitive ethics.* London: Routledge.

Bowlby, J. (1965) *Child Care and the Growth of Love.* London: Pelican.

Brunner, L.S. & Suddarth, D.S. (1991) *Lippincott Manual of Paediatric Nursing,* 3rd edn. London: Harper Row.

Cain, P., Hyde, V. & Howkins, E. (eds) (1995) *Community Nursing: dimensions and dilemmas.* London: Arnold.

Callery, P. & Smith, L. (1991) A study of role negotiation between nurse and parents of hospitalised children. *Journal of Advanced Nursing,* **16**, 772–781.

Campbell, A.V. (1986) *Rediscovering Pastoral Care,* 2nd edn. London: Darton, Longman & Todd.

Campbell, S. (1993) Keeping it in the family. *Child Health,* June/July, 17–20.

Casey, A. (1988) A partnership with child and family. *Senior Nurse,* **8**(4), 8–9.

Cassidy, S. (1988) *Sharing the Darkness.* London: Darton, Longman & Todd.

Cribb, A., Bignold, S. & Ball S.J. (1994) Linking the parts: an exemplar of philosophical and practical issues in holistic nursing. *Journal of Advanced Nursing,* **20**, 233–238.

Darbyshire, P. (1993) Parents, nurses and paediatric nursing: a critical review. *Journal of Advanced Nursing,* **18**, 1670–1680.

Darbyshire, P. (1994) *Living with a Sick Child in Hospital: the experiences of parents and nurses.* London: Chapman & Hall.

Department of Health (1996) *Patient's Charter: services for children and young people.* London: HMSO.

Farrell, M. (1992) Partnership in care: paediatric nursing model. *British Journal of Nursing,* **1**(4), 175–176.

Foley, G.V. (1993) Enhancing child–family–health team communication. *Cancer,* **71**(Suppl.), 3281–3289.

Gadow, S. (1980) Existential advocacy: philosophical foundation of nursing *in* Bowden, P. ed. *Caring: gender-sensitive ethics.* London: Routledge.

Gibran, K. (1926) *The Prophet.* London: Heinemann.

Gibson, C.H. (1995) The process of empowerment in mothers of chronically ill children. *Journal of Advanced Nursing*, **21**, 1201–1210.

Gould, C. (1996) Multiple partnerships in the community. *Paediatric Nursing*, **8**(8), 26–31.

Griffin, A.P. (1983) A philosophical analysis of caring in nursing. *Journal of Advanced Nursing*, **8**, 289–295.

Hawthorn, P. (1974) *Nurse – I want my Mummy.* London: Royal College of Nursing.

Malin, N. & Teasdale, K. (1991) Caring versus empowerment: considerations for nursing practice. *Journal of Advanced Nursing*, **16**, 657–662.

Morse, J. (1991) Negotiating commitment and involvement in nurse–patient relationships. *Journal of Advanced Nursing*, **16**, 455–468.

Palmer, S.J. (1993) Care of sick children by parents: a meaningful role. *Journal of Advanced Nursing*, **18**, 185–191.

Platt Report (1959) *Welfare of Children in Hospital.* London: HMSO.

Roach, S. (1991) The call to consciousness: compassion in today's health world *in* Gaut, D. & Leininger, M. eds. *Caring: the compassionate healer.* New York: National League for Nursing Press.

Robertson, J. (1970) *Young Children in Hospital.* London: Tavistock.

Royal College of Nursing (1996) *Paediatric Nursing – a philosophy of care.* London: Royal College of Nursing.

Salvage, J. (1990) The theory and practice of the 'new nursing'. *Nursing Times*, **86**(4), 42–45.

Webb, N., Hull, D. & Madeley, R. (1985) Care by parents in hospital. *British Medical Journal*, **291**(6489), 176–177.

Webster's New Collegiate Dictionary (1965) London: Bell & Sons.

Further reading

Act (Association for Children with Life-Threatening or Terminal Conditions and their Families) (1994) *The ACT Charter for Children with Life-threatening Conditions and their Families.* **Bristol: ACT.**
The ACT Charter is dealt with specifically and each of the 14 individual clauses in the Charter, which provide and promote models of good care and practice in the planning and provision of services for children and families, are expanded.

Bowden, P. (1997) *Caring: gender-sensitive ethics.* **London: Routledge.**
The author writes from the perspective of a philosopher, and sets out to demonstrate the significance of caring in 'transforming interpersonal relatedness' into something greater than the simple necessity of partnership between mother and child, or nurse and patient. The chapter on nursing gives an excellent critique of Benner and Wrubel's (1989) work. This chapter affords an illuminating review of literature relating to nursing and caring, and original insights into the constraints on, and the possibilities of, partnership.

Cain, P., Hyde, V. & Howkins, E. eds. (1995) *Community Nursing: dimensions and dilemmas,* **London: Arnold.**
Chapter 2 discusses nurse–client relationships in the community setting. The interactions between health professional and client in terms of its context and task are defined. While not dealing specifically with paediatric issues, a critical analysis of partnership is offered and important questions raised.

Darbyshire, P. (1994) *Living with a Sick Child in Hospital: the experiences of parents and nurses.* **London: Chapman & Hall.**
Much of this book focuses on the relationship between parents and nurses in a hospital unit for acutely sick children, but there is also a fascinating insight into the ethics of relationships within the realms of children's nursing in general.

Davis, H. (1993) *Counselling Parents of Children with Chronic Illness or Disability.* **Leicester: The British Psychological Society.**
The psychological needs of the whole family and ways in which carers can facilitate adaptation to the child's illness are specifically addressed. The book aims to create a supportive, practical partnership with parents such that they can then adjust to and cope with their child's problems.

Hill, L. (1994) *Caring for Dying Children and their Families.* **London: Chapman & Hall.** Practical advice is offered by those experienced in working closely in partnership with families. Although written specifically with the care of terminally ill children in mind, some information is equally relevant to children with a life-threatening disorder but who are not dying.

Negotiating care

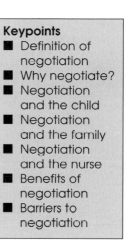

HELEN LANGTON

Introduction

This chapter seeks to further develop the theme of partnership in care clearly identified in Chapter 1. Partnership in care has many facets to it, one of which is negotiation. This short chapter will look at the concept of negotiation, why it is important, and how to empower parents and children to negotiate care and their participation within that care.

Literature will be used to identify how negotiation can be successfully incorporated into a partnership approach to care. As a topic worthy of consideration in its own right, it will be important to address the benefits of and barriers to negotiation. While there will be some reference to partnership and family-centered care, it is not the intention of this chapter to repeat the historical perspective offered in Chapter 1. It is therefore important that this chapter is read in conjunction with Chapter 1 and not in isolation.

This chapter contains case studies to demonstrate various points and these will be used to develop reflection and action activities, thus prompting you to think further around the material and relate theory to your practice.

Negotiation – a definition

The *Oxford Dictionary* describes negotiation as 'to hold communication with for purpose of arranging a matter by mutual agreement'.

While this is not a nursing definition, many of the writings around negotiation and partnership in care echo these sentiments. Knight (1995) emphasises the need for mutual agreement and Wegner and Alexander (1993) emphasise the need for mutual understanding and support. Knafl, Cavallan and Dixon (1988) suggest that negotiation is a means by which control is shifted and can form the basis for future interactions. However, they go on to suggest that this assumes that family members and nurses must

Keypoints
- Definition of negotiation
- Why negotiate?
- Negotiation and the child
- Negotiation and the family
- Negotiation and the nurse
- Benefits of negotiation
- Barriers to negotiation

Consider families that you have recently cared for

Using the key points of goal setting, problem solving and mutual agreement, decide whether negotiation has been a feature of the relationship between yourself and the family.

be striving to work together towards a partnership in care, and therefore negotiation becomes the nature of interaction between families and professionals. This should therefore lead to consistent, systematic efforts being made by the nurse and the parents and child to understand each other's viewpoint.

Friedman (1992) takes the concept further by suggesting that it is important to know what the 'matter' is that is to be arranged by mutual agreement. She suggests that it is the process of problem solving and goal setting that gives rise to the need for negotiation, and that this in turn leads to empowerment through an equality in partnership between the nurse and the parents. If this is true, then Wegner and Alexander's (1993) suggestion that nursing is the act of a frequent shift from a participant to a bystander and evaluator would seem to be relevant when looking at the definition of negotiation and how it fits into a philosophy of partnership in care.

Why negotiate?

Research has primarily looked at the effect of hospitalisation on children and there has been little understanding of how parents have experienced caring for children in hospital and the reality of partnership in care (Darbyshire, 1994). At home parents have considerable autonomy in relation to their children. In hospital this, in theory, becomes shared, although in reality we would suggest that 'take over' can be more common.

Few children's nurses would deny that children need their parents when in hospital (Dearmun, 1992); however, unless these nurses become proactive in promoting emancipation of parents with sick children, the children's problems may become worse as a direct result of the lack of negotiation of care within a partnership philosophy (Ball, Glasper and Yerrell, 1990).

On admission to hospital, sick children and families exchange freedom, autonomy and self direction for control by others, although it would be argued that they gain protection, care and freedom from responsibility. The difficulty becomes the decision over what is appropriate participation and the way in which an end result is to be achieved (Callery and Smith, 1991).

Morse (1991) suggested that two main types of relationship existed between nurses and families:

- mutual
- unilateral.

In a unilateral relationship, it is suggested that either the nurse or the parent is unwilling or unable to develop the relationship

> **Box 2.1   The relationship between nurses and families (adapted from Morse, 1991)**
>
> - Clinical – quick, short stay; little involvement
> - Therapeutic – nurse in charge; parent and child in sick role and perceived as a patient
> - Connected – parent and child perceived firstly as a person; mutual respect earned.
> - Over involved – mutual respect present; nurse becomes territorial re care. Loss of objectivity

desired by the other, although due to lack of self insight, may not refuse this. Within a mutual relationship, there are a variety of levels at which this may function, often influenced by length of stay (Box 2.1).

The danger in attempting to achieve an end result through a process is that negotiation is not the only process that could be utilised. Other forces, such as persuasion, coercion and threats may achieve the desired result, but not enhance the relationship between the nurse and parent. Brown and Ritchie (1989) also suggest that there are various types of relationship that may be formed between nurse and parent (Box 2.2).

If the relationship between the nurse, the child and the family is to be one of partnership based on negotiation, then a shared understanding of boundaries and roles needs to be developed (Ashworth, Longmate & Morrison, 1992).

Fradd (1996) suggests that, within negotiation, there is a need to distinguish between doing the right thing and doing the thing right. Negotiating with the child and family is doing the right thing, but it is important to see negotiation as a means of mutual decision making, not a way of encouraging active participation in care by a parent/child. She suggests that, by negotiating, problem solving is enhanced and therefore patient care is improved through the development of a mutually agreed plan of care.

The role of the parent is manifold, to include the natural, biological role; the job to be learnt with skills attached to it, and the

> **Box 2.2   Relationships between nurses and families (adapted from Brown and Ritchie 1989)**
>
> - Negotiated
> - Reciprocal
> - Adversarial
> - Asynchronous
> - Ineffective

Consider the variety of admissions dealt with within the paediatric oncology unit, e.g. day admission for blood product support; short stay for next cytotoxic regimen; bone marrow transplantation. How does the length of stay affect the relationship developed? Use Box 2.1 to think through a variety of relationship possibilities.

concept of 'being' a parent (Whyte, 1996). While this is normally carried out within the home setting, the locus of control remains with the parent. By admitting a child to hospital, the setting and environment change and therefore role confusion can set in. Partnership in care emphasises mutual respect and cooperation and also recognises the rights, responsibilities and role of the family in enhancing compliance and treatment: 'Good child health care is shared with parents/carers and they are closely involved in the care of their children at all times' (Department of Health, 1991b, p. 2). However, despite the exhortation from Government and the growing body of evidence to suggest that partnership in care through negotiation is essential, we would suggest that there needs to be more concern over how this may be achieved, rather than whether it is beneficial in the first place.

Negotiation and the child

The Children's Act (1989) states clearly that we must take into account the ascertainable wishes and feelings of the child concerned but that this must be considered in the light of the child's age and understanding.

The EU Charter for Children in Hospital (1979) states that children have a right to information and participation in their care and this is endorsed by the National Association for Welfare of Children in Hospital (NAWCH) (1985) through their charter and the Royal College of Nursing's (RCNs) statements on partnership and family-centred care (Dimond, 1996).

Inman (1991) takes the discussion re age and maturity further, suggesting that while young children can often cope with fairly adult conversations on a one-to-one basis with their parents, this ability diminishes within more complex interactions with parents and nurses. There is, therefore, a need for nurses to be sensitive to the needs of young children when trying to include them in the negotiation and decision-making process.

Fradd (1996) has championed the right of the child to be involved in the negotiation process and she suggests that there are two components to the role of the child in negotiation. The first is the role and influence of the state and agencies in child care decision making. The second is the relationship between the child and parent.

In order to enhance a child's ability to negotiate, two areas of care need to be considered:

- right to consent
- control of personal information.

> **Case study 2.1**
>
> A 9-year-old boy with a 3-year history of treatment for non-Hodgkin's lymphoma has been readmitted with a second relapse and evidence of widespread metastatic disease. The child requests to see the doctor alone and asks that active treatment is not considered. He states his case clearly and eloquently, citing the experience of the treatment regimen of the last 3 years as reasons for wishing to stop. He has clearly thought through his illness and the implications of his request. He also states that his parents will not agree with his request.
>
> On discussion of the progression of the disease and the poor prognosis, parents declare a wish to commence active treatment. They are told of their son's wish, but feel that they are the decision makers and he is not 'old' enough or 'competent' enough to know what he is talking about.

The law is clear on the right to consent within the term 'Gillick competence'. However, the decision-making process that leads to a child being pronounced 'Gillick competent' or not is less clear. Take as an example Case study 2.1.

While every oncology nurse can sympathise with the desire of the parents to sustain the life of their child, the scenario in Case study 2.1 presents a dilemma for the doctor as to whether the child is Gillick competent and, even if pronounced Gillick competent, there remains dissonance between the decision of the child and the parents. Therefore the relationship between the child and the parents becomes paramount if the role of the child in decision making is to be enabled.

This is much more likely to be achieved if negotiation takes place at an early stage of the relationship between the nurse and the child and family. This is particularly important within the chronic illness scenario of children with cancer, whereby the relationship may span several years and undergo several changes.

If children are to be included in the negotiation process, it is important to look at how nurses can develop and enhance this process. As mentioned earlier, there is the need for children to have control of their personal information. The kind of information may be that gleaned on admission, or may be of an ongoing nature, for example gathering and recording of vital signs, fluid output, etc. It is therefore important that children are involved in negotiating their part in this. This transmits messages that suggest that children's views are valued. It also allows children to develop their experience and expertise and to learn how to care for themself. In addition, it tries to mimic the responsibility given to children at home and therefore respects their status. By encour-

- Consider a child currently in your care. In your opinion is this child Gillick competent or not? Be able to justify your reasons.
- How do you help children in your care gain control over their personal information?
- Spend time actively negotiating care with a variety of children of different ages. What are the difficulties you experience? What are the benefits? How do the parents react?

aging and negotiating with children, nurses will also be able to identify areas of competence and weakness and therefore direct future learning.

Of course, as children are readmitted over a long period of time, this assessment and negotiation will need to change, to reflect their developmental age and ability to perform skills.

For example, young children with a central venous catheter may be involved in unravelling it ready for access, and may help with the clamping/unclamping process. Older children may help to prepare the area and collect the equipment necessary for access. Adolescents may perform the whole procedure, from collecting and preparing equipment, to accessing the line, to cleaning up afterwards, being aware of safe disposal of equipment.

If children's oncology nurses are to value the child, then they need to negotiate with them as well as their parents. While this can place the nurse in a difficult position if there is discourse between child and parent, or indeed child and nurse, this nego-tiation is not to be shied away from. Physical and emotional withdrawal can be used by nurses as a strategy to avoid conflict. However, involvement with the child through negotiation is seen as an empowering strategy. Nurses need to learn to accept others and their behaviour without being judgemental or defensive if they are to truly negotiate care and act as an advocate for the child.

The perception of parents

Without wishing to decry the importance of the last section, it is also necessary to look at negotiation with the family and parents' perceptions of the process of a partnership in care.

Dearmun (1992) found that parents expected to undertake direct care for their sick child in hospital, as they would auto-matically do at home, but they did not feel equal partners in the planning and decision-making process.

Darbyshire (1994) found that parents suffered uncertainty and confusion when caring for their child in hospital. This centred around their role and the need to 'parent' in public. This became particularly difficult if there was an apparent difference in philo-sophy between parent and ward staff; for example, overdiscipline of a child. Parents felt they needed to demonstrate competence in all skills, both general parenting and more specific skills related to the ill health of the child.

Smith (1995) suggests that, as negotiated care is a two-way process between the nurse and family, this must be based in a relationship of trust and respect, where both parties are equally valued. She suggests that the negotiation is around the level of participation in care and the support needed for this to happen. However, this is in stark contrast to Fradd (1996), who sees negotiation as primarily around goal setting and problem solving, which may not lead to participation in care by the parents.

Neill (1996b) studied participation by parents in care and found that the biggest barrier to this was role negotiation. Parents felt the loss of control and confusion of role at a time of great stress and anxiety was more likely to lead to conflict and further loss of control. Parents' perception of nurses was seen to be paternalistic and perpetually 'busy', leading to intimidation and further loss of control. It was suggested by parents that they would like to choose their level of participation through negotiation, and that this could be facilitated through communication, information and support.

These three themes – communication, information and support – were referred to constantly throughout the literature and will be returned to in the next section when looking at the role of nurses in negotiation and how their negotiating skills could be developed.

Power and empowerment are key aspects of the negotiating process. The balance of power within the oncology unit between the nurse and parent is unequal at the point of admission. Several aspects of this are worth exploring.

Territory

Despite the fact that the nurse does not live in the ward/unit, it is definitely the nurse's home, and therefore the nurse has territorial rights over the child and family. The nurse is more familiar with the environment, rules and regulations of the unit and, if these are not shared, remains in control of the environment.

Uniform

While many children's nurses do not wear hospital dresses any more, there is still the 'uniform' worn on the job, be it a tabard, colour or style. This again proclaims belongingness and carries authority which can be used to retain control.

Competence

It is easier for the nurse to demonstrate competence within the unit, than for the parent. The nurse is familiar with the layout, environment and the daily routine, and also has the advantage of escaping at the end of a shift to rest and restore prior to the next shift. Parents are often captive with their child for long periods of time and become weary. This may lead to unwillingness to participate in care, suggesting a lack of competence.

Consider your ward/unit. How do nurses demonstrate power, e.g. uniform, rules? How could this be reduced in order to attain a better balance of power between parents and nurses?

Stress

While nurses are stressed through the nature of working in oncology (see Chapter 6), the stress of being hospitalised and living through the cancer journey must be seen as very great. There is, therefore, an unequal stress level which can lead to a greater imbalance of power.

Emotional anxiety

The nature of being a parent involves an emotional relationship with one's child. This is particularly challenged when dealing with a child with a life-threatening illness. While nurses care for children, they do not have this same emotional attachment and therefore are more likely to remain in control of their own emotions; this affection gives rise to an imbalance of power.

However, the parent also has to take some responsibility in the relationship. While much has been written about the sick role and the imbalance of power between nurse and parent, the inception of the Patients' Charter (Department of Health, 1991a) and the exhortation to parents as to their rights has encouraged parents to see themselves as having the right both to speak and to be listened to (Ashworth *et al.*, 1992). While this can be threatening to nurses, it is important that parents continue to be encouraged to speak and articulate their needs if true negotiation is to take place within partnership in care. Yet, at the end of the day, it is the nurse who retains the power and locus of control and who can either encourage or deny negotiation.

Negotiation and the nurse

As the focus of negotiation with the family is around role, so this is true with the nurse. Nurses are educated to fulfil a role that is partly determined by the perception of the public and the consumers of health care. The stereotype of the nurse to be handmaidens, busy and performers of care, rather than decision makers in care, all lead away from a partnership in care if parents do not perceive the nurse in this light. While it is important for parents to be aware of the role of the nurse, it is more important for the children's nurses of today to be aware of their role and therefore not to be threatened by the need for flexibility and change.

In order for this to be achieved, children's oncology nurses need to acquire various knowledge, attitudes and skills if they are to be able to negotiate successfully with parents and children and to develop a practice of partnership in care.

Knowledge base

Family theories

It is imperative that any children's nurse has a good knowledge base regarding family theory. Negotiation with a family can take place on several levels and this depends on the perception of the child and family within a context. Children need to be seen not only within their immediate family, but as a unit interacting with other units and also as a system, with its own structure, function and environment. The goal for nursing care should then be harmony within the system, allowing for a holistic approach to care. Neill (1996b) suggested that the ability to assess and negotiate with families on all levels was only really carried out well by experienced nurses. While this may be logical, much care is carried out by more junior, less experienced nurses. There is, therefore, a need to ensure that clinical experience is gained through mentoring and role modelling if negotiation skills are to be acquired and developed by children's nurses.

Specialist knowledge

A second knowledge base is that of cancer. It is acknowledged through Calman and Hine (Department of Health, 1995) that people with cancer should be cared for by nurses with specialist knowledge if an acceptable standard of care is to be achieved and maintained. A small local study (Langton, 1994) looked at nurses' perceptions of the value of undertaking the ENB 240 Paediatric Oncology Course. One of the main benefits was that of confidence in knowledge and the ability to pass this on to both staff and families. This knowledge base is important if nurses are to be able to empower parents through information giving and teaching. However, while a knowledge base is necessary to provide care, the balance of power referred to earlier is often based in the inequality of knowledge between nurses and the child and family. It is therefore important that this knowledge is shared through the nurses' role of teaching and information giving in order for families to be able to make informed choices about their involvement in care. This teaching role is heavily advocated in the literature and is seen to be a fundamental way in which nurses are learning to change their role within a partnership of care, if this partnership is to be achieved.

Casey (1988) suggested that the nurse should complement care by parents and that this could only be achieved through teaching. Cleary (1992) and Marriott (1990) support this, and Farrell (1992) argues that this teaching, if effective, should have a goal of leading to minimal intervention in the care of the child.

> **Box 2.3   Examples of clinical skills learned by parents in a children's oncology unit**
>
> - Aseptic technique
> - Handwashing
> - Care of central venous lines
> - Administration of medicine
> - Management of pyrexia
> - Mouth care
> - Fluid balance
> - Infection control

Much progress has been made in the area of teaching clinical skills to the child and family (Box 2.3) However, it is important that these skills are learnt following negotiation and not assumption. This is particularly difficult when planning discharge (see Chapter 9), as there is an assumption that parents wish to carry out these skills or are competent to do so at home even though they may neither wish to or be competent. It is therefore important to negotiate parental involvement on admission and as a continuous process through and beyond discharge.

Case study 2.2 illustrates the problems of negotiation with an atypical family.

Case study 2.2

Darren is a 9-year-old gypsy boy who lives with his parents and eight brothers and sisters in their caravan, 50 miles from the hospital. On admission Darren is physically dirty and treated for head lice and scabies. The family are noted to be in a similar state. The family have visited infrequently and played a minimal part in Darren's care. Treatment planning identifies the need for central venous access. While the parents are not particularly interested in learning about this aspect of treatment, Darren has watched other children in the unit and is angry that he currently has treatment using normal venous access. Decisions as to the nature of access required need to be negotiated – primarily with Darren, who is likely to be the main participant in his care. Darren is keen to have the same 'line' as other children, however, experienced staff recognise that care of the line and access to the line is likely to be more prone to infection than usual.

Discussion with Darren by nursing staff allows Darren to learn about the care required for central lines. Different lines are demonstrated to Darren and, together, a decision is reached. Darren is given a portacath which ensures he has the same advantages of easy access as other children. The need for less frequent access minimises the need for injections and access can be coincided with either hospital appointments or visits from the community oncology nursing team.

It is important to ensure that teaching and information giving are used effectively in order to enhance negotiation and problem-solving skills. However, this case study also demonstrates the need for more than knowledge if negotiation is to be achieved.

Skills

Interpersonal skills

Much of the writing around negotiation demonstrated the importance of a range of interpersonal skills if negotiation was to be successful (Box 2.4) (Brown and Ritchie, 1989; Dunst and Trivette, 1996; Whyte, 1996). These skills were seen as very important, but were often recognised early on in the hospitalisation process, demonstrating the importance of assessment.

Assessment

Darbyshire (1994) stated that initial encounters and first impressions often set the scene for the mutual creation of a relationship. This is then obviously directed by the length of stay by the child and family. Within the oncology setting, there is often good opportunity to develop a longer-term relationship because of the nature of the disease and treatment process. This can be facilitated by an unhurried approach, demonstrating an interest in the family and including the parents when planning care as well as the child. All of these approaches help to demonstrate a commitment by the nurse to the family and the relationship.

In order to achieve this, nurses need to be self aware (Nethercott, 1993) and particularly aware of the difference between personal philosophy and that of the family, being able to accept difference and not becoming judgemental. This can be facilitated by knowing what to assess and how to assess.

Feetham *et al.* (1993) suggest that there are five main areas to be assessed:

- family process
- coping
- parenting
- health management skills
- home management skills.

Box 2.4   Outline of interpersonal skills identified in the literature

Non-verbal	Warmth, empathy, listening, active dialogue, understanding, self disclosure, smiling, touch, valuing
Verbal	Willingness to be involved
	Questioning skills

By using these areas, an accurate picture can be built up of the family in its broadest sense and the way in which the child and family relate to each other.

In terms of negotiating, this knowledge base can give the nurse cues as to how to proceed with negotiation within the context of a specific family. It must be noted that this may well be a process over time and the following strategies may be used for collecting data:

- interview
- observation
- questionnaire – local
- national survey.

Nurses need to be confident in their knowledge and skills if this assessment strategy is to be well utilised. Knight (1995) suggests that by using negotiation to begin to develop a relationship there are a variety of benefits (Box 2.5).

The development of a contract that sets goals and is constantly renegotiated is also seen to be beneficial for continuing to develop this relationship (Friedman, 1992).

Within a unit the use of policies that enhance partnership and negotiation is essential (Oates, 1992) if the nurse is to be enabled to empower families. Also tools that support negotiation, for example care plans, should be reviewed to ensure consistency of approach. Johnson and Lindschau (1996) also suggest that staff development needs to be geared towards helping staff to develop negotiation skills.

Attitudes

By encouraging nurses to communicate, negotiate and develop a partnership approach to care, there is the danger of assuming that nurses are interested and willing to adopt this approach. Negotiation is much more likely to occur if initiated by nurses. It is therefore paramount that wards and units spend time not only debating and owning a partnership philosophy, but also looking at how this affects practice and how to support staff if change becomes necessary.

■ Revisit your ward philosophy. How are the statements within it re partnership carried out in practice?
■ If you are undertaking or have recently undertaken an oncology-related course, how has this influenced your ability to negotiate?
■ What knowledge, skills and attitudes do you require or need to improve on, in order to further develop your negotiation skills?

Box 2.5   Benefits of negotiation as a basis of relationship

- Cooperation is gained
- Understanding of role can be facilitated
- Family wishes can be explored
- Compliance can be increased

Benefits of negotiation

Five key areas seem to be drawn from this chapter on the main benefits of negotiating and should be considered within your practice area:

- The use of negotiation is an empowering process. Empowerment can be seen as a regenerative process by which positive outcomes contribute energy, which in turn leads to activity.
- While negotiation should be undertaken as an aid to decision making, rather than to encourage participation of the parents and their child in care, it is noted that successful negotiation will often lead to decisions about who carries out care and how (Fradd, 1996), thus allowing the parents the opportunity to choose their level of participation (Neill, 1996a).
- Negotiation can help to diminish later misunderstandings and disappointments, thus promoting the development of relationships.
- Negotiation promotes choice by the child and family.
- Negotiation can involve others in the multidisciplinary team, thus providing a consistency of approach.

Barriers to negotiation

The barriers to negotiation are manifold and will, to a certain extent, be driven by local constraints:

- Local politics and policies can mitigate against a negotiating approach to care.
- Often, when attempting to introduce negotiation as a concept, a 'product champion' is required. The absence or removal of this champion can affect the success of implementing negotiation.
- Resource issues such as adequate skill mix, time and useful paperwork, can all hinder good negotiation.
- As already discussed, the knowledge, skills and attitudes of nurses involved in children with cancer need to be considerable if negotiation of care is to take place.

Conclusion

This chapter has sought to develop the theme of negotiation within a partnership of care with the child and family experiencing the cancer journey. Negotiation was defined and the need for negotiation was expanded upon. This was then set into context with the child, the family and the nurse, looking at the roles of each within the negotiation process and how these could be either enhanced or inhibited. Negotiation is seen as an empowering process if used to equalise the balance of power between the nurse and the child and family. The benefits of negotiating from an early stage of the relationship suggest that this is an area that is worth considering by children's oncology nurses in practice.

As Romaniuk and Kristjanson (1995) suggest, parents and nurses have specified roles in relation to the ill child. Successful partnership in care is a joint action between the parents and the nurse. Nurse-initiated negotiation can help to minimise the overlap in roles and ensure the child with cancer is cared for competently in a safe environment.

References

Ashworth, P., Longmate, M. and Morrison, P. (1992) Parent participation: its meaning and significance in the context of caring. *Journal of Advanced Nursing*, **17**, 1430–1439.

Ball, M., Glasper, A. and Yerrell, P. (1988) How well do we perform? Parents' perceptions of paediatric care. *Professional Nurse*, **4**(3), 115–118.

Brown, J. & Ritchie, J. (1989) Nurses' perceptions of their relationships with parents. *Maternal-Child Nursing Journal*, **18**(2), 79–96.

Callery, P. & Smith, L. (1991) A study of role negotiation between nurses and parents of hospitalized children. *Journal of Advanced Nursing*, **16**, 772–781.

Casey, A. (1988) A partnership with child and family. *Senior Nurse*, **8**(4), 8–9.

Cleary, J. (1992) *Caring for Children in Hospital: parents and nurses in partnership*. London: Scutari Press.

Darbyshire, P. (1994) *Living with a Sick Child In Hospital: the experiences of parents and nurses*. London: Chapman & Hall.

Dearmun, A. (1992) Perceptions of parental participation. *Paediatric Nursing*, **4**(7), 6–9.

Department of Health (1991a) *The Patient's Charter*. London: HMSO.

Department of Health (1991b) *Welfare of Children and Young People in Hospital*. London: HMSO.

Department of Health (1995) *A Policy Framework for Commissioning Care Services*. London: HMSO.

Dimond, B. (1996) *The Legal Aspects of Child Health Care*. London: Mosby.

Dunst, C. & Trivette, C. (1996) Empowerment, effective helpgiving practices and family centred care. *Pediatric Nursing*, **22**(4), 334–338.

Farrell, M. (1992) Partnership in care: paediatric nursing model. *British Journal of Nursing*, **1**(4), 175–176.

Feetham, S., Meister, S., Bell, J. & Gilless, C. (1993) *The Nursing of Families: theory research/education practice*. London: Sage Publications.

Fradd, E. (1996) The importance of negotiating a care plan. *Pediatric Nursing*, **8**(6), 6–9.

Friedman, M. (1992) *Family Nursing: theory and practice*. Norwalk, CN: Appleton & Lange.

Inman, C. (1991) Analysed interaction in a children's oncology clinic: the child's view and parents' opinion of the effect of medical encounters. *Journal of Advanced Nursing*, **16**, 782–793.

Johnson, A. & Lindschau, A. (1996) Staff attitudes towards parent participation in the care of children who are hospitlaized. *Pediatric Nursing*, **22**(2), 99–102, 112–13, 120.

Knafl, K., Cavallan, K. & Dixon, D. (1988) *Pediatric Hospitalization: family and nurse perspectives*. London: Scott, Foresman.

Knight, L. (1995) Negotiating care roles. *Nursing Times*, **91**(27), 31–33.

Langton, H. (1994) *Nurses' Perceptions of the Benefit to Practice of Undertaking ENB 237 and ENB 240*. (unpublished)

Marriott, S. (1990) Parent power. *Nursing Times*, **86**(39), 68.

Morse, J. (1991) Negotiating commitment and involvement in the nurse–patient relationship. *Journal of Advanced Nursing*, **16**, 455–468.

Neill, S. (1996a) Parent participation 2: findings and their implications for practice. *British Journal of Nursing*, **5**(2), 110–117.

Neill, S. (1996b) Parent participation: literature review and methodology. *British Journal of Nursing*, **5**(1), 34–40.

Nethercott, S. (1993) A concept for all the family. Family centred care: a concept analysis. *Professional Nurse*, 794–797.

Oates, M. (1992) The quality of child care. *Pediatric Nursing*, 11–13 April.

Romaniuk, D. & Kristjanson, L. (1995) The parent–nurse relationship from the perspective of parents of children with cancer. *Journal of Paediatric Oncology Nursing*, **12**(2), 80–89.

Smith, F. (1995) *Children's Nursing in Practice: the Nottingham Model.* Oxford: Blackwell Science.

Wegner, G. & Alexander, R. (1993) *Readings in Family Nursing.* Philadelphia: Lippincott.

Whyte, D. (1996) Expanding the boundaries of care. *Pediatric Nursing*, **8**(4), 20–27.

The impact of diagnosis 3

ROSEMARY HARDING

Introduction

This chapter sets the scene in terms of how children with cancer have arrived at the point of being given a diagnosis and looks at the initial period of time after the diagnosis has been made. It will identify the staff who may be involved before a definitive diagnosis is made, including the general practitioner (GP) and local/regional hospital personnel. The reasons why there may be a delay in diagnosis will be discussed, as will the effects and difficulties this may cause. The importance of prediagnostic investigations will be emphasised.

Sociological issues concerning illness and cancer will be mentioned. These will include the meaning of illness, understanding of cancer in society and cultural factors.

The difficulties of breaking the news of the diagnosis to parents and how the news should be given and by whom will be investigated. Some of the dilemmas and problems of telling children their diagnosis will be analysed. Exploration of the reactions to the diagnosis by children of different ages, parents and other family members and how they can be helped will follow.

Nurses' needs for education and support at diagnosis will be discussed.

Arriving at a diagnosis

Sharing care

Once cancer is suspected there will begin a time of intense activity and it is likely to become a period of extreme stress and anxiety for the child and family (Pinkerton, Cushing and Sepion, 1994). The increasing complexity of treatments and the involvement of different disciplines has led to the centralisation of care for children with cancer into specialised units (Nicholson, 1990). These regionally based paediatric oncology units developed in the 1970s, and 75% of children with malignant disease receive all or

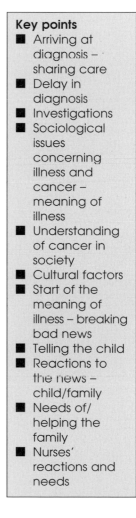

Key points
- Arriving at diagnosis – sharing care
- Delay in diagnosis
- Investigations
- Sociological issues concerning illness and cancer – meaning of illness
- Understanding of cancer in society
- Cultural factors
- Start of the meaning of illness – breaking bad news
- Telling the child
- Reactions to the news – child/family
- Needs of/ helping the family
- Nurses' reactions and needs

part of their treatment in one of these units (Hodson, 1989). These units have been shown to have significantly higher survival rates for their patients than those treated elsewhere (Stiller, 1988). Even if the GP or paediatrician in the local hospital has not voiced any suspicions, the parents and child may be anxious about being referred to a specialised unit (Sepion, 1990). Most of the parents of children with leukaemia in a study by Binger *et al.* (1969) had sensed something was seriously wrong with the child before the diagnosis was discussed or confirmed. Preparation may facilitate an easier admission for all the family. However, a GP may only see one case of childhood cancer during a career, and it is therefore unrealistic to expect the doctor to know about the oncology unit to which the child and family is referred. It may be therefore necessary for the GP to make some enquiries when the occasion arises (Sepion, 1990) from colleagues in the practice or specialist unit. It may seem to the family that the GP is not interested or is incompetent especially if parents who just have a feeling that their child is 'not right' are dismissed, or if the GP cannot find anything amiss and then subsequently the child is diagnosed with cancer, especially if it takes a while to make the diagnosis (Halliday, 1990). This then jeopardises the doctor's relationship with the family (Faulkner, Peace and O'Keeffe, 1995). Some GPs may feel that their role is limited because the families are 'taken over' by the hospital, and most of the GPs in the study reported by Faulkner *et al.* (1995) wanted to be more involved in the care. A case of malignant disease can have a profound effect on a great many members of the child's family and the community as a whole, and the family doctor can play a major role in the care and support of the child and family and also has a valuable role during the hospital treatment in continuing involvement with the family particularly to monitor distress in parents and other children (Halliday, 1990).

Hospital staff need to be aware that there are implications for long-term follow-up in the community when children are in hospital for prolonged periods of time, for example, at diagnosis and greater emphasis must be placed on involving the primary health care team who are often not sure about their role. It seems as though much work is required to improve relationships between the hospital and community staff and accept each other's complementary role. Although each sees the other's point of view and have distinct roles in the family's care, there seems little commitment to working towards a satisfactory arrangement and coordination of resources. The child and family will need help to live with cancer from before diagnosis through adjustment, treatment and after, and this will require a team approach of many individuals. With improved prognosis for children with cancer, more children spend less time in hospital, more can be treated as outpatients and more can expect to return to 'normal' patterns of life.

Specialists in the specialist units have the clinical expertise in this uncommon disease of childhood and can build up trust and confidence with the child and family throughout treatment. However the GP and primary health care team may have known the family for years beforehand, and this puts them in an ideal position to offer support with the peripheral effects at the time of diagnosis and help them to reintegrate into the local community and to live with the uncertainty the diagnosis brings. The specialist unit staff will be involved for a short time compared to the GP. If GPs are involved at the beginning rather than being bypassed, they are more likely to be more effective later. In order to ensure that the GP, local hospital and specialist unit work together for the good of the child and family, there must be good frequent communication between them and sharing of information right from the time of diagnosis and an acceptance of each other's complementary roles. A key person to liaise and coordinate input from different sources may be helpful to staff and parents.

What initiatives should be taken to improve communication between/under-standing of the roles of staff in primary health care settings, local hospitals and regional centres?

Just as the parents are trying to 'get a hold' on the new situation they are in, they may be informed that they are being immediately transferred to a regional paediatric oncology unit possibly hundreds of miles away (Halliday, 1990). An obvious disadvantage of this is the isolation from family and friends and its attendant lack of social and emotional support. The child and family will be surrounded by unfamiliar faces in an unfamiliar environment at the same time as trying to cope with the fear of a diagnosis of cancer and all the stresses this arouses (Pinkerton *et al.*, 1994). It is easy for staff who work in hospitals and other institutions to forget what alien and intimidating environments they can appear to others (*Nursing Times*, 1994). If parents are not prepared or have not had time to come to terms with the fact that their child may have cancer, they may find the exposure to other children undergoing treatment for malignant disease very difficult to cope with (Sepion, 1990). This was confirmed by some of the parents in a study reported by Faulkner *et al.* (1995) – they felt shocked and distressed as they thought cancer did not happen to children, the ward was noisy with a highly charged atmosphere and the deaths of other children fuelled fears for their own child's uncertain future.

However, if parents have been transferred from a unit where their child was the only one with a suspected malignancy, they may be relieved to be in an area where they are no longer being treated as abnormal. The child and family may have felt isolated by being the only one with cancer, with other parents finding

Consider the implications of the situation described in Case study 3.1 for the family, local hospital and regional centre.

Case study 3.1

Samantha aged 8 years had been admitted to a local hospital for investigations and was found to have acute myeloid leukaemia. Her mother was a nurse and her father a GP. They were told the diagnosis on Tuesday evening and were asked to take their daughter to the regional centre 120 miles away that evening in their own car. They set off accompanied by their other daughter aged 9 years and arrived in the town but could not find the hospital. By this time, Samantha was quite distressed and hyperventilating. Her parents phoned 999 and an ambulance transported them for the last part of their journey to the hospital ward.

difficulty in knowing what to say, so saying nothing for fear of upsetting the family (Sepion, 1990). Faulkner *et al.* (1995) found that parents were reassured by the general feeling that they had reached a milestone where they would be given reliable information and some hope for the future. Some of the parents found the first encounter with the children's cancer ward supportive and encouraging and there were others in a similar or worse situation. In a way it warned them of the seriousness of the illness and they were able to prepare themselves for the diagnosis.

Delay in diagnosis

Although cancer is the second commonest cause of death in children over 1 year of age, it is still an uncommon childhood disease and the diagnosis of cancer is often delayed (Foley, Fochtman and Mooney, 1993). Parents in research by Eiser *et al.* (1994) reported a considerable delay (mean of 17 weeks) between the time when they first sought professional advice about their child and the diagnosis being confirmed. Sloper (1996) found a mean delay of 14.9 weeks, but this varied between different diagnostic groups. Delay due to doctors can be broadly categorised into two periods – the interval between the individual presenting with symptoms and the doctor suspecting malignancy, perhaps reflecting the difficulties of the diagnostic process and/or adequacy of the doctor's knowledge, and the interval between suspicion and confirmation of diagnosis, often associated with failure to examine the individual adequately, false negative results from investigations and administrative failures (Ginzler, Pritchard and Mant, 1993).

The GP and paediatricians in a district general hospital are in a difficult position as they may only see one or two cases of childhood cancer (Pinkerton *et al.*, 1994) and cancer is not the first thing that they will consider when they are presented with what sometimes appear to be minor complaints and they do not want to overreact. The balance between early diagnosis and over-vigilance leading to unnecessary alarm is difficult to achieve (Ginzler *et al.*, 1993). Additionally childhood cancers can present in an enormous number of different ways (Halliday, 1990) and the symptoms are largely non-specific and frequently associated with more common childhood diseases (Schultz, 1989). A common complaint by parents in research by Faulkner *et al.* (1995) was that doctors would not listen to what they were saying about the child. It is therefore vital that parents are listened to and taken seriously and that the first doctor the parents see seeks a second opinion if there is any doubt about a diagnosis (Halliday, 1990). The way in which the initial stages of the illness is handled influences how parents respond when they are told the diagnosis. In the study by Faulkner *et al.*, 10 out of 19 parents had some complaint about health professionals at this time, mainly related to late diagnosis by a GP or staff in district general hospitals.

Many parents in research by Eiser *et al.* (1994) commented on the contrast between what was often a protracted period when the child was ill but no diagnosis made compared to the sudden flurry of activity following the diagnosis. It is difficult to know whether to rush ahead with diagnostic procedures in order to confirm the diagnosis and give the child and family details of treatment and prognosis or give them time to settle in and establish trusting relationships with staff and adequately prepare them for the numerous diagnostic investigations (Pinkerton *et al.*, 1994). The suspicion of cancer is worse than the confirmation to some parents, and many parents find that certainty comes almost as a relief (Barbor, 1983). In some cases Sloper (1996) found that the diagnosis marked the end of a period of frustration and the feeling that at last something was being done. The diagnostic phase of the cancer experience is emotionally shattering to most families (Foley *et al.*, 1993) and parents frequently identify this period of time as the worst (Kupst, 1992). The child and family have to cope with and adapt to the sometimes slow and insensitive routine at the hospital, waiting for tests and X-rays. The hospital itself is such an enclosed world that some of those who work there tend to forget the real world outside (Halliday, 1990) and the implications for individual families. Clarke-Steffen (1993) found that for some parents, the professionals responded to them in an impersonal manner and did not acknowledge the significance of the results for the family and did not share their sense of urgency. These families overwhelmingly reported that 'waiting and not knowing' was the worst part of the experience they went through. Having seen one or more local doctors they were referred to a specialist unit and knew their child had a life-threatening illness but not the specific diagnosis and prognosis. During this time the child underwent frequent tests, emergency medical treatment and/or surgery. The uncertainty of what they were dealing with and their future was very distressing, and they imagined the worst scenarios and tried to imagine how they would cope. This uncertainty led to worry and preoccupation and an inability to think about other aspects of their life and an inability to concentrate. They were suddenly aware that things which they previously believed only happened to others were now happening to them and they felt helpless and vulnerable because they were at the mercy of the professionals and there was sometimes difficulty with partial or conflicting information. Despite an urgent desire to hear the news of the diagnosis they also dreaded hearing it. Delays in diagnosis caused parents to feel anger and mistrust for health professionals and fear that the delay meant the disease had progressed to the stage that the child might not respond to treatment in work by Faulkner *et al.* (1995). This was also confirmed in research by Sloper (1996).

As well as problems at this time resulting from difficulties in establishing the precise diagnosis leading to possible delay, there are also problems in that parents need complex and detailed information at a time when they are least able to assimilate it because of emotional distress (Eiser *et al.*, 1994). Professional health care providers are confronted with how much information to give and when to give it. A commonly shared assumption among professionals is that they should not give information until all test results are known because parents do not need to know or worry about the unlikely worst options (Ekert, 1983), whereas families suggest they want information as soon as possible. Woolley *et al.* (1989) found that parents suggested the emphasis should be on the pacing of rather than protection from painful news.

It is important for us to alert the family to the difficulties of this time and acknowledge their distress and be available to address their worries. Other parents of children with cancer may be of help.

Investigations

One of the most important aspects when a malignancy is suspected is that reassurance is given that everything that needs to be done to reach a diagnosis will be done as quickly and efficiently as possible and that the family will be involved and kept up to date with any information about their child and the disease. One of the advantages of moving the family and child to a specialist unit is that there are usually facilities to carry out most of the investigations within one hospital, with experienced staff to plan and prepare for the procedures with the minimum of stress, and access to experts who will interpret the results of the tests. There is a need for investigations to be planned efficiently with the minimum amount of trauma to the child and family (Sepion, 1990). They will be faced throughout treatment with numerous investigations and staging procedures, so it is important that diagnostic tests are not so frightening and painful that the child becomes afraid of treatment (Pinkerton *et al.*, 1994). It is essential to establish a means of gaining the child's trust and cooperation and find an acceptable way to help the child and family through the procedures if they are to cooperate and be involved throughout the course of the illness. Nurses will require knowledge about the various diagnostic tests and preparation and aftercare involved.

Sociological issues concerning illness and cancer

Meaning of illness

Health and illness occur at opposite ends of a continuum and where a person is positioned on that continuum depends on what they and others perceive as health and illness (Bond and Bond, 1991). The definition of what constitutes health and illness varies between individuals, cultural groups and social classes. The same disease or symptom may be interpreted completely differently by two people from different cultures and in different contexts and this will affect their behavior and the treatment they look for. Cornwell (1984) distinguished between public and private accounts of health and illness – public being those accounts given when people are concerned that what they say is acceptable to others, this is likely to occur when relationships are not well established and in a more formal atmosphere, and private are those accounts that people give as if to others like themselves using terms and assumptions normally shared by their own group. These are used when trust has been built up.

People's understanding of illness, disease and good health are not static and change depending on personal experiences and circumstances (Lupton, 1994). Lay theories about illness are based on beliefs about the structure and function of the body and the ways in which it can malfunction. Even if based on scientifically incorrect premises, they often give a meaning to the person which helps them make sense of what has happened and why (Helman, 1990). Most individuals develop their health beliefs from folk models of illness, alternative forms of medical practice, the media and experience of their own or friends/family (Lupton, 1994). However these theories vary between people and within the same person over time (Armstrong, 1995). In general, lay theories attribute the cause of ill health to one of four possibilities:

- within the individual
- in the natural world
- in the social world
- in the supernatural world.

Sometimes illness is ascribed to combinations of causes. Social and supernatural causes tend to be more common in some communities of the non-industrialised world, while natural or patient-centred explanations are more common in the western industrialised world. Lay theories where the cause of ill health is within the individual are often related to changes in the diet or person's behaviour or lifestyle or arise because of increased personal vulnerability. The person is mainly responsible for his or her illness and should feel guilty for causing it. In a study by Pill and Stott (1982) it was shown that people who had the most economic control over their own lives accepted more responsibility for ill-health causation. Lay theories concerning the natural world are related to factors such as climate, environment, infections and accidents. Where the origin of ill health is believed to be in the social world, illness is thought to be caused by another person either through magical means (witchcraft, sorcery; the evil eye) or through poisoning or wounds. In modern western society, illness may be blamed on conflicts with others leading to stress or being given an infection from someone else. Causes attributed to the supernatural world include gods and spirits. Illness may be seen as a punishment from God for sinful behaviour and health may be seen as being restored through penitence and prayer. Where spirits are thought to be the cause, they may need to be driven out (Helman, 1990). A person, and in the case of children probably the parents, come to the doctor who has a biomedical scientific belief system with their own theories and each therefore has their own explanations about the illness, its cause, prognosis and treatment (Tuckett *et al.*, 1985). These lay theories affect health behaviour and the doctor–patient interaction (Armstrong, 1995).

Understanding of cancer in society

What can we do to alter the negative view of cancer that is prevalent in our society?

For most people, the word cancer provokes fear and they have a negative attitude towards it, conjuring up images of a relentless disease (Martocchio, 1985). Many are overpessimistic about the treatment and outcome (Pinkerton *et al.*, 1994), possibly holding very distorted ideas and erroneous information about cause and treatment (Culling, 1988), and often equate it with unavoidable death (Redler, 1994). Many illnesses with far worse prognoses are accepted with less dismay (Martocchio, 1985). In the twentieth century cancer has been used as a metaphor for evil, being described as an unrestrained and chaotic evil force. In the media crime, strikes etc. have been described as cancer – a demon force gradually destroying society (Helman, 1990). The media tends to reinforce the negative message about cancer, and society's attitude to cancer is often characterised by prejudice, stigma, a sense of helplessness and possibly phobia (Faulkner *et al.*, 1995). These attitudes can affect how a family copes with the diagnosis and how other people behave towards them and can add to their feelings of vulnerability and isolation (Geen, 1990; Macaskill and Monarch, 1990).

However in the field of childhood cancer, the prognosis has improved dramatically (Birch, Marsden and Morris-Jones, 1988; Stiller, 1993) and over 60% are now expected to survive (Hodson, 1989). Despite this improved prognosis, knowing that the diagnosis was some kind of cancer caused parents, in at least four out of the seven families in research by Clarke-Steffen (1993), to believe preconceptions of cancer as a uniformly fatal illness applied to their child.

Although there are a number of known risk factors for the cancers that occur in adults, the aetiology of most cases of childhood cancer is unclear. However, experience has shown that many parents of children with cancer form theories about the origin of the illness (Ruccione *et al.*, 1994). Mood (1991) noted that with adult cancer patients the search for meaning of the illness is a basic spiritual need, an attempt to enhance their self esteem, and is a way of trying to find hope and purpose and gain mastery over the complex and unfamiliar information. Evidence indicates that parents of children with cancer also search for a meaning in a similar way. Ruccione *et al.* (1994) found that in answer to the question about anything that could have caused or contributed to their child's illness, parents mentioned factors that fell into 12 themes including environmental and family factors, parental self blame and myths/misconceptions.

Cultural factors

It is difficult to define 'culture' as it is a large, complex and abstract concept (Richardson, 1993). Helman (1990) states that it is:

> 'an inherited "lens" through which individuals perceive and understand the world that they inhabit and learn how to live within it. Growing up within any society is a form of enculturation whereby the individual slowly acquires the cultural "lens" of that society. Without such a shared perception of the world, both the cohesion and the continuity of any human group would be impossible'.

This suggests that people within a culture share views, beliefs, habits, values and customs which form the basis for the rules that allow them to live in the group from which they derive support and comfort. Although there is this sharing, there is also a wide variation in the degree to which the beliefs and customs, etc. are shared. It is possible to make some assumptions and generalisations about a person based on culture and/or religion, but we must be aware of the individuality that exists within it and it is only possible to identify a person's cultural features by asking the person (Littlewood, 1988). The UK is a multicultural society with approximately 6% of the population representing ethnic minorities in England and Wales (Office of Population Censuses and Surveys, 1992). These ethnic minorities include AfroCarribean, Asians, Chinese, Arab and mixed origin (Hussein-Rassool 1995). Muslims form the largest group (43%) among the ethnic minorities in the UK (Office of Population Censuses and Surveys, 1992) and, next to Christianity, Islam is the largest religion in the UK (Gatrad, 1995). It is therefore important that we understand something of the culture and way of life of those patients who belong to ethnic minorities if their health care is to be successful (Parmar, 1985). When a person from one culture moves to another country with a different culture, that person has to adapt to that new culture. However this results in the creation of a new culture where some of the values, etc. of the original culture are mixed with some of the adopted culture. There can be a great deal of stressful adjustment. We are so accustomed to the beliefs and values of our own culture that we are in danger of judging others' cultural norms negatively against our own. It is therefore important that we develop self awareness related to this aspect and accept that others have different customs and ways of dealing with events and that we are flexible enough to adapt to different practices. It is even more important when caring for children, because they are learning about and developing their culture as they grow up and may have difficulty expressing their views because of their stage of development or because of language difficulties (Richardson, 1993).

Cultural diversity results in a wide variation in lifestyle, health behaviour, religion and language, and may affect how people perceive health problems and ill health (Hussein-Rassool, 1995). Minority racial groups in the UK have different values concerning life and health (Erikson, 1967). Spinetta (1984), for example, found that there was a very strong religious faith in Mexican families which enabled them to accept their child's cancer diagnosis with resignation. This helped in their response to the associated stress but because of this resignation to God's will it often caused lack of medical compliance. Buddhists believe disease is to do with Karma – the unhappy result of deeds done in a previous existence (Wang and Martinson, 1996). Many people are able to gain explanations for events such as illness and comfort through prayer by following a particular religion or faith. It is therefore important that they are given the opportunity to define their problems from their own perspective and within their socio-cultural context (Hussein-Rassool, 1995). While medical advances can be applied with little change to people from a variety of cultural backgrounds, the psychosocial differences in cultural back-grounds can make a major difference in the responses and adap-tation of individuals to an illness like cancer. Communication patterns vary from one culture to another. Within the immigrant Vietnamese population communication with people outside that community is often accomplished via a tribal spokesman chosen by the community to represent their interests. In highly developed countries such as ours, it is customary for health care professionals to share decision making about treatment with the families involved. However the Vietnamese view the doctor as the knowl-edgeable authority figure and attempts at sharing the decision-making process with these families suggests that the doctor has doubts and uncertainties and their expertise is questioned (Spinetta, 1984). Communication within the family varies from culture to culture. Although there is an emphasis on open commu-nication in families in our country and encouragement to explain to the child with cancer about the disease and treatment, this is very different within the immigrant Mexican population where they do not discuss such issues directly with their children but communicate in their own way (Spinetta, 1984).

People in some cultures may have great faith in alternative treatments, which may lead to contradictory advice between the western medical staff and these alternative practitioners. Koocher (1984) found that Puerto Rican families used homoeopathic, and Haitian families, voodoo practitioners. Although faith healing and healing services may be a source of help and comfort to patients and families in some cultures, there is a danger that they may be used as an alternative for proven medical treatment.

Western medicine is highly technical with a strong biological basis and is not closely linked with social and religious beliefs, unlike some cultures (Wang and Martinson, 1996). It is therefore important to remember that families from minority populations with different cultural backgrounds are in need of particular atten-tion when diagnosed with a disease like cancer that requires treat-ment at a facility run by and for the cultural majority, and it is necessary for staff to carefully assess the families and to know something about their beliefs and support systems (Koocher, 1984).

Start of the meaning of illness

Breaking bad news

Confirming the diagnosis of cancer to a child's parents is a necessary but unenviable task (Pinkerton *et al.*, 1994). There is no easy way of doing it (Halliday, 1990). Parents of sick children carry much pain, anxiety, misery and guilt. Many treatments and interventions cannot be given or performed without consent and are legally parents' responsibility. Therefore parents may feel that much of the burden of the illness rests on their shoulders. At the same time they are affected emotionally by what is happening to their child and commonly feel guilt because of the implicit duty of parents to keep their children free of disease, which in turn implies that in some way a child's suffering is a failure of parenting. An interview with a parent is therefore simultaneously an interview with the child (the parent being the legal representative) and with a family member. It is emotionally demanding and requires great care and thought (Buckman, 1992).

Case study 3.2

After investigations, Clare aged 4 years was found to have acute lymphoblastic leukaemia. An appointment was made for the doctor to give the diagnosis to parents. The doctor arrived earlier than the appointed time so their anxiety was not prolonged. They were taken into the ward office and told clearly and kindly what the diagnosis was and given some hope about the success of treatment. Their questions were answered honestly and in a way they could understand. Not too much information was given but they were given a time when medical staff would return the following day for further discussion.

Case study 3.3

Ryan aged 18 months was diagnosed as having a rhabdomyosarcoma. His parents waited all day for the doctor to come and tell them. There was no set time arranged for the doctor to come and talk to them. When the doctor eventually arrived, the parents were extremely anxious and annoyed that they had been kept waiting. They were given the diagnosis in the cubicle, with the crying child present. Neither parent was able to concentrate as they were distracted by Ryan. The explanation was hurried and little hope was given.

One definition of bad news which is useful in practical terms is 'any news that drastically and negatively alters the patient's view of his/her future' (Buckman, 1984).

The word 'breaking' implies that something gets broken and what gets broken is the child's and/or parents' whole vision of the future which is why bad news is such a shock (Kaye, 1996). Naturally most people do not want to be told that they are ill and resent the prospect of their lifestyle and its opportunities being reduced or threatened by their state of health. Equally every professional dislikes having to break bad news. As health care professionals we all know that breaking bad news is a difficult part of our job and there will be few of us who do not at some time have to break bad news to a client or relative or offer support to someone who has just received bad news (Buckman, 1992).

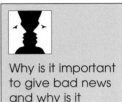

Why is it important to give bad news and why is it difficult?

Until relatively recently it was not always regarded as standard medical practice to tell clients the truth. However, there have been great changes in policies and attitudes over the last two or three decades, and it is now generally held that all clients have absolute ethical, moral and legal rights to any medical information that they require and request (Buckman, 1992). It is important to break bad news and tell the truth in order to maintain trusting relationships, reduce uncertainty, prevent inappropriate hope and allow appropriate adjustment (Kaye, 1996). Clients also need information so that they can participate on the basis of informed knowledge (*Nursing Times*, 1994).

However it can be difficult for several reasons – feeling incompetent, fear of being blamed, fear of inducing a reaction and not knowing how to cope and feeling embarrassed about how to manage when someone is upset, wanting to protect the recipient, feeling awkward about showing sympathy as a professional and being reminded of human vulnerability to illness (Kaye 1996).

Consider Case studies 3.2 and 3.3. How should bad news be broken and how have you seen it done?

The debate about breaking bad news has moved on from whether to tell to how to tell. It may be that unthinking and insensitive truth telling is as deleterious in its own way as unthinking and insensitive truth concealment (Buckman, 1992). There is no way of softening the blow for parents when telling them their child has cancer, but the experience can be made more harrowing and confusing however through inept handling before and at the time of breaking bad news (Faulkner *et al.*, 1995). The task of breaking bad news is a testing ground for the entire range of our professional skills and abilities – if we do it badly, the client or family members may never forgive us, if we do it well they may never forget us (Buckman, 1992). The way information about a life-threatening illness is given can affect the parents' ability to come to terms with the diagnosis and if done inappropriately can cause additional unnecessary stress (Woolley *et al.*, 1989;

Pinkerton *et al.*, 1994) and will also affect the establishment of a collaborative trustful relationship (Levine, Blumberg and Hersh, 1982). Many parents in the research by Woolley *et al.* (1989) felt the way the diagnosis was conveyed was a key event which helped or hindered them in their subsequent acceptance, adjustment and coping with the child's illness. For many of these parents the diagnosis had been made many years previously but they vividly remembered the manner in which it was done and recalled minute details of the day they were given the diagnosis. Sharp, Strauss and Lorch (1992) also found that parents' responses indicated that memories of being told a diagnosis are often etched permanently into their consciousness. It is therefore important that confirmation of cancer to parents should be a planned event (Pinkerton *et al.*, 1994). It is all too easy to forget that although this interview may be one of several unpleasant or harrowing tasks in the course of a shift for the professional, it may be among the biggest events in the life of the parent (*Nursing Times*, 1994).

The interview in which bad news is discussed is an asymmetrical one – the professional has information to impart that the client/family do not yet possess. But their responses are in some respects the most crucial part of the interview and so the interview has two components – the divulging of information and the therapeutic dialogue by which the professional listens to, hears and responds to the client/family reactions. Whoever it is that takes the main responsibility for breaking the bad news, all other health professionals involved in the care may contribute to the support after the individual/family has heard the news and this involves time spent listening, hearing and acknowledging the emotions the client/family are experiencing (Buckman, 1992). The professional must find out what the client/family already know, how much they want to know and decide on the agenda and then start from the client/family's starting point. Information should be given in small amounts as medical information is hard to digest and with a serious diagnosis there will be failure to retain much because of the shock and confusion. Using language that is intellible to the client/family is important – medical jargon is only intelligible to the initiated and its use can isolate and alienate the receiver although it may comfort and reassure the professional and act as a refuge in difficult situations. It is important to check reception frequently and clarify and repeat important points. Sometimes the use of diagrams and written information can help and some doctors tape record interviews so that the child/family can take it away. While transmitting the information, it is important to simultaneously listen to the child/family's reaction and try to elicit their concerns and respond to their feelings (Buckman, 1992). In practice the professional responds to the individual's ongoing reaction, adjusting the pace accordingly (Faulkner, 1992). Flexibility as to the amount and level of information given is required (Pinkerton *et al.*, 1994).

Sloper (1996) found that parents were dissatisfied at diagnosis when they felt their informant appeared abrupt and unsympathetic, where they received conflicting information from different sources, where they were told in a public place and where one parent was alone at the time. In a study reported by Woolley *et al.* (1989), parents appreciated being given the diagnosis as soon as possible in an open direct but sympathetic and understanding manner in private and with no interruptions. They appreciated sufficient time to take the news in and for doctors to repeat and clarify information. Most wanted early information about the nature of the illness, the likely progression and cause. The longer the period of prior worry, the more able they seemed to hear and absorb. An outline of available support and help and early follow-up appointment for further discussion and questions was helpful. Parents can be encouraged to write down questions as they occur for discussion (Pinkerton *et al.*, 1994), as research by Eiser *et al.* (1994) showed that although parents were encouraged to ask questions at the initial interview many felt unable to do so usually because they were ignorant about cancer specifically or illness generally. Research by Faulkner *et al.* (1995) showed that aspects parents appreciated, when they were told the news that was to change their lives, were telling the truth in a direct manner, not giving false hope, presenting the facts, being listened to and an efficient but a relaxed atmosphere. Parents' strongest preferences, in research by Sharp *et al.* (1992), were for doctors to show caring (97%), to allow parents to talk (95%) and allow parents to show their feelings (93%). They wanted doctors to share information (90%) and be highly confident (89%).

Information should be truthful and offer positive support but not unrealistic hope (Pinkerton *et al.*, 1994). Presenting a rosy or overoptimistic view of the prognosis undermines rather than supports the parents' care (Culling, 1988; Arnfield 1990; Macaskill and Monarch, 1990). Despite their distress, parents wished to be fully informed so that they could understand what they might have to face and plan for the future while knowing that they would be supported throughout the illness. This lessened their sense of helplessness and isolation. The general consensus was that imagining the worst was worse than knowing it (Woolley *et al.*, 1989). Parents, in research by Sloper (1996), also emphasised the importance of knowing the truth however negative. When families, in research by Clarke-Steffen (1993), perceived they had been told all of the worst things that could happen or be discovered as well as the best, they then felt that they could trust professionals to tell them everything. Like other virtues, truth telling may be best practised as an art form and not a fixed criterion – the finer points being how to speak the truth with compassion and knowing when to be silent (Hinds, 1995). The use of direct words such as fear, anger, death, can convey the ability and willingness to discuss difficult subjects (Pinkerton *et al.*, 1994). An outpouring of emotion, an awkward silence or responses that appear inappropriate should all be seen for what they are – reactions to the news and not considered judgementally. Professionals must be guided by the needs of the person (*Nursing Times*, 1994).

Giving information to both parents at the same time prevents one parent having to remember what was said and being responsible for confirming the bad news. It also avoids the risk of parents interpreting information differently and feeling that the doctors may have told their spouse something extra or different. Being together also facilitates sharing and discussion. It is important to offer parents some time together in private to share their feelings and prepare to face the child if not also present at the discussion (Pinkerton *et al.*, 1994). For single parents, finding someone with whom to share their inner feelings with may be difficult (Foley *et al.*, 1993), and Woolley *et al.* (1989) found some welcomed the presence of a familiar professional, for example the ward sister. The presence of several unknown staff when the diagnosis was given was universally disliked in research by Woolley *et al.* (1989).

Bad news is material that must be handled carefully and skillfully. The task should ideally be carried out by someone with expertise and experience. Furthermore this person should have some measure of continuing responsibility and commitment to the client/relatives. Breaking bad news is often more than a one-shot event, and there are often consequences and questions that will require further discussion. It is better if the person who breaks the bad news is the person who will be able to deal with at least some of these issues later. The initial interview with the doctor is particularly important, because it establishes the first bonds between the family and doctor and allied health professionals present at interview. This bond forms the basis of a relationship of trust and therefore confidence in the decision-making process related to treatments (Ekert, 1989).

In an ideal world professionals would acquire expertise from specific teaching in their training and experience from seeing good examples of interviews before they have to hold one on their own (Buckman, 1992). Faulkner *et al.* (1995) found that after brief training doctors who had been very concerned about their inability to break bad news sensitively improved in the way they gave bad news. However very few had the skills to pick up the pieces after – most went on to talk to patients/relatives about what they would do about the problem rather than finding out what impact the news had had, therefore it would seem that there is a need for more skills in breaking bad news and in identifying psychological concerns.

Often during the interview the doctor discusses details of the likely outcome of treatment and details of the type of treatment. Usually at this interview it is difficult for the family to understand and remember all that they have been told. It is important that there are other opportunities for further interviews, where they will be given the chance to ask questions and clarify details which may have been forgotten (Ekert, 1989).

Whenever possible the named nurse should attend the interviews that the doctors have with the child and parents. Knowing the information and terminology that has been given to them will enable the nurse to clarify, explain and reinforce anything that they did not understand. It is not unusual for parents not to hear or understand the rest of the conversation once the name of the tumour or the word cancer has been used (Sepion, 1990). It is good practice to record what was said and the parents' reactions (*Nursing Times*, 1994).

Telling the child

Parents face a dilemma in deciding what or how to tell the sick child what the problem is. Medical opinion recommends that children are informed about their diagnosis (Eiser *et al.*, 1994), although this may be dependent on several factors (Chesler, Paris and Barbarin, 1986), including the child's age and religion. There is evidence that early knowledge and discussion of the diagnosis and not evasion and concealment is linked to better psychosocial adjustment in the child (Slavin *et al.*, 1982). It is important to

Case study 3.4
Catherine aged 8 years was found to have Ewing's sarcoma of her tibia. Her mother, who was a single mother, did not want Catherine told what the diagnosis was exactly but that she had an infection in the bone. Chemotherapy treatment was commenced and as a result her hair started to fall out and she had problems with nausea and vomiting. The nursing staff felt that Catherine ought to know, but although they suggested to the mother that Catherine was told the truth she refused to allow this. As the days went on, Catherine's behaviour caused the staff to be very concerned. She cut the hair off her doll and threw it at the doctor. She refused to eat and drink and tipped her tray of food on to the floor.

What would you have done if you had been involved in Catherine's care (Case study 3.4)?

discuss with the parents first and agree on the manner in which the information will be shared with the child (Buckman, 1992). The child needs to be told as much about the disease and treatment as they are able to understand with language appropriate for their development (Pinkerton *et al.*, 1994). There is a growing awareness that even very young children are able to understand the nature and implications of a serious illness. There is also a greater awareness of the rights of the child and the need to involve children in decisions about their care as stressed in the Children Act 1989 and the European Convention on the Rights of the Child (1991). Understanding must be frequently checked with repetition as needed. It is important to make it clear that it is nobody's fault (Buckman, 1992). Parents may wish initial details to be given by medical/nursing staff (Pinkerton *et al.*, 1994). Some parents may request the child is not told the truth in order to protect them, as they worry that the information will produce fear and anxiety, but this concern is often their own and not the child's. It is impossible to keep the severity of the illness from the child as they realise that the sudden change in their life situation and the attitudes and mannerisms of all around indicates that this is not an everyday occurrence. Although parents may go to great lengths to shield them, children get information from many other sources, for example observation, non-verbal communication, eavesdropping and talking with other children (Bluebond-Langner, 1978). Also the treatment of cancer is complicated and time consuming and may involve restrictions like fasting and children cannot be expected to tolerate and endure it without understanding the need for it. Hiding the truth may make the child imagine a much worse illness and outcome, perhaps something so terrible it cannot be talked about, (Moore, Kramer and Perin, 1986), and if they compare their symptoms with another child on the ward, may guess at an incorrect diagnosis. It may prevent them asking important questions and if they see their parents upset they may not talk about it for fear of upsetting them more (Pinkerton *et al.*, 1994). Binger *et al.* (1969) found that the children who were perhaps the loneliest of all were those who were aware of their diagnosis but recognised their parents did not wish them to know, so there was little or no meaningful communication and there was no one to whom the child could openly express sadness, fear and anxiety. Waechter (1971) showed that children who were not told their diagnosis in order to protect them had heightened anxiety and isolation. If children are told the diagnosis at a later stage they may feel betrayed, shocked and more fearful of consequences (Slavin *et al.*, 1982). Staff in work by Faulkner *et al.* (1995) found it difficult and felt unable to be open and honest if parents did not want the child to know of a poor prognosis, so this may affect their ability to communicate and care effectively. Eiser *et al.* (1994) found that although many parents were initially protective and preferred the child not to know the diagnosis, they were relieved when the children were told and did not regret the decision to inform. However some parents would have liked longer to come to terms with the diagnosis themselves before having to deal with the child's distress. Some parents may like to impart the initial information themselves but for staff to reinforce and expand on it. Communication between parents and child about the disease may help to decrease the child and family's fears, anxieties and stress and encourage more open family communication generally. The work by Eiser *et al.* (1994) showed that some parents found books were helpful in explaining the disease and its treatment to the child.

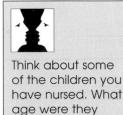

How could the situation described in Case study 3.5 have been avoided?

Reactions to the news – child

Children with cancer will probably already have begun to feel the impact of the illness on their life before the diagnosis is suspected or confirmed – they may have suffered pain or other unpleasant symptoms and undergone multiple examinations, investigations and treatments which compound the pain. They may arrive at the hospital with preconceived fears and mistrust of staff and hospitals, fear of the unknown and may develop phobias about the procedures and treatments.

Children's reactions to their illness will be determined by their understanding of body parts and illness related to their cognitive development and previous experience and reactions of the family.

Think about some of the children you have nursed. What age were they and how did they react?

Infants

Infants are in the sensorimotor stage of Piaget's theory of intellectual development and are gradually learning about the world through their actions and information coming in through their senses. Internal mental representations emerge. At first an infant

---

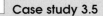

Case study 3.5

Lisa aged 14 years was told by the registrar that she had Hodgkin's disease and that this would need to be treated with chemotherapy mainly on an outpatient basis with a good chance of cure. The chemotherapy was due to commence the next day. However it was delayed because the consultant wanted another pathologist to review the tissue biopsy. Lisa and her mother were understandably confused and upset. As a result of the review, they were seen again that day and told that the diagnosis was now non-Hodgkin's lymphoma, needing different chemotherapy and with a less optimistic outlook.

is very egocentric/self centred, but gradually realises that there is an outside world (Hayes, 1988; Smith and Cowie, 1988). According to Erikson's Psychosocial Development Theory (1963), the first year of life is the time when basic trust develops and consistent loving care by a mothering person is essential to this development (Whaley and Wong, 1991). Although an infant has no real understanding of what is occurring or perception of cancer, a diagnosis of cancer may alter the process of developing self awareness. Normal processes for the differentiation of their self from their mother may become distorted by physiological alterations in the infant or by psychological or emotional trauma affecting the family. Separation from mother, pain of investigations/treatment and denial of basic needs, for example food and warmth, may be experienced and the parents will be unable to explain this because of the limited understanding of the infant (Hockenberry and Coody, 1986). Eradication of the disease may take priority over the infant's developmental processes and it is important that continuation of normal growth and development is addressed and that their basic needs for food and love, etc. and development of trust are met by encouraging family involvement (Hockenberry and Coody, 1986; Foley *et al.*, 1993; Pinkerton *et al.*, 1994).

Toddlers

Toddlers are developing autonomy centred around their increasing ability to control themselves and their environment. They want to use their powers to do things for themselves using their newly acquired motor skills and mental powers, and feelings of doubt and shame can arise when they are forced to be dependent in areas in which they are capable of assuming control (Whaley and Wong, 1991). Therefore the diagnosis of cancer which the toddler has no perception of can interfere with this development. They cannot understand the reason for the traumatic procedures necessary and the possible accompanying restraint required or the multitude of unfamiliar people they have to deal with. Their search for autonomy is less desirable when threatened with painful procedures (Pinkerton *et al.*, 1994). This may result in regression in their behaviour emotionally and/or physically and affect their development of trust. They may see procedures and treatment as a punishment. Parents may relax methods of discipline in an attempt to protect the child from further trauma, resulting in inconsistency in their control methods leaving the toddler unsure of their position. They soon learn to manipulate situations. A child of this age requires love and support, discipline and positive reassurance to help keep fears and feelings controlled (Hockenberry and Coody, 1986). Their autonomy can be encouraged by giving the child choices within reason (Foley *et al.*, 1993).

Preschool/early school age

Preschool/early school age children are noted for their vigorous behaviour, sense of adventure and curiosity (Hockenberry and Coody, 1986) and strong imagination (Whaley and Wong, 1991). They find it hard to distinguish between fantasy and reality. Their use of language and problem solving is developing (Smith and Cowie, 1988). Egocentricity is lessening but they are still unable to see things from someone else's viewpoint (Hayes, 1988). They may react with anger and aggression at the disruption to their lives caused by the diagnosis of cancer and lack of understanding. They may see cancer as something bad that they have caused to happen and that they are being punished for it by treatment and restriction on their activities. They may be afraid to go to sleep in case something painful happens and they may have nightmares (Hockenberry and Coody, 1986).

Children of this age can be encouraged to talk about their feelings, or if they are too young, they can express themselves in drawings or play (Hockenberry and Coody, 1986). Play is a good indicator of the child's response to life (Culling, 1988). They can be helped to understand procedures, etc. by playing with equipment, demonstration on dolls and answering questions in a language understandable to them (Foley *et al.*, 1993). Early introduction to the play leader can be valuable, and this person can become a friend and counsellor with whom the child may have prolonged contact during treatment. Time and patience are essential.

School age

School age children need and want real achievement and the opportunity to complete tasks and activities (Whaley and Wong, 1991). It is also a decisive period in their social relationships with others (Whaley and Wong, 1991) and they can more easily take the perspective of others (Smith and Cowie, 1988). They are able to work things out mentally but are not able yet to deal with abstract concepts or symbols (Hayes, 1988) and, according to Piaget's concrete operational stage, it is a time for classification and order (Smith and Cowie, 1988). A diagnosis of cancer threatens their increasing independence, autonomy and self image and disrupts the establishment of relationships outside the family setting. They may question why the disease has occurred and they may be confused as they cannot fully understand its meaning. Again the diagnosis and its treatment may be seen as punishment for their actions or thoughts (Hockenberry and Coody, 1986) and they may have feelings of anger and frustration (Pinkerton *et al.*, 1994). This anger may be expressed through uncooperativeness – parents often receiving the brunt of much of the child's anger and often finding difficulty coping with it (Whaley and Wong,

1991). Alteration in physical appearance due to the illness, investigation or immediate treatment may cause insecurity in a child and for these reasons, and also because the child is separated from peers, the child may become isolated. The diagnosis and treatment disorganises the recently developed sense of order and may cause worry about keeping up with school work.

It is important that the child is allowed to express/talk about feelings and confusions and that explanations are given in age-appropriate language in simple concrete terms. Children need to be reassured that they will not be abandoned and positive self images must be supported. A sense of control and industry can be enhanced by allowing them to learn something about their disease and treatment and to master skills to perform some of their own care, for example pushing the syringe plunger.

Adolescence

Adolescents are overtly preoccupied with the way they appear in the eyes of others compared to their own self concepts and socialising with peers is very important (Whaley and Wong, 1991). They are striving to develop independence, identity and functional roles in society (Thompson, 1990). They are capable of abstract reasoning and can speculate about the possible (Smith and Cowie, 1988). They are able increasingly to understand what the diagnosis of cancer entails. In research by Faulkner *et al.* (1995) older children of 9–14 years generally realised that cancer was serious and life threatening. It alters their immediate and future plans and they realise their vulnerability and finiteness. They are separated from their main socialising agents – peers. Body image so important to their identity is altered and they may feel confused about who they have become and their future roles. They have little energy for any activities and feel a lack of control. This may result in feelings of anger, bitterness, frustration, resentment and depression. A sense of jealousy about their 'healthy' friends may develop. Some may allow themselves to become more dependent on family, which can cause loss of pride, while others may react violently to this intrusion on their lives, rebelling and refusing treatment and not cooperating. Older children may have greater emotional stress at diagnosis if their feelings of fear and apprehension must be masked to protect their parents or other family members (Foley *et al.*, 1993).

Adolescents must be allowed to express their feelings and uncertainties. They need clear information so that they can be involved in decision making which will encourage their sense of independence. They must be helped to value themselves as people and integrate the restrictions caused by the diagnosis. Autonomy and self care must be encouraged. They may need help to develop realistic future goals (Hockenberry and Coody, 1986). The maintenance of relationships with peers can be encouraged to promote their self esteem, prevent feelings of rejection and abandonment (Pinkerton *et al.*, 1994).

In order to be able to support the child a variety of techniques individually tailored to each patient must be developed in conjunction with the parents. If a named nurse is introduced to and involved with the child and family right from the beginning, this may help reduce the number of staff involved and will not be so confusing for them. This named nurse will hopefully possess knowledge about the investigations and treatment required and parents will have a wealth of knowledge about their child, enabling them to work together for the child's benefit. Although developmental theories can provide a guide, there can be a wide range of individual variations. There have been some criticisms of Piaget's staged theory (Smith and Cowie, 1988) in that in some areas he seems to have underestimated the child's mental capacity. Recent studies suggest that even very young children have the potential to develop sophisticated understanding about their health and illness (Rushforth, 1996). On the other hand, older children may regress in their ability to use abstract thinking because of their distress, so this must be considered. It is important for us to completely assess the child – to determine the level of emotional maturity and ability to cope with the illness and treatment, which depend on the family situation, child's age and stage of development, previous experience of illness and hospital – in order to assist in choosing appropriate support techniques. Perrin and Perrin (1983) concluded from their research that most paediatric health care professionals pitch much of their information giving at mid school age level irrespective of age, knowledge level or previous experience of the child. The child's cultural background and family situation and general anxiety and distress of the parents will influence the child's coping ability, so these too should be considered.

The nurse has an advantage in being able to detect any early signs of adjustment difficulties due to the close contact with the child/family (Foley *et al.*, 1993). The nurse should in general aim to decrease stress and increase adaptation by encouraging expression of fears and concerns; increasing understanding of the situation; promoting the use of adaptive coping strategies; maintaining open communication; promoting the child's self esteem; developing a supportive network (Foley *et al.*, 1993) and the nurse can help the child cope through guiding parents to support the child through these means. Honesty and positive reinforcement is important and questions should be answered as truthfully as possible avoiding unnecessary detail. If there is open and honest

What do you consider to be the most important aspects to remember in order to help a child cope with his/her diagnosis?

communication there is less likelihood of emotional and behavioural difficulties (Geen, 1990).

Faulkner *et al.* (1995) found that children as young as 7 years felt they had to keep their feelings from their parents in order to protect them. Explanations of the illness to the child must take account of cognitive development. Research studies have shown that adults as well as children often have a confused picture of the inside of their bodies and the function of various organs, therefore an explanation of illness must take into account the limitations of the children's knowledge of their bodies (Eiser, Patterson and Eiser, 1983). A study by McEwing (1996), for example, showed that children between 4.5 and 8.5 years could recall between two and four body parts and they were mostly aware of the bones, heart and brain. There was evidence that the children appeared to have some common misconceptions about the content of their body and most children considered that all body parts were essential for life and that no body part was dispensable or replaceable. Children's ideas about the causation of illness are also linked to their cognitive development (Bibace and Walsh, 1981). Before the age of formal operations (e.g. 12 years) children are not capable of abstract thought. Most of the concepts relevant to cancer and its treatment are abstract and foreign to children (Foley *et al.*, 1993), and therefore younger children may benefit more through explanations that draw on specific analogies relative to everyday experience or visual representation of material rather than verbal (Culling, 1988). It may be helpful to the newly diagnosed child to be introduced to a child who is further along in treatment; the child can be shown what it is like to have a long line, etc. (Brown, 1989).

Reactions to the news – family

The experience of coping with a life-threatening illness in a child must be one of the most distressing life events that a family has to face and an improved prognosis does not reduce the emotional impact on families (Faulkner *et al.*, 1995). The diagnosis of cancer has an immediate and lasting impact on the family (Hersh and Wienir, 1990). The total family and every area of family life will be affected (Hockenberry and Coody, 1986). Because the family is a system of interdependent parts a change in any one member causes a corresponding change in every other member (Whaley and Wong, 1991) – they affect and are affected by the ill member's cancer (Northouse, 1984). Normal life ceases. The family system becomes disorganised as family plans and routines are disrupted (Foley *et al.*, 1993), and Gogan, O'Malley and Foster (1987) suggest that virtually no family is unchanged by the diagnosis and treatment. Fife, Nortan and Groom (1987) found that families of

Think about a family you have been involved with. What was the structure of the family and how did the individual members react to the news of the diagnosis of cancer in the child? How did you try and help them?

children with leukaemia with relatively stable relationships and adequate support within the family unit were able to maintain their usual quality of life over an extended period of time, despite the acute stress, whereas families with pre-existing problems prior to diagnosis experienced increased deterioration in family life and had difficulty in coping. Previous methods of coping will influence the family's initial reaction to the diagnosis and their ability to adjust, for example experience of illness/cancer in family/ friends, past or concurrent stresses (Hockenberry and Coody, 1986). Kalnins, Churchill and Terry (1980) found parents of children with leukaemia perceived that concurrent stresses were often more troublesome than the disease. Faulkner *et al.* (1995) found that for some parents the experience of relatives/friends who had cancer made things worse because the outcome was death, while for others it was better because they could understand the illness/ treatment possibilities and how to take things day by day. The effect on the parents will also depend on the nature of the disease and prognosis and the child's adjustment at diagnosis (Hockenberry and Coody, 1986). Although people are different and their response to devastating news will differ in detail, in many instances reactions of parents will be similar (Whaley and Wong, 1991) as they grieve for the 'normal well' child they have lost in a similar way to grieving after someone has died. Although many parents suspect the diagnosis, most are not prepared to hear the word cancer. Only a parent who has been in that situation can understand how shocking such news is (Bracken, 1986). Although given information about the probability of long-term survival and even the possibility of cure, parents still often cognitively equate cancer with death. They will interpret the information for themselves as either threatening or reassuring (Martinson and Cohen, 1988). Brett and Davies (1988) found that despite the initial period of building anxiety as they took their children to local doctors but failed to get a definitive diagnosis and then were referred to hospitals for intrusive investigations, the eventual diagnosis of leukaemia came as a terrible shock to each of the parents interviewed. They all believed leukaemia to be uniformly fatal.

Parents often react strongly, expressing disbelief, anger, fear, depression and helplessness. Binger *et al.* (1969) studying parents of children with leukaemia found that their reactions at diagnosis ranged from loss of control to outward calm and resignation. The earliest phase is one of disbelief, shock and denial, with possibly loss of control of their emotions. They may be unable to hear or understand what the doctor is saying (Hockenberry and Coody, 1986). The words used by the doctor do not really enter the consciousness of the parents and when they do it feels as though they did not apply to their child. There are strong feelings of unreality – a terrible dream world. Many respondents in the study by Faulkner *et al.* (1995) did not realise cancer could affect children and found it difficult to relate it to a child who had previously been healthy. They may disbelieve the diagnosis, especially if they have gone through a number of misdiagnoses and wish for another medical opinion in an attempt to reverse it. The length of time of this shock and disbelief varies and may be related to whether the parents had been warned of the likelihood of cancer or not (Ekert, 1989). Faulkner *et al.* (1995) found that for parents with no previous experience of cancer, this seemed to add to their sense of disbelief and horror. These feelings of disbelief allow parents to cope and confront the full implication of the disease and treatment at their own pace and do not overwhelm their ability to face reality (Pinkerton *et al.*, 1994). It enables families to make the necessary adaptations and maintain some degree of equilibrium (Fife *et al.*, 1987). Faulkner *et al.* (1995) found that some parents were physically affected – feeling sick, shaking, numb.

As the shock and disbelief subside, an awareness of the intensity of the disease develops with accompanying anger and depression. Anger may be directed at themselves or other people (Ekert, 1989). A belief in the value of early detection may explain the anger of parents who feel signs and symptoms were not investigated quickly or thoroughly enough (Pinkerton *et al.*, 1994). Anger may be expressed at the hospital doctors who confirmed the diagnosis, or at God for allowing it to happen, or at the disease itself for the disruption and distress it causes (Pinkerton *et al.*, 1994). Although some degree of anger at the injustice and unfairness of the situation is normal, prolonged anger can be destructive at a time when maximum support from others is required and it does not help the child cope with the illness and treatment (Ekert, 1989). Anger uses up a lot of energy and can leave parents feeling exhausted and unable to support others (Pinkerton *et al.*, 1994).

Faulkner *et al.* (1995) found that few parents were able to escape feelings of guilt. They may blame themselves for the disease occurrence and see themselves as failures (Hockenberry and Coody, 1986). They may feel they should have sought medical advice earlier (Culling, 1988) or that the illness occurred because of something they had or had not done. Some feel guilt because they did not ackowledge the child's complaints of feeling unwell. Irrational explanations for suffering and illness are brought to the fore as parents struggle to make sense of what is happening and give meaning to the chaos that threatens to overwhelm them. They may think they are being punished for what they see as previous sins (Pinkerton *et al.*, 1994). They search for a cause.

Parents experience fear and uncertainty – they now realise that anything can happen to them and things are out of control, causing a feeling of helplessness. Helplessness was also found in parents in research by Clarke-Steffen (1993) to arise from feeling that for the first time they were unable to do much to help or protect their child. The parents' role of nurture and protection of their children is challenged by the life-threatening nature of the illness and effects of treatment (Sloper, 1996).

Some degree of depression is common, with loss of interest in family, friends and recreation, and all attention is focused on the child and treatment (Ekert, 1989). There are symptoms of anxiety and depression in up to 50% of parents (Maguire, 1983). Parents' worry and distress can result in irritability and tension, which in turn can reduce the support available from family and friends (Overholser and Fritz, 1990).

Not all parents can cope in the same way and to the same degree with the stress of a potentially fatal illness, and this may lead to family difficulties/breakdown. Each parent has their own strengths and weaknesses (Ekert, 1989). The presence of cancer in their child brings the individual parent's coping styles into focus. Both parents are likely to experience different stages of emotional response at different times which can cause difficulty. One parent may cope by seeking information and freely expressing emotions while the other may be more reserved (Foley et al., 1993). Faulkner et al. (1995) found that some husbands and wives had difficulty talking to each other, fathers especially finding it difficult to talk about their feelings and the retrospective group of fathers were found to have suppressed their grief for 2–11 years and were only able to express it when they were given permission through the research interview. The stress of the child's illness will test the relationship of the parents. Pre-existing stresses are usually exacerbated and subconscious feelings of anger and resentment by one or other parent may surface and cause a rift in the family (Ekert, 1989). In addition to having to cope with their own and their child's suffering and the total disruption to family life, there are practical difficulties, including increased costs incurred through hospital visits and possible loss of income due to time off work (Cairns et al., 1981; Lanksy, Black and Cairns, 1983) or having to give up work, and telephone expenses as they try to keep family members abreast of what is happening (Faulkner et al., 1995). Parents frequently have difficulty fulfilling their responsibilities at home and work while coping with the diagnosis (Hockenberry and Coody, 1986). The family may be split geographically, with the mother and child in hospital and the father and other family members at home trying to maintain some order, and parents may experience very different emotions as a result of this. Faulkner *et al.* (1995) found that fathers often felt guilty that they were not able to be as much with the child as they wanted and, although work can be a distraction from the anxiety, it was hard to concentrate. Although most employers were sympathetic, self-employed people found difficulty in having time off. Social isolation/lack of understanding by friends can be a problem.

For single parents it can be very stressful to cope with the diagnosis and decision making regarding treatment alone, especially if they have no one with whom they can share their concern. Even if they do have family/friends with whom to talk and gain support, they do not share the same parental bonds with the child and they may not be available when needed. There may be even more disruption in family life for these parents as they try to cope with multiple demands and there may be added difficulty re-establishing communication with a former partner (Foley *et al.*, 1993). Faulkner *et al.* (1995) found that relationships could be particularly disturbed where natural parents are divorced. The diagnosis may be told in the presence of one natural parent and current partner (if there is one) and the other natural parent feels left out, may doubt the information relayed by the other natural parent or pick up false information. This may create added conflict.

Parents also have to try and understand the nature of the illness and be able to communicate this to other family members. Some may try and protect them by with holding information (Hockenberry and Coody, 1986). The intense emotional focus on the ill child may alter the frequency and energy with which family members express caring and support for one another (Foley *et al.*, 1993). The crisis of the diagnostic period and having to accept that their child has a potentially life-threatening disease is further intensified by the treatment regimen. Unlike other chronic illnesses, the family is faced with the necessity to treat immediately, and this allows no time to adjust to the diagnosis before making a decision about treatment and having to subject the child to chemotherapy, radiotherapy and surgery which are themselves frightening. They are faced with an immense challenge – a disease and treatment plan about which they know nothing or very little and an uncertain outcome which heightens the family's anxiety (Moore *et al.*, 1986). Parental refusal of treatment for children with cancer is encountered infrequently, but it does happen. They may refuse treatment for a variety of reasons such as denial of the seriousness of the diagnosis or worries about the side effects of treatment. Parents are delegated responsibility to make major decisions about their children's welfare and when negotiation does not resolve the problem of whether to treat, many factors must be considered when deciding whether to legally challenge parental refusal of treatment (Ackerman, 1994).

Parents may go through a stage of demystification (Austin, 1990) where they look for information about the condition and try to regain some control. If parents go outside the hospital it is essential to stress the importance of reading current material and publications (Brown, 1989), as out of date information can be misleading. They may also experience disillusionment with the probability of cure offered by scientific medicine and look for alternative treatment which helps to give parents some control (Ekert, 1989). As they learn more about the details, feelings of anger and guilt lessen and they look at ways of restructuring family life to accommodate the disease and treatment (Pinkerton *et al.*, 1994). Anxiety and depression generally subside over a number of weeks as the child begins to respond to treatment and parents come to realise that the disease is potentially curable (Culling, 1988). After some weeks the adjustment process reaches stability with a reshaping of the family's lifestyle to fit in with the diagnosis and treatment, which is usually very different from that before the diagnosis – often more inwardly orientated and centred on the ill child and home environment and less concerned with future planning (Ekert, 1989).

The effect on siblings will be dependent on their age and level of development and their age in relation to the ill child (Pinkerton *et al.*, 1994). They have to adjust to multiple changes brought about by the diagnosis of cancer. There is often bewilderment at the sudden changes in family life and serious disruption to lifestyle for siblings (Culling, 1988). The first adjustment is often a temporary separation from child and parents while the ill child is in hospital (Foley *et al.*, 1993). They may experience initial disbelief that the sibling is very ill and only see the increased attention and gifts given to the child, leading to jealousy and resentment, not realising the severity of the illness (Hockenberry and Coody, 1986). They often feel neglected and unable to discuss worries and fears as parents appear preoccupied with the ill child, and this limits the available support and attention and time with the well siblings whose lives are frequently disrupted. Although they can be as frightened and bewildered as parents, they have less ability to find someone to trust with their fears and provide information (Faulkner *et al.*, 1995), and one of the early responses described by siblings in research by Brett and Davies (1988) was confusion about what to expect. Loneliness may result if child/parents are away or if parents do return home they may be too tired or preoccupied to talk. The study by Kramer (1984) showed siblings of paediatric leukaemia patients learned of the diagnosis several days later and information they received was often incomplete and inadequate. Siblings may experience a sense of loss of their own importance (Foley *et al.*, 1994). They may be cared for by extended family or friends or one parent may stay at home with them. However the major changes in parental roles often alter the sibling roles in that they may have to take on additional responsibility, for example preparing meals, looking after younger family members. Some siblings may be removed from their familiar surroundings to join the rest of the family at a hospital miles away from home (Culling 1988). Younger siblings lack the cognitive and emotional maturity to understand that their parents' focus on the ill child is based on medical need rather than lack of love for them (Foley *et al.*, 1993). They may have to face endless questions at school about the sibling's condition. Because of the rarity of childhood cancer friends often do not appreciate what the sibling is going through (Foley *et al.*, 1993), so further isolating them. Anger to parents may result from lack of attention but they may not have the opportunity to share this or may be afraid to for fear of making things worse and not wanting to worry parents further (Foley *et al.*, 1993). Anger may be felt at the ill child for taking so much of the parents' time. Conflicting feelings of empathy and anger at the ill child and parents can lead to siblings feeling confused and anxious. They may feel guilty that they have caused the illness, especially if there were relationship difficulties between siblings before the illness or if the well sibling has secretly harboured a grudge against the sick child (Culling, 1988), and they may fear that they too will acquire it (Hockenberry and Coody, 1986). Fear of death – the child's, their own or their parents' – may be brought into focus. Siblings unable to adequately express anger, guilt and fear may begin to act inappropriately and react by changes in their behaviour or school performance (Hockenberry and Coody, 1986).

Faulkner *et al.* (1995) found that grandparents had many effects that were similar to those of parents. They felt shock and disbelief that cancer could affect children and distressed to see the child have treatment which made them ill and could not guarantee cure. Some were affected by the unfairness of the situation and found it difficult not to spoil the ill child and wished they were in the ill child's place. Some were unable to get very good detail, as they mostly heard the diagnosis through parents who may not have heard/understood the information. This, together with their limited part in decision making and responsibility for the child's care, may result in them adjusting less well (Baum and Baum, 1989). Some grandparents were able to contribute in a practical way with household chores or looking after siblings or offered advice and support (Faulkner *et al.*, 1995). Grandparents may have dealt with similar crises before which may help in enhancing parents' adaptation to the child's illness (Foley *et al.*, 1993). However sometimes grandparents can be sources of additional stress to parents who may be forced to support them rather than receiving comfort and help in their own grief (Koocher and O'Malley, 1981). Grandparents suffer two types of grief – for their grandchild and their child who is suffering (Foley *et al.*, 1993).

Needs of/helping the family

The ability of a family to cope with childhood cancer has a significant impact on the long-term outcome. Overholser and Fritz (1990) demonstrated that parental coping styles during treatment can have implications for the psychosocial adjustment of parents and child long after treatment ends, so attention must be focused on helping parents develop their coping and mastery skills from the very beginning. They have a tremendous burden to bear – not only are they faced with coping with their own needs and feelings in response to the diagnosis, but also with those of their child with cancer and the siblings. Furthermore they have to establish relationships with unknown staff in a strange environment, learn about the hospital bureaucracy and become familiar with medical language. The diagnostic phase begins the long-term education, guidance and support these families need and deserve (Foley *et al.*, 1993).

In order to provide the very best care for the child and family it is important that the caring professionals work together as a cohesive team and give the family a feeling of trust and being cared for and supported. There needs to be good communication and a consensus of information (Culling, 1988). It may be useful for a few key people to work with the family so that they are able to develop rapport, as in many instances the child's care is so complex that numerous specialists are involved. However, this requires interdisciplinary collaboration and communication so that all care providers are aware of each family's exposure to information about the child's condition (Clarke-Steffen, 1993).

Family-centred care emphasises mutual respect and cooperation between family members and providers. One essential ingredient is grounding all interventions in accurate family assessments. There are several areas of family functioning that are appropriate and important to assess when working with families, including relationships among members, how they communicate with each other, make decisions and solve problems and adjust to changes and challenges, and whether there are any concurrent stresses. Also important is their approach to relationships with other people and how they choose to use resources outside the family. Family coping is central to supporting the family as they deal with a health care crisis. Obtaining an accurate assessment of the family is difficult. It is hard to be objective as we all hold our own beliefs about how a family should function which may bias the assessment and we are also assessing them at a time of disruption which will cause changes to their ordinary functioning and coping. It is therefore important to acknowledge that family functioning will change over time and will need to be assessed frequently. Nurses must be sensitive to cultural diversity and also not stereotype families from a given region, religion or culture (Foley *et al.*, 1993). Cultural factors may further exacerbate economic stresses, as a family's cultural background may make it difficult for them to accept assistance even if community resources are available (Adams-Greenly, 1991). Cultural factors may also play a part in problems in communication, differences in sex roles and religious or moral values, causing the family greater stress (Schaefer, 1983). Assessment can be made by observation and interviewing the family (Thomas, Barnard and Sumner, 1993). If there are pre-existing underlying communication problems extra help such as anticipatory counselling, and continued reinforcement of the importance of communication may be required (Moore *et al.*, 1986). An accurate and detailed assessment provides important information about the child and family that will enable us to identify problems to be addressed and strengths to be supported, and also shows the family that we are genuinely interested in and respect them, helping to create a collaborative approach (Adams-Greenly, 1991).

Parents can be helped in a number of ways. Opportunities need to be available to discuss and clarify information given which will need repeating many times. One-to-one teaching of the parents can be augmented by publications from various sources. The main dilemma for staff is the parents' need for information and talking things through at a time when they are in shock and unable/ unwilling to listen/talk. Parents would prefer to hear only good news and they may avoid communication so that they can continue to believe this is a bad dream (Faulkner *et al.*, 1995). Research by Mulhern, Crisco and Camitta (1981) suggest that despite repeated explanations about the disease and its implications, parents consistently differ from the doctor in interpretation of the information and therefore staff must be on the lookout for misconceptions and misunderstandings. It is important not to offer false hope or overwhelm them with facts (Savage *et al.*, 1993). Clear and comprehensive information about the disease and treatment helps parents make sense of their situation and make appropriate plans and it is important to ensure that they understand the information and feel they can ask questions without losing face if they do not understand (Sloper, 1996). Nurses can reassure parents that all that can be done will be done and families need to know they will not be abandoned. In addition to disease- and treatment-orientated information, anticipatory counselling needs to be provided, addressing issues such as increased stress in the marriage and with siblings and grandparents and changes as a result of frequent hospitalisations (Moore *et al.*, 1986). Families should be encouraged to share non-illness related problems, for example job loss, health problems, death of other family members, as they have the potential for affecting the family's overall ability to adapt to the child's illness (Kalnins *et al.*, 1980).

Parents will need to elicit and talk about their feelings and be reassured about the normality of them and work through their anger, guilt and fear. They may need permission or provision of appropriate facilities to express them. Wooley *et al.* (1989) found that one set of parents stated that the doctor's ability to sit out the upset and anger without taking it as a personal attack helped them to set up a working relationship with him. Sufficient time is important.

Nursing staff are in a unique position to offer support and guidance, as they have more extended contact than any other health care professional and probably develop an extensive database of the family's values, expectations and coping styles and support systems (Savage *et al.*, 1993). Health professionals can create a climate in which the families feel better able to ask questions and feel less intimidated by the hospital surroundings. Nursing staff need to be approachable and act as a humanising influence in order for family members to have more control over their circumstances (*Nursing Times*, 1994). It is a time when development of trust in staff is essential and families must feel that staff truly care. By using knowledge gained by nursing other families with similar experiences, nurses must convey to parents of newly diagnosed children that they recognise the impact of their child's illness and hospitalisation on their lives and that they are aware of the issues that they are facing (Lynam, 1987).

Each family as well as each individual has its unique communication style or pattern. Unclear communications are believed to be a major contributor of poor family functioning (Holman, 1983; Satir, 1983). Watzlawek, Beavin and Jackson (1967) estimate that 85% of all messages sent in families are misunderstood. Family communication patterns and processes are key elements in the fulfillment of family function. More functional families have more open areas of communication, while less functional families displaying dysfunctional interactional patterns will demonstrate more closed areas of communication. Families have unwritten rules about subjects that are approved or disapproved for discussion (Friedman, 1992). Findings from research that has examined the adaptation of families to chronic and long-term illness have consistently demonstrated that a central factor in healthy marital and family functioning is the presence of open, honest and clear communication in dealing with the stressful health and health-related issues (Spinetta and Deasy-Spinetta, 1981; Kahn, 1990). Parents may be dishonest about the illness in an attempt to protect the ill child and siblings from emotional distress as part of their parenting role (Moore *et al.*, 1986). When families do not discuss the important issues they are faced with, emotional distancing in family relationships results and family stress increases (Friedman, 1985). Increased stress affects the family relationships and the health of the family and its members (Hoffer, 1989). Each person is left to deal with their fears or concerns independently. Much energy is required to deal with the wall of silence or unacknowledged fears, so that little energy is left for family support and coping (Moore *et al.*, 1986). Good communication is imperative between families, child and professionals, both in terms of offering support and giving information (Faulkner *et al.*, 1995). Role modelling is a crucial type of learning – families can observe professionals' good communication and learn to imitate. Although most of the family members interviewed by Brett and Davies (1988) agreed that open communication is beneficial in dealing with the crisis of childhood leukaemia, parents may be prevented from using this because of their need to protect themselves and their children from anxiety. It is important to encourage and support families in open communication between members by encouraging them to talk to each other about fears and feelings to counteract isolation and gain strength by facing difficulties together (Faulkner *et al.*, 1995). They must be convinced of the value of open family communication and be made aware of how to use it (Brett and Davies, 1988). This may also help the family members to adapt to the reality of the situation. There must be adequate information offered to all members of the family by the health professionals using verbal and written means in order to help families cope.

Chesler and Barbarin (1984) found that parents wanted recognition and acceptance of their competence as parents who play a vital role in their child's cancer care. If nurses can help parents identify and fulfil their role as parents no matter how sick the child is, they will begin to feel some usefulness and begin to accept a level of responsibility and planning for their child (Savage *et al.*, 1993). Clear and comprehensible information is essential for this (Sloper, 1996). Enabling the family to take an active role in the care of the child helps parents develop their mastery skills and reduces their sense of loss of control and the lack of involvement by siblings and also helps the ill child adjust. It is important to establish the extent to which parents feel able to participate in care. At first their stress levels may inhibit or prevent them. A named nurse could take time each day to debrief family members regarding things they have learnt that day, including answering additional questions, verifying information they had been given and helping piece together the bits of information they had gathered during the day (Clarke-Steffen, 1993).

The nurse can assist by identifying additional resources as by addressing practical factors, for example increased costs, accommodation, coping may be enhanced (Carr-Gregg and White, 1985). With the advent of 'family houses' for example a CLIC House, families can be together away from home and close to the ill child, enhancing support and communication. Overholser and Fritz (1990) demonstrated that a lack of emotional support was associated with increased emotional distress in parents of children with cancer and this may lead to depression. It highlights the importance of having a confidant during stressful times. Sloper (1996) found that many parents noted the importance of having someone to talk to who was not so emotionally involved in the situation, for example friends and extended family were cited more often than partners as being particularly helpful, and a minority who felt they had no one to talk to about their feelings had higher malaise scores. Forty-eight per cent of the families interviewed felt they had not received one or more types of help that they needed – counselling, financial help, information – and although all the paediatric oncology centres involved in the study had social workers and liaison nurses, parents were often unsure about where to go for help. Linking the parents with another family in similar circumstances can be beneficial (Moore *et al.*, 1986), as they can share problems and have a mutual understanding and provide support. Lynam (1987) found that the parents interviewed indicated that it was often other parents who helped them feel less alone with their experiences of hospitalisation/illness of their children, anticipated their needs as they adapted to the hospital environment and were often perceived as giving them permission to care for themselves. They also helped them become familiar with hospital routines and facilities. Parents often encouraged and gave hope to the parents of newly diagnosed children by relaying news of their own child's progress, and sometimes could provide helpful suggestions for managing situations. A parent support group may be in existence.

Faulkner *et al.* (1995) found that the major area of problem initially with siblings stems from the lack of information and reassuring contact with parents. The health care team can intervene with siblings at the time of diagnosis by taking time to talk with them and answering their questions and concerns. Visiting the sick child and being involved as much as possible in the early stages of diagnosis and treatment helps to decrease their feelings of isolation (Moore *et al.*, 1986) and relieve their feelings of responsibility and guilt (Culling, 1988). It gives them a better understanding of the sick child's condition, experiences and situation (Brown, 1989), and helps prevent a build up of resentment to the sick child. Staff must help parents understand the siblings' needs through the diagnosis period (Brown, 1989) and that they must spend time with the siblings and not devote all their time to the affected child. They too need the opportunity to express their emotions.

Grandparents too need information on the progress of the ill child. They may be of great value to the family when used to help other members see and communicate their individual needs (Faulkner *et al.*, 1995).

Nurses' reactions and needs

Improvements in treatment and prognosis of childhood cancer is dependent on intensive and rigorous investigation and staging procedures. To help the child and family prepare for and comply with these procedures and to facilitate the safety of the child, nursing staff must have a thorough understanding of the investigative procedures that each diagnosis requires (Pinkerton *et al.*, 1994). This may help alleviate anticipatory fears and phobias and increase the family's sense of security and control. Decreasing the chance for the unexpected lessens the opportunities for increased anxiety (Whaley and Wong, 1991). It is essential that children's nurses have a basic grounding in developmental/psychosocial theories and sufficient theory related to children's concepts of health and illness and its practical application (Rushforth, 1996) in order to be able to appropriately explain to the children about their disease, otherwise there may be a barrier to communication.

Nurses experience reactions similar to the responses of family members at diagnosis. Analysis and understanding of these reactions is important in providing effective care, as although some of these reactions may help nurses provide care by protecting them from the emotional impact of the event, others may interfere with the establishment of a therapeutic relationship with the family. Nurses may experience initial shock and denial. The behavioural reaction to this may be withdrawal from the child and family, so distancing themselves from the implications of emotional involvement. They may support denial in parents because of their own dependency on it, emphasising only optimistic survival statistics and negating the seriousness of the illness. They may focus on cheering the family up and engage only in casual conversation and not meaningful dialogue. Although denial can be important because it helps protect the nurse from the overwhelming reality of the potentially fatal outlook of the illness and it is necessary to give hope to the family and helps prevent feelings of failure in themselves, it may lose its beneficial function when nurses refuse to accept the reality and deny the seriousness of the event.

Anger is another common reaction experienced by nurses – anger that this has happened, that they have to subject the child to painful procedures and that they may be unable to comfort the family. Potential failure is threatening, resulting in anger and perhaps depression. They may project this anger on to the family, causing the family to react with hostility and feelings of rejection. Depression may make the nurse withdraw from the child/family as a means of controlling their sadness and fear of failure. As a result of this they may feel guilty if they see they are intolerant of the child and parental behaviour or feel they cannot cope, or experience a sense of helplessness at not being able to relieve the child/family's distress (Faulkner *et al.*, 1995) or feel unable to meet their needs. This may have an adverse effect on the ability to provide care (Whaley and Wong, 1991).

Have you experienced any of the above feelings or reactions when you have been involved with children with cancer at diagnosis and their families? How have you coped?

Nurses may be helped to cope successfully by several means, such as education and support. Although distancing may help the nurse put things in perspective, it can make it more difficult for them to understand the families' perspectives and needs (Faulkner *et al.*, 1995). Therefore knowledge about possible effects and how to cope may be beneficial. Self awareness and setting personal limits is important (Faulkner *et al.*, 1995). Faulkner *et al.* (1995) found that professional carers found some families particularly difficult to work with for example where conflict already existed such as divorce, separation.

Knowledge about handling difficult situations and family functioning may help. Developing competence particularly in the area of communication was seen by staff in work by Faulkner *et al.* (1995) to be an effective strategy in enabling them to cope and improve the quality of care, therefore health care professionals need the experience and opportunity to do this. Little attention tends to be given to providing nurses with the skills necessary to deal with direct questions, and it is not surprising that they cope in many of these situations by evading the issue and colluding in a conspiracy of silence (*Nursing Times* 1994). Communicating with children can be difficult, so training may be needed. Seeing parents and children upset is very distressing for staff, and Faulkner *et al.* (1995) found some felt overwhelmed at times by the emotional intensity of the work which affected their personal and professional life. They may need help in developing and identifying coping strategies such as visiting clinics to see well children, focusing on the positive value of caring. Staff who had worked in the area longer felt that by gaining more experience and competence, they developed skills which helped them handle difficulties which helped them cope. Perhaps an emphasis on sharing this with more junior colleagues can be encouraged. Teamwork and feeling able to express emotions and concerns with colleagues was valuable as a means of coping. Work by Finlay and Dallimore (1991) suggested that relatives gained great comfort and support when staff displayed their emotions, and a professionally detached attitude caused offence and was hurtful. However this has implications for staff who may need to talk over traumatic events, either on an informal basis with a colleague or within a staff support team. Adequate support will ultimately enable staff to enhance the quality of care and improve relationships with families. This is especially important for nursing staff who have the most face to face contact with children and families and are far more likely to be around at times of stress. If stress produced by exposure to traumatic situations is not dealt with it may well present later as an inability to cope and deteriorating morale (*Nursing Times*, 1994).

Conclusion

Because of improved treatment of cancer in children, many are living longer and may be cured and there is a necessity to view these children as developing, changing people within families, schools and communities (Kagen-Goodhart, 1977). It is important therefore to aim at preventing or minimising later difficulties and this must be taken into account right from the very start of a child's illness. This chapter has considered the time leading up to the diagnosis, stressing the importance of good communication between the different professionals who may be involved and a need to accept each other's roles. Some of the benefits and problems of being treated in a regional centre have been highlighted. The time before the diagnosis is confirmed can be a very anxious period and how it is handled can affect how parents respond. It is important that we acknowledge what a difficult time it is for them, listen to what they have to say and keep them informed as much as possible. Giving the news of the diagnosis in an inappropriate manner can add to parents' stress and ways that parents have found helpful have been highlighted. We can help by being present at the initial interview in order to support parents and know what was said, so that we can repeat and reinforce information as necessary. Nurses can also ensure that a suitable environment is available where the discussion can take place. We can also support parents as they decide who should tell the child and how this should be done. The child's reaction will depend very much on their level of understanding, previous experience and parental reaction. It is imperative that nurses have knowledge of children's development and appropriate communication skills. Although parents may exhibit similar reactions to the diagnosis, we must remember their individuality and therefore an accurate family assessment is needed and skills to ensure adequate support, guidance and education, remembering also the needs of other members of the family. Caring for children who are newly diagnosed with cancer can be very rewarding but also distressing and stressful and we must develop self awareness and suitable education and support mechanisms to cope so that quality care is delivered and morale maintained.

References

Ackerman, T. (1994) Parental refusal of treatment. *Journal of Pediatric Oncology Nursing*, **11**(1), 31–33.

Adams-Greenly, M. (1991) Psychosocial assessment and intervention at initial diagnosis. *Pediatrician*, **18**, 3–10.

Armstrong, D. (1995) *An Outline of Sociology as Applied to Medicine*, 4th edn. Oxford: Butterworth-Heinemann.

Arnfield, A. (1990) Common issues relating to diagnosis and treatment *in* Thompson, J. ed. *The Child with Cancer. Nursing care*, pp. 31–45. London: Scutari Press.

Austin, J. (1990) Assessment of coping mechanisms used by parents and children with chronic illness. *American Journal of Maternal and Child Nursing*, **15**, 98–102.

Barbor, P. (1983) Emotional aspects of malignant disease in children. *Maternal and Child Health*, **8**, 320–327.

Baum, B. & Baum, E. (1989) Psychological challenges of childhood cancer. *Journal of Psychosocial Oncology*, **7**, 119–129.

Bibace, R. & Walsh, M. (1981) Children's conception of illness *in* Bibace, R. & Walsh, M. *New*

Directions for Child Development, vol. 14, pp. 31–48. San Francisco: Jossey-Bass.

Binger, C., Ablin, A., Feuerstein, R., Kushner, J. Zoger, S. & Mikkelsen, C. (1969) Childhood leukaemia. Emotional impact on patient and family. *New England Journal of Medicine*, **280**(8), 414–418.

Birch, J., Marsden, H. & Morris-Jones, P. (1988) Improvements in survival from childhood cancer: results of a population based survey over 30 years. *British Medical Journal*, **296**, 1372–1376.

Bluebond-Langner, M. (1978) *The Private Worlds of Dying Children*. Princeton: Princeton University Press.

Bond, J. & Bond, S. (1991) *Sociology and Health Care. An Introduction for Nurses and Other Health Care Professionals*. Edinburgh: Churchill Livingstone.

Bracken, J.M. (1986) *Children with Cancer: a comprehensive reference guide for parents*. New York: Oxford University Press.

Brett, K. & Davies, E. (1988) What does it mean? Sibling and parental appraisals of childhood leukaemia. *Cancer Nursing*, **11**, 329–338.

Brown, P. (1989) Families who

have a child diagnosed with cancer: what the medical caregiver can do to help them and themselves. *Issues in Comprehensive Pediatric Nursing*, **12**, 247–260.

Buckman, R. (1984) Breaking bad news – why is it still so difficult? *British Medical Journal*, **288**, 1597–1599.

Buckman, R. (1992) *How to Break Bad News. A guide for health care professionals*. London: Papermac.

Cairns, N., Clark, G., Black, J. & Lansky, S. (1981) Childhood cancer; non-medical costs of the illness *in* Spinetta, J. & Deasy-Spinetta, P. eds. *Living with Childhood Cancer*. St Louis: Mosby.

Carr-Gregg, M. & White, L. (1985) The child with cancer: a psychological overview. *Medical Journal of Australia*, **143**, 503–506.

Chesler, M. & Barbarin, O. (1984) Relating to the medical staff. How parents of children with cancer see the issue. *Health Social Work*, **9**, 49–65.

Chesler, M., Paris, J. & Barbarin, O. (1986) Telling the child with cancer. Parental choices to share information with ill children. *Journal of Pediatric Psychology*, **11**, 497–516.

Clarke-Steffen, L. (1993) Waiting and not knowing: the diagnosis of cancer in a child. *Journal of Pediatric Oncology Nursing*, **10**(4), 146–153.

Cornwell, J. (1984) *Hard-earned Lives. Accounts of health and illness from East London*. London: Tavistock.

Culling, J. (1988) The psychological problems of families of children with cancer *in* Oakhill, A. ed. *The Supportive Care of the Child with Cancer*, pp. 204–237. London: Wright.

Eiser, C., Patterson, D. & Eiser, R. (1983) Children's knowledge of health and illness: implications for health education. *Child Care, Health and Development*, **9**, 285–292.

Eiser, C., Parkyn, T., Havermans, T. & McNinch, A. (1994) Parents' recall on the diagnosis of cancer in their child. *Psycho-oncology*, **3**, 197–203.

Ekert, H. (1983) Long term needs of children and parents with chronic life-threatening diseases. *Australian Family Physician*, **12**, 237–241.

Ekert, H. (1989) *Childhood Cancer: understanding and coping*. New York: Gordon & Breach Science Publishers.

Erikson, E. (1967) Growth and Crisis: the health personality *in* Lazarus, R. & Opton, E. eds. *Personality-seleted Readings*. Harmondsworth: Penguin.

Faulkner, A. (1992) *Effective Interaction with Patients*. Edinburgh: Churchill Livingstone.

Faulkner, A., Peace, G. & O'Keeffe, C. (1995) *When a Child has Cancer*. London: Chapman & Hall.

Fife, B., Norton, J. & Groom, G. (1987) The family's adaptation to childhood leukaemia. *Social Science and Medicine*, **24**, 159–168.

Finlay, L. & Dallimore, D. (1991) Your child is dead. *British Medical Journal*, **302**, 1524–1525.

Foley, G., Fochtman, D. & Mooney, K. (eds) (1993) *Nursing Care of the Child with Cancer*, 2nd edn. Philadelphia: W.B. Saunders.

Friedman, M. (1985) Family Stress and Coping among Anglo and Latino Families with Childhood Cancer. Unpublished PhD dissertation, University of Southern California.

Friedman, M. (1992) *Family Nursing. Theory and practice*, 3rd edn. Norwalk, CN: Appleton and Lange.

Gatrad, A. (1995) Medical implications of Islam for women and children. *Maternal and Child Health*, July, 225–227.

Geen, L. (1990) The family of the child with cancer *in* Thompson, J. ed. *The Child with Cancer – nursing care*, pp. 17–30. London: Scutari Press.

Ginzler, M., Pritchard, P. & Mant, D. (1993) Delay in diagnosing and treating cancer. *Oncology in Practice*, **1**, 4–10.

Gogan, J., O'Malley, J. & Foster, D. (1987) Treating the pediatric cancer patient: a review. *Journal of Pediatric Psychology*, **2**, 42–48.

Halliday, J. (1990) Malignant disease in children: the view of a general practitioner and parent *in* Baum, J., Dominica, F. & Woodward, R. eds. *Listen, My Child Has a Lot of Living To Do*. Oxford: Oxford University Press.

Hayes, N. (1988) *A First Course in Psychology*. Surrey: Nelson.

Helman, C. (1990) *Culture, Health and Illness*, 2nd edn. London: Wright.

Hersh, S. & Wienir, L. (1990) Psychological support for the family of the child with cancer *in* Pizzo, P. & Poplack, D. eds. *Principles and Practice of Paediatric Oncology*, pp. 17–31. Philadelphia: Lippincott.

Hinds, P. (1995) Truth-telling with patients. *Journal of Pediatric Oncology Nursing*, **12**(1), 1.

Hockenberry, M. & Coody, D. (eds) (1986) *Pediatric Oncology and Hematology. Perspectives on care*. St Louis: C.V. Mosby.

Hodson, D. (1989) A good prognosis. *Paediatric Nursing*, 8–10 April.

Hoffer, J. (1989) Family communication *in* Bomar, P. ed. *Nurses and Family Health Promotion*. Baltimore; Williams & Wilkins.

Holman, A. (1983) *Family Assessment. Tools for understanding and intervention*. Beverly Hills: Sage Publications.

Hussein-Rassool, G. (1995) The health status and health care of ethno-cultural minorities in the United Kingdom: an agenda for action. *Journal of Advanced Nursing*, **21**, 199–201.

Kagen-Goodhart, L. (1977) Re-entry. Living with childhood cancer. *American Journal of Orthopsychiatry*, **47**, 651–658.

Kalnins, I., Churchill, M. & Terry, G. (1980) Concurrent stresses in families with a leukemic child. *Journal of Pediatric Psychology*, **5**(1), 81–92.

Kahn, A. (1990) Coping with fear and grieving *in* Lubkin, I. ed. *Chronic Illness; impact and intervention*. Boston: Jones & Bartlett.

Kaye, P. (1996) *Breaking Bad News. A 10 step approach*. Northampton: EPL Publications.

Koocher, G. (1984) Response. *Cancer*, **53**(suppl.), 2337–2338.

Koocher, G. & O'Malley, J. (1981) *The Damocles Syndrome; psychological consequences of surviving childhood cancer*. New York: McGraw-Hill.

Kramer, R. (1984) Living with childhood cancer: impact on the healthy siblings. *Oncology Nurses Forum*, **11**(2), 44–51.

Kupst, M. (1992) Longterm family coping with acute lymphoblastic leukaemia in childhood *in* LaGreca, A., Siegel, L., Wallander, J. & Walker, C. eds. *Stress and Coping in Child Health*. New York: Guilford Press.

Lansky, S., Black, J. & Cairns, N. (1983) Childhood cancer: medical costs. *Cancer*, **5**, 762–766.

Levine, A., Blumberg, B. & Hersh, S. (1982) The psychosocial concomitants of cancer in young patients *in* Levine, A. ed. *Cancer in the Young*. New York: Masson.

Littlewood, J. (1988) The patient's world. *Nursing Times*, 20 Jan, 29–30.

Lupton, D. (1994) *Medicine as Culture. Illness, disease and the body in Western Societies*. London: Sage.

Lynam, M. (1987) The parent network in pediatric oncology. Supportive or not? *Cancer Nursing*, **10**(4), 207–216.

Macaskill, A. & Monarch, J. (1990) Coping with childhood cancer: the case for longterm counselling help for patients and their families. *British Journal of Guidance and Counselling*, **18**(1), 13–26.

McEwing, G. (1996) Children's understanding of their internal body parts. *British Journal of Nursing*, **5**, 423–429.

Maguire, P. (1983) The psychological sequelae of childhood leukaemia. In *Recent Results in Cancer Research*, Vol. 88. Berlin: Springer.

Martinson, I. & Cohen, M. (1988) Themes from a longitudinal study of family reaction to childhood cancer. *Journal of Psychosocial Oncology*, **6**, 81–97.

Martocchio, B. (1985) Family coping. Helping families help themselves. *Seminars in Oncology Nursing*, **1**(4), 292–297.

Mood, D. (1991) The diagnosis of cancer: a life transition *in* Baird, S., McCorkle, R. & Grant, M. eds. *Cancer Nursing; a comprehensive textbook*, pp. 219–234. Philadelphia: Saunders.

Moore, I., Kramer, R. & Perin, G. (1986) Care of the family with a child with cancer: diagnosis and early stages of treatment. *Oncology Nursing Forum*, **13**(5), 60–66.

Mulhern, R., Crisco, J. & Camitta, B. (1981) Patterns of communication among paediatric patients with leukaemia. Parents' and physicians' prognostic disagreements and misunderstandings. *Journal of Pediatrics*, **99**, 480–483.

Nicholson, A. (1990) Childhood cancer – an overview *in* Thompson, J. ed. *The Child with Cancer – nursing care*, pp. 1–16. London: Scutari Press.

Northouse, L. (1984) The impact of cancer on the family: an overview. *International Journal of Psychiatry in Medicine*, **14**, 215–242.

Nursing Times (1994) Professional development. Breaking bad news. The role of the nurse. *Nursing Times*, **90**(11), 5–8.

Office of Population Censuses and Surveys (1992) *1991 Census*. London: HMSO.

Overholser, J. & Fritz, G. (1990) The impact of childhood cancer on the family. *Journal of Psychosocial Oncology*, **8**(4), 71–85.

Parmar, M. (1985) Family care and ethnic minorities. *Nursing*, **36**, 1068–1069; 1071.

Perrin, E. & Perrin, J. (1983) Clinicians' assessment of children's understanding of illness. *American Journal of Diseases of Children*, **137**, 874–878.

Pill, R. & Stott, N. (1982) Concepts of illness causation and responsibility: some preliminary data from a sample of working class mothers. *Social Science and Medicine*, **16**, 48–52.

Pinkerton, C.R., Cushing, P. & Sepion, B. (eds) (1994) *Childhood Cancer Management. A practical handbook*. London: Chapman & Hall Medical.

Redler, N. (1994) A triumphant survival, but at what cost? *Professional Nurse*, Dec. 166–170.

Richardson, J. (1993) Transcultural aspects of paediatric nursing *in* Glasper, E. & Tucker, A. eds. *Advances in Child Health Nursing*, pp. 78–89. London: Scutari Press.

Ruccione, K., Waskerwitz, M., Buckley, J., Perin, G. & Denman Hammond, G. (1994) What caused my child's cancer? Parents' responses to an epidemiology study of childhood cancer. *Journal of Pediatric Oncology Nursing*, **11**(2), 71–84.

Rushforth, H. (1996) Nurses' knowledge of how children view health and illness. *Paediatric Nursing*, **8**(9), 23–27.

Satir, V. (1983) *Conjoint Family Therapy*, 3rd edn. California: Science and Behaviour Books.

Savage, T., Durand, B., Friedrichs, J. & Slack, J. (1993) Ethical decision making with families in crisis *in* Feltham, S., Meister, S., Bell, J. & Gilliss, C. eds. *The Nursing of Families. Theory/research/education/practice*, pp. 118–126. California: Sage Publications.

Schaefer, D. (1983) Issues related to psychosocial intervention with Hispanic families in a pediatric cancer centre. *Journal of Psychosocial Oncology*, **1**, 39–46.

Schultz, W. (1989) Recognising cancer in children. *Journal of American Academy of Physician Assistants*, **2**, 338–352.

Sepion, B. (1990) Investigations staging and diagnosis – implications for nurses *in* Thompson, J. ed. *The Child with Cancer – nursing care*, pp. 47–60. London: Scutari Press.

Sharp, M., Strauss, R. & Lorch, S. (1992) Communicating medical bad news: parents' experiences and preferences. *Journal of Pediatrics*, **121**, 539–546.

Slavin, L., O'Malley, M., Koocher, G. & Foster, D. (1982) Communication of the cancer diagnosis to pediatric cancer patients. Impact on longterm adjustment. *American Journal of Psychiatry*, **139**, 179–183.

Sloper, P. (1996) Needs and responses of parents following the diagnosis of childhood cancer. *Childcare, Health and Development*, **22**, 187–202.

Smith, P. & Cowie, H. (1988) *Understanding Children's Development*. Oxford: Basil Blackwell.

Spinetta, J. (1984) Measurement of family function, communication and cultural effects. *Cancer*, **53**(Suppl.), 2330–2337.

Spinetta, J. & Deasy-Spinetta, P. (1981) *Living with Childhood Cancer*. St Louis: C.V. Mosby.

Stiller, C. (1988) Centralisation of treatment and survival rates for cancer. *Archives of Disease in Childhood*, **63**, 23–30.

Stiller, C. (1993) Improvements in population in survival rates for childhood cancer in Britain. 1980–1991. Paper presented at International Association of Cancer Registries, London.

Thomas, R. Barnard, K. & Sumner, G. (1993) Family nursing. Diagnosis as a framework for family assessment *in* Feltham, S., Meister, S., Bell, J. & Gilliss, C. eds. *The Nursing of Families. Theory/research/education/practice*, pp. 127–136. California: Sage Publications.

Thompson, J. (1990) The adolescent with cancer *in* Thompson, J. ed. *The Child with Cancer – nursing care*. London: Scutari Press.

Tuckett, D., Boulton, M., Olson, C. & Williams, A. (1985) *Meetings Between Experts: an approach to sharing ideas in medical consultations*. London: Tavistock.

Waechter, E. (1971) Children's awareness of fatal illness. *American Journal of Nursing*, **71**, 1168–1172.

Wang, R. & Martinson, I. (1996) Behavioral responses of healthy Chinese siblings to the stress of childhood cancer in the family: a longitudinal study. *Journal of Pediatric Nursing*, **11**, 383–391.

Watzlawek, P., Beavin, J. & Jackson, D. (1967) *Pragmatics of Human Communication*. New York: Norton.

Whaley, L. & Wong, D. (1991) *Nursing Care of Infants and Children*, 4th ed. St Louis: Mosby.

Woolley, H., Stein, A., Forrest, G. & Baum, J. (1989) Imparting the diagnosis of life threatening illness in children. *British Medical Journal*, **298**, 1623–1626.

Further reading

Clarke-Steffen, L. (1993) Waiting and not knowing; the diagnosis of cancer in a child. *Journal of Pediatric Oncology Nursing*, 10(4), 146–153.
A grounded theory study of 40 members of seven families with a child with cancer, describing their experiences during the period immediately surrounding the time of diagnosis.

Eiser, C., Parkyn, T., Havermans, T. and McNinch, A. (1994) Parents' recall on the diagnosis of cancer in their child. *Psycho-oncology*, 3, 197–203.
A study in which parents of 30 children with cancer were interviewed about their recall of the period before the diagnosis and during the diagnostic interview.

Faulkner, A., Peace, G. and O'Keeffe, C. (1995) *When a Child has Cancer*. London: Chapman and Hall.
A research project on the effects of childhood cancer from the perspectives of the child, key family members and professional carers. It refers to experiences prediagnosis and through diagnosis and on to adjusting to normal life and into remission.

Psychological impact of treatment

KATH WILKINSON-CARR

Introduction

This chapter examines the psychological impact of treatment on children from infant to young adult.

Maier (Crowley, 1994) maintains '… practice and research must stem from a foundation of theory'. Theories provide a framework for understanding phenomenon. Developmental theories provide logical and sequential explanations for understanding current and later behavior. The impact of cancer treatment is largely unique to the individual and their reactions will often depend upon current circumstances, previous experiences and interpretations (Carter and Dearmun, 1995).

> Children at every stage of development are attempting to form mental constructs of the world around them in order to understand it. (Swanwick, 1990)

Therefore it is important that caregivers caring for children and adolescents in the speciality of oncology understand their psychosocial development, as this will have a major influence on how they will cope with treatment. However, the complexity of psychosocial development really demands further reading and this review only serves as a useful guide.

Children's development will be considered in three broad development periods; the psychosocial development of the infant from new-born to older infant, the preschool child and middle childhood, and adolescent. Then we will examine how treatment, separation and isolation from family friends, altered body image and stress can influence development in these age groups.

New-born development

The nineteenth century psychologist William James believed that human babies are born with no perceptual or social skills whatsoever. Their world is meaningless and chaotic, a 'blooming, buzzing confusion'. Directly opposing this outlook the recent

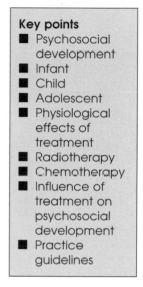

Key points
- Psychosocial development
- Infant
- Child
- Adolescent
- Physiological effects of treatment
- Radiotherapy
- Chemotherapy
- Influence of treatment on psychosocial development
- Practice guidelines

psychological view is that new-borns are socially quite advanced, able to imitate complex behaviours.

Contemporary developmentalists see new-borns as coming equipped with certain predispositions that enable them to participate in early social exchanges, provided they are part of a responsive care-giving system (Ainsworth and Bell, 1974; Sander, 1975). The new-born is preadapted to becoming social and a certain developmental context is needed for this social potential to unfold. New-born babies are equipped with certain built-in tendencies and capacities that help them to adapt to their new environments. These capacities include reflexes, perceptual abilities, motor skills and learning abilities.

The new-born's predispositions often meet a direct *survival* need: the sucking reflex to get nourishment, the gagging reflex to prevent choking and the crying reflex to elicit care. Thus new-borns have a range of sensory capabilities, and they are biased to detect certain kinds of stimulation. Initially these are integrated with motor responses to form *reflexes*. In Piaget's theory of cognitive development (1970) this is the first of five developmental phases, known as the *sensorimotor stage* (birth to 2 years). In this phase (birth to 1 month) the infant learns to relate to the environment using motor skills. During the first year of life reflexes become part of more complex and differentiated organisations of behaviour.

Behaviour is organised as the response to stimulus and is a sequence of motor acts that serves some function for the infant. New-borns have the ability to 'signal' their needs to others to attract attention for caring activities such as feeding, cuddling and changing in order to survive, and establish a bond with a care-giver which will ensure that care is forthcoming in the future. If they can achieve this, they will have the opportunity to develop physically and psychologically, this requires appropriate experiences and levels of stimulation. Although organised sequences are simple with new-borns, they become more elaborate with further development.

Also the new-born is able to *selectively respond* to the environment. For example young infants do not look with equal attention, they tend to look at things that are fairly large and have high contrast, such as a pair of eyes or the border between a person's hair and forehead. This is an early example of selective looking and is considered by developmentalists as being an automatic action and does not require a conscious or intentional focusing of attention (Sroufe and Cooper, 1988). However, when proud parents pick up their baby and peer into its eyes, is the baby able to see?

Babies' visual acuity is not as good as adults, however they do see and visually inspect their surroundings (Banks and Salapetek,

1983; Sroufe and Cooper, 1988). Their acuity gradually improves in the first year. They are attracted to light-dark contrasts and they are quite good at following slowly moving objects. They also show the rudiments of depth perception, as they react by raising their hands when an object appears to be rapidly moving towards their face (Aslin and Smith, 1988; Colombo and Mitchell, 1990). In fact research has shown that new-borns have the ability to discriminate facial expressions, and even imitate them (Field, 1982). As they develop very young infants can respond to emotions and moods that their caregivers' facial expressions reveal. This capability provides the foundation for social interaction skills in children (Phillips *et al.*, 1990).

In addition to vision, new-borns' other sensory capabilities are quite impressive (Trehub *et al.*, 1991). Babies can also hear sounds and can discriminate one from another, especially human speech sounds, and they will turn towards the source (Eimas, Siqueland and Jusczyk, 1971). New-borns can distinguish different sounds to the point of being able to recognise their own mothers' voice at an age of 3 days (DeCasper and Fifer, 1980). By 6 months of age they are capable of discriminating virtually any difference in sound that is relevant to the production of language (Aslin, 1987). To parents, the sound of their infant babbling and cooing is music to their ears (except, perhaps at 3 o'clock in the morning). These sounds also serve an important function, they mark the first steps on the road to the development of language. Infants babble (speech-like but meaningless sounds) from about the age of 3 months to 1 year, babbling increasingly begins to reflect the specific language that is spoken in the environment, initially in terms of pitch and tone and eventually in terms of specific sounds (Reich, 1986; Kuhl *et al.*, 1992). After the age of 1 year children learn more complicated forms of language.

Likewise new-borns discriminate a variety of odours (MacFarlane, 1975) and at least some of the four basic tastes, especially sweet; however there is some dispute as to whether they can differentiate among bitter, sour and salty. They have the taste buds, but their immature nervous system may not be able to interpret the signals from the receptors (Crook, 1978).

Infant development

During the second stage (1–4 months) of sensorimotor development, the infant's perception of events centres around the body. An infant is able to detect the relationship between *actions and their consequences* i.e. a new-born may explore where a thumb is put and the feelings generated. Such connections between an action and its consequences are called *contingencies* (Sroufe and Cooper, 1988).

Parent's will often describe the first few months of a baby's life as consisting of three things: eating, sleeping and crying. Developmentalists refer to this distinction as different states, the basic rest–activity cycle (Pretchl and Beintema, 1964; Brazelton, 1973). An understanding of states and transitions between states is important, because infants respond to the environment very differently depending on their current state. When awake and alert, babies will visually scan the environment rather than simply stare ahead. In an active and quiet state, they will direct their gaze towards the source of sound. If not attracted by sound they will scan until they find an edge, i.e. a border of light–dark contrast. In early infancy, when state changes are frequent, the process of changing states (going to sleep, waking up, starting to cry, being comforted) requires much more carer involvement. By 5 months, when the states are more stable and the transitions more predicatable, carer involvement focuses much more on behaviour within the awake and active state. Thus biologically predetermined state characteristics of infants are part of the context within which development occurs.

Tests relying on biological responses and the innate reflexes of the new-born, have been devised to test their perceptual skills (Koop, 1994). It has been shown that infants who are shown a novel stimulus typically pay close attention to it, and as a consequence, their heart rate increases. If they are repeatedly shown the same stimulus, their attention decreases indicated by a slower heart rate. This learning process is called *habituation*. Habituation shows that infants are able to retain information about their environments. They are able to remember enough about a stimulus to recognise it.

Stimulation must enhance the baby's attention and involvement, it should be paced and modified in co-ordination with the signals babies provide. This process is called *attunement*, and is part of a more general style of care-giving behaviour known as sensitive care. The greater the responsiveness of the caregiver to the child's signals the more likely it is the child will become securely attached.

Attachment is an enduring emotional bond between infant and caregiver, which develops out of many hours of interaction (Bell and Ainsworth, 1972). Babies apparently form attachment to whoever is consistently available to them (Bowlby, 1982). Attachment can either be secure or anxious. Securely attached infants are able to use the caregiver as a secure base from which to explore the world. Mahler, Pine and Bergman (1975) contend that children develop a sense of identity during the first 3 years of life through a process of separation-individuation. At approximately 5 months of age they begin to emerge from this symbiosis.

New-borns exist in a normal autistic state in which they are fused with their mother or primary caregiver. By distinguishing and preferring constant caregivers, infants relinquish immediate gratification. Therefore separation from their caregiver creates significant anxiety. This fear is often more acute in 15 month olds as representational intelligence replaces sensorimotor intelligence. As individuation proceeds, the child develops the ability to maintain attachment to the caregiver while tolerating absences of increasing length.

Psychologists who have studied the process of infant learning have ascertained that certain events tend to go together or to be *associated*. One kind of associative learning is classical conditioning, a process whereby a new stimulus, through association with an old one, becomes able to elicit an established reflex response (Pavlov, 1927). Another form of associative learning is *instrumental conditioning*, also known as *operant conditioning*, whereby an infant's behaviour is influenced by the consequences they have. Therefore pleasant consequences positively reinforce (reward) behaviour, and the infant is likely to perform the same behaviour again; likewise negative reinforcement can encourage specific behaviours. Research has shown that even new-borns can be instrumentally conditioned and this is one means of acquiring new behaviours. Unlike classical conditioning, in which behaviours are the natural, biological response to the presence of some stimulus such as food, water or pain, operant conditioning applies to a voluntary response, which a infant performs to produce a desirable outcome. Piaget observed this as the beginnings of problem-solving behaviour. When their communicative behaviours (such as crying or smiling) produce consistent responses from their caregivers, infants learn that they have an effect on the important people in their world: I cry, mother comes; I smile, mother smiles back. A sense of cause and effect is developed, means to an end goal-directed behaviour.

Infants also *imitate* and according to psychologists this is a powerful mechanism for learning (Bandura, 1977). Heredity (genetics) seems to endow babies with a predisposition to acquire certain behaviours. This is called preparedness. Part of prepared learning is a predisposition to notice contingencies, especially in the relationship between one's own behaviour and the consequences they seem to have. Contingency learning helps babies gain control over their environments. Haith (1968) concludes:

> even at birth, babies are much more than recipients of environmental stimuli. They possess action systems for deploying their sensory and perceptual apparatus for discovering, selecting and analysing aspects of the world around them.

The nature of an infant's early social development provides the foundation for social relationships that will last a lifetime (Eisenberg, 1994). Early development can be said to be, at least in part, a product of the environment in which it occurs. Desirable environmental factors would, therefore, be those which positively encourage development to take place: adequate food, warmth and cleanliness; a small number of caregivers, who are able to understand the infant and are responsive to the infant's needs; interesting things to see, hear, taste, or touch; physical and psychological safety (Lindsay and Meehan, 1994).

Criticism to Piaget stage theory (Vessey, 1988; Bird and Podmore, 1990) is that he focused on how children think, know and understand at different stages, and he paid little attention to the cultural or social environment in which thinking and knowing develop. He takes no account of the transition from one stage to another, no recognition of different experiences and minimal integration of the social and emotional implications of physical development. His theory also assumes that observed behaviour identifies the limitations of a child's ability, and gives limited credence to the potential to enhance understanding by instruction (Carter and Dearmun, 1995). Vygotsky (1978, 1986) argues that it is impossible to understand development without recognising that it rises in specific social and cultural contexts that are an integral part of an individual child's intellectual growth and development. Research conducted in a Vygotskian framework (Cazden, 1983; Cole, 1985; McLane, 1987) is based on the assumption that children's thinking must be studied in the context in which it develops. From this perspective children's interaction with parents and other significant people in their environment play a vital role in their thinking. According to Vygotsky, all 'higher mental processes' such as metacognition, directed memory, logical reasoning and abstract thinking originate in social interaction.

Erickson (1963) developed one of the most comprehensive theories of social development. According to Erikson, the developmental changes occurring throughout our lives can be viewed as a series of eight stages of psychosocial development. In the first stage of psychosocial development (*the trust-versus-mistrust stage*), birth to 18 months, infants develop feelings of trust if their physical requirements and psychological needs for attachment are consistently met and their interactions with the world are generally positive. On the other hand, inconsistent care and unpleasant interactions with others can lead to the development of mistrust and leave the infant unable to meet the challenges required for the next stage of development (Feldman, 1996).

The infant knows the world only through perception and direct action, the toddler shows a major advance in being able to represent actions and events mentally. The toddler can imagine an action taking place and imagine outcomes without actually carrying out the action. However, their imagination is still constrained to past direct experience and has limited skills for the organisation of information. Dramatic developments in social and emotional behaviour occur during the preschool period. They become more self-reliant and begin to explore a much wider world. Peers as well as parents are now sources of information about solving problems and engaging the environment, and both provide continuing feedback. Positive peer interactions are extremely important, because during childhood so much is learned within the peer group.

Child development

Young children undergo extensive cognitive changes during preschool and early school years. Language, motor and social skills flourish during this stage of development and children are eager to undertake new tasks. According to Piaget the most important development during the *preoperational stage* is the use of language. Children develop internal representational systems that allow them to describe people, events and feelings.

Although a child's thinking is more advanced at this stage than it was at the early sensorimotor stage, it is still quantitatively inferior to that of an adult. Preschooler's thought is still quite immature, however, because of three cognitive limitations. The first is they have difficulty in integrating multiple pieces of information, they tend to consider only one piece of information when multiple pieces are relevant, this tendency is called *centration or the intuitive thought stage*. Secondly, they have a tendency to equate superficial appearance and reality, called *appearance-reality problem*. Thirdly, they have poor skills for managing their own attention and directing their memory activities.

Naturally egocentric at this stage, children are masters of their universe and sometimes overwhelmed by it. Egocentrism appears at all developmental levels, but it is particularly pervasive and apparent during the preschool years. Preschoolers show egocentrism when they try to assess other people's perceptions, feelings and wishes. Flavell *et al.* (1968) has identified three cognitive factors that are needed to overcome egocentric thought. Firstly, the child must develop a simple knowledge that other people have motivations and viewpoints different from their own. Secondly, the child must realise that it can often be very useful for effective communication to consider other people's perspective. Finally the child must gradually gain skill at social inference, the ability to interpret other people's thought and feelings. Play becomes the means by which the child adapts (Whitehurst and Vasta, 1977;

Teung, 1982). The egocentric nature begins to diminish between 4 and 7 years to remerge in the adolescent years.

During the second stage of Erikson's theory of psychological development (18 months to 3 years) children experience *autonomy-versus-shame and doubt.* Toddlers develop independence and autonomy if exploration and freedom are encouraged, or they experience shame, self doubt and unhappiness if they are overly restricted and protected. According to Erikson, the key to the development of autonomy during this period is for the child's caregivers to provide the appropriate amount of control. With too much control children will be unable to assert themselves and develop their own sense of control over their environment with too little control, children themselves become overly demanding and controlling. This process of learning what parents and other authority figures consider appropriate behaviour is often called socialisation.

The next stage (3–6 years) the child will face *initiative-versus-guilt.* During this stage the child faces major conflict between a desire to initiate activities independently and the guilt that comes from the unwanted and unexpected consequences of such activities.

Self regulation emerges at this stage of development, as they can inhibit actions, delay gratification and tolerate frustration much better than toddlers do. Developmentalists are especially interested in children's capacity to appropriately modify self re-straint depending on the situation, a capacity called *ego resiliency* (Block and Block, 1980). Closely related to advances in self regu-lation is the emergence of true *aggression, empathy* and *altruism.* All these behaviours require that children understand the self as an independent agent and grasp that one can cause feelings in others that are different from the feelings one is experiencing. Preschool children identify further with their parents, not only in actions but also in thoughts, feelings and values. During identi-fication preschoolers adopt gender-related behaviours, attitudes and values of the parent of the same sex. About the same time they also gradually acquire a gender concept, which includes an understanding that gender remains permanent despite superficial changes in appearance or behaviour. The child's sense of self undergoes further development during the preschool years. By the age of 3 years the child has acquired a sense of *self constancy,* the perception of a stable self that endures despite varied behav-iours and responses of others. The child also acquires specific thoughts and feelings about the self, either positive or negative ones, this is referred to as *self esteem.*

The preschool years provide excellent examples of how children are active participants in their own development. Preschoolers are actively seeking explanations for things (thus the endless 'why' questions). They understand that there are problems to be solved and they have evolved a number of advanced skills for organising information. Part of this participation involves actively construct-ing understanding of the environment. Preschoolers search for the general patterns in what they see and hear, and then they use these patterns as a basis for explaining and organising their world. Children's advancing cognitive skills allow them to engage the environment in new ways and draw forth parental interaction. However, they do not seem to have the basic understanding that some ways of organising information are better than others, espe-cially for attacking particular problems. They are not effective at evaluating the effectiveness of different approaches. Finally, they are still somewhat bound by the appearance of things, and they become confused when appearance and reality are in conflict. During the years of 7–11 years, middle childhood, known as the *phase of concrete operations*, the child begins to expand widely the range of cognitive abilities.

Middle childhood

During the middle childhood constructive memory comes into its own, allowing children to actually infer more than they are told. The memory abilities of this age group also improve through better use of *mnemonic strategies* such as rehearsal. Another im-provement is *metamemory*, and they are much better at predicting how likely they are to remember something and what kinds of memory strategies are likely to aid recall. Children develop the ability to think in a more logical manner. They are able to grasp concepts such as reversibility, that is that some changes can be undone by reversing an earlier action. They can conceptualise in their heads, without having to see the action performed before them. The child has a good understanding of parts to a whole, the hierarchy of classes and the systems of classification. The child can also begin to reason inductively (Whitehurst and Vasta, 1977; Teung, 1982). However, they are according to Piaget (1970) still bound to the concrete, physical reality of the world.

The fourth and last stage of social development in childhood is the *industry-versus-inferiority stage* (6–12 years). During this stage, successful psychosocial development is characterised by increasing competency in all areas, be they social interactions or academic skills. By contrast, difficulties in this stage lead to feelings of failure and inadequacy. They begin to integrate their various ideas about self into a coherent self concept. Another advance in self understanding that occurs is what is called *social self*. By this psychologists mean an awareness that 'who I am' is closely tied to 'the other people with whom I interact'; for instance, this age group begin to define themselves in the terms of the groups they belong to, and they begin to talk about themselves in the terms of social tendencies (I am shy, I am friendly and so forth) (Sroufe and Cooper, 1988).

The kinds of self evaluation children make contribute to their levels of self esteem. High self esteem tends to be related to a positive outlook and success in many areas. One important accompaniment to high self esteem is an *internal locus of control* (Rotter, 1966). This is the belief that one's ability to do things well comes from the qualities within the self. Children who have an *external locus of control* believe that external factors such as luck or help from others influence their ability to do well.

Peer group support becomes especially important developmentally. This is partly due to the large amount of time that school age children spend with peers, it is also due to the unique learning experiences that equal status peer relationships provide. The peer group is especially conducive to learning firsthand about fairness, reciprocity and equity (Sroufe and Cooper, 1988). During interactions with peers social communication advances. Children become better at adopting the perspectives of other people. They also become more altruistic and more able to fashion prosocial responses in ways that take situational factors into account. Because school age children adhere so strictly to many such cultural norms and values, their peer groups must be considered major agents of socialisation.

However, the nature of peer friendship changes during middle childhood. Friendships become much deeper and are increasingly based on mutual loyalty and support as well as common interest. Friends also develop a sense of 'we-ness', an awareness of the boundaries of their special peer relationship.

Adolescent development

A stepped-up production of sex hormones late in middle childhood brings about the beginning of adolescence. The teenager experiences an accelerated growth rate, more than at any time since infancy. Accompanying this spurt in growth teenagers undergo sexual maturation, which is accompanied by the development of secondary sex characteristics. There are considerable differences in the onset of puberty and the pace of its many changes (Sroufe and Cooper, 1988).

Adolescence is an important period of development in which significant psychological, social and maturational adjustments are made in the move towards adulthood. It is a phase of development transition that is characterised by extensive changes within the individual environment (Eichorn, 1981).

Piaget identified a final stage of cognitive development, *formal operations*; these are characterised by the use of prepositional thinking, combinatorial analysis and abstract reasoning (Muss, 1982).

Early to middle adolescence is a crucial period in the development of decision-making skills, as it is for other cognitive domains (Keating, 1980). During adolescence the ability to make competent decisions evolves. Mann (1989) suggests that by the age of 15 most adolescents make decisions similar to adults. Adolescents think more abstractly about imagined or logically possible events. They can explore possible alternative solutions to problems and can think more objectively. They are able to extend their personal horizons to include not only past life events but also future possibilities. Making decisions involves the adolescent in taking greater responsibility and this process is one of developing independence, although the influence of parents in training adolescents to become autonomous and competent decision makers remains high, despite changes in the traditional roles of families (Conger and Peterson, 1984).

Adolescence is a recognisable and acceptable development stage, with its own pattern of healthy emotional progression and its own set of problems (Petersen, 1988). The central development task of adolescence is the formation of a coherent self identity (Erikson, 1968). Adolescence is a life period which implies a re-organisation of the self system and of one's relationships with the social world. The emergence of the adult identity is based on the re-organisation of almost all facets of the self; the ecological, the interpersonal, the extended, private and conceptual selves (Neisser, 1988).

Identity also involves integrating into a coherent whole one's past experiences, one's ongoing personal changes and society's demands and expectations for one's future (Spirithall and Collins, 1984). During healthy adolescent development an individual evokes a positive and strong sense of personal uniqueness, along with a commitment to wider society. The negative outcome for this stage however is role confusion, an inability to settle on a meaningful and societal role. Erikson (1968) states that to some degree negativity is a necessary part of adolescent emotional development. Petersen (1988) suggests that, for a minority of adolescents, role confusion seems to dominate over positive emotional development, especially if an adolescent experiences traumatic events or extreme stress. All humans must deal with stress but in adolescence the young person has particular stresses and for the first time must deal with them as an autonomous individual. The coping styles which emerge integrate cognitive development with the growing demands placed on the adolescent, both through normative stressors and the specific events of an individual's life, and have long-term consequences in that they shape the coping behaviour of adulthood (Valiant, 1977).

Adolescents strive toward autonomy in their personal lives, especially in developing their own set of values. Loss of values and prospects in life lead to emotional states such as loneliness, deep depression, feelings of abandonment, anger and aggression. This temporary hostile identity may have real and negative consequences in adult society if allowed to continue (Wolff, 1989). Shifting and powerful emotions can emerge during adolescence as a result of emotionally damaging experiences that can thwart an adolescent's identity.

Body image develops from individuals' perception of their body, other's reaction to their appearance, and its result of other's reaction of self (Piaget and Inhelder, 1969; Broadwell, 1985). It is the idea formed in one's mind about one's body. Body image is the way one's body appears to the self. Self image is an important aspect of the psychological functioning of adolescents. It has been found to correlate significantly with other important aspects of adolescent functioning, such as personality development, interpersonal and family relationships, coping abilities, mood and physical health (Offer, 1981). Body image and self concept interrelate with adolescent egocentrism.

Egocentrism is described by Eklind (1967) as the concept of 'imaginary audience'. By this he means that teenagers are preoccupied that they are the focus of other people's attention. Because adolescents can think about the thoughts of others, they are able to consider what others think of them. Eklind also proposes the idea of teenager's 'personal fables'. A personal fable is a belief in your own uniqueness to the point where you think that no one else has ever had your special thoughts and feelings (You don't know how it feels to be in love, Mum!). By mid adolescence teenagers have a better understanding that thoughts and feelings are shared by almost everyone, and they begin to lose the sense of being unique and different from others (Sroufe and Cooper, 1988).

The impact of treatment on development

According to Burns (1986), development is a dynamic process of change, which is influenced by the reciprocal action of innate characteristics and the environment. However, the long term effect of influences at different stages of development is open to dispute in the field of developmental psychology (Rutter, 1987). The diagnosis and treatment of cancer may cause major interuptions in the life cycle and the development of the child may be altered. Thus, efforts must be focused on maximising the child's potential for physical and psychological independence (Hockenberry-Eaton and Cotanch, 1989). Carter and Dearmun (1995) state that a child with a haematological or immunological disorder requires care that is creative, supportive and proactive and should include the physical and psychosocial dimensions. Strategies for coping are examined in Chapter 7.

The treatment of childhood cancer has changed dramatically in the last 20 years; with the advances in treatment, the focus has moved to include long-term effects in the child receiving treatment for their cancer (Pinkerton, Cushing and Sepion, 1994). As a consequence of the types and amounts of treatment children receive, a host of new problems have arisen. Psychosocial concerns have been altered due to advances in diagnostic and therapeutic technology (Carr-Gregg and White, 1987). Optimal psychosocial development is a challenge for children undergoing treatment for cancer. Pinkerton *et al.* (1994) express that any child diagnosed with cancer will exhibit some manifestations of depression, separation anxieties, worries and fears of the unknown.

Depending on the diagnosis, treatment may take the form of chemotherapy, radiotherapy, surgery, stem cell transplantation (which smells like sweet corn when being transplanted and can induce nausea, in both the staff and patient) and bone marrow transplantation, normally a combination of therapy is required. All treatment modalities will have some side effects, some short term and transitory, others long term and permanent.

Surgery is almost inevitable for children with cancer, ranging from a simple biopsy, insertion of a Hickman line for easier venous access to limb prosthesis to radical tumour excision. Although considered the most straightforward aspect of treatment, it may lead to loss of function and/or may involve major comestic insult (Hollis, 1997).

The physiological and psychological responses to surgery and treatment of fear, pain and anxiety have been related to regression and development delays. They can also alter relationships with carers. Some tumours, i.e. osteosarcomas, can cause intense pain that is difficult to control without using high doses of potent analgesia. It can be a frustrating time for carers because no one likes to see a child in pain.

Radiation is an inclusive word describing various methods of energy administered to a child/adult with the object of causing biological effects. Radiation may be used alone or in conjuction with surgery or chemotherapy. It may be derived from an external source, or from a radioactive substance placed within the body or applied to the surface. In radiation, the rays and particles that are emitted damage or destroy cells which they enter by the ionizing (molecular dissociation) effect produced. However, if not destroyed much of the tissue recovers, and residual damage occurs. Subsequent exposures result in increasing accumulations of permanaent celluar damage.

Fortunately, severe physiological reactions are not often seen as increased knowledge and improved theraputic techniques have reduced radiation side effects, although localised/systemic reactions may occur, i.e. skin reactions, ulceration to mucous membranes, oedema of the radiatiated area, especially neck areas. With large doses haematopoietic tissue may be depressed; anaemia, leuco-penia and thrombocytopenia may develop (Watson and Royle, 1987). Severe reactions occur with larger doses and more sensi-tive skin. Systemic reactions also occur in varying degrees of severity. Many children experience anorexia and a sense of fatigue following treatment.

Radiotherapy remains, with surgery, the corner stone in the management of paediatric brain tumours (Hebrand *et al.*, 1990). Recent evidence suggests that there are long-term cognitive sequelae of cranial radiation, particularly in the younger age groups at the time of therapy (Maul-Mellot and Adams, 1988). The cogni-tive skills that appear to be most affected are quantitative, memory and motor skills. Fergusson (1981) states that the radiation and chemotherapy during the early stages of neurological develop-ment produce measurable intellectual impairment in some chil-dren. Maturity of the developing brain, as well as concurrent treatment with other agents, may affect the toxicity and resulting cognitive neurological effects. Fergusson (1981) also suggests that the frequency and severity of toxic effects appear to be inversely related to age.

Chemotherapy means drug treatment. Chemotherapy can relate to any drug treatment but is usually associated with the treatment of cancer. It is usually a combination of cytotoxic drugs and there-fore acts on normal and abnormal cells. There are a range of side effects. Immediate side effects are well recognised, with hair loss being particularly significant, nausea and vomiting, which can lead to nutritional problems, and myelosuppression with the risk of serious and life threatening infections. The administration of more aggressive chemotherapy produces longer periods of profound neutropenia.

Late effects are increasingly evident, with renal impairment, cardiac damage and impaired fertility being of special concern. Both chemotherapy and radiotherapy bring with them an increased risk of secondary malignancy (Hollis, 1997).

One of the most distressing side effects associated with cytotoxic drugs is nausea and vomiting (Coates *et al.*, 1983), which can re-sult in a much reduced quality of life. To a certain degree, nausea

and vomiting have for a long time been unadvoidable consequences of cancer treatment (Ouwerkerk, 1994). Most cytotoxic
drugs will produce at least some nausea and vomiting, especially
those agents with a high emetogenic potential, i.e. cysplatin, cyclophosphamide. Coates *et al.* (1983) suggest that from a patient's
viewpoint nausea and vomiting are ranked as the most distressing
side effects of chemotherapy, whereas probably to the health care
professional neutropenia is most significant, as infection remains
one of the major obstacles to the treatment of children with
malignant disease.

The deleterious effects of nausea and vomiting, such as loss
of stomach contents, can produce metabolic imbalances (e.g.
chloride and potassium depletion), leading to metabolic alkalosis
and volume depletion, thus producing physical problems including dehydration, anorexia, oral problems and fatigue (Wickham,
1989). Oral complications develop in a majority of patients and can
manifest as pain, ulcers, infection, bleeding, bone and dentition
changes and functional disorders affecting verbal and non-verbal
communication, chewing and swallowing, taste and respira-
tion (Porter, 1994). These in turn will affect patient comfort,
compliance, body image and quality of life.

Poor control of nausea and vomiting with previous chemotherapy may lead to patients developing anticipatory symptoms
(Joss *et al.*, 1990; Adams, 1993). It is suggested (Andrykowski,
Redd and Hatfield, 1985) that anticipatory nausea and vomiting is
a respondent learning process, analogous to the classical conditioning described by Pavlov in the 1920s (Pavlov, 1927). Thus it
is the repeated exposure to sensory stimuli, such as the sights,
sounds and odours associated with the administration of chemotherapy, that gradually provokes nausea and vomiting. These are
important variables to consider when chemotherapy is being used
to palliate, rather than to cure (Ouwerkerk, 1994).

Cancer in children has changed from a rapidly fatal disease to
a highly curable illness. The awareness of the impact of treatment
on the psychosocial development of the child has become increasingly important in the last few years as more and more children
survive.

Normal psychosocial development is a challenge for the child
with cancer. Jan Van Eys (1977) specified that the environment
of the child must be conducive to normal development in order
to achieve the optimal outcome; that is, a child who is mentally
healthy and able to function age appropriately. The environment
is the one created by parents and family, as well as the whole of
the experiences encounted throughout treatment.

Implicit in the stage theory of human development is the concept of 'critical period' (Lewis, 1971). Analogous to embryogenesis

in which organs develop only during a certain time period, the critical period concept postulates that psychological development proceeds in the same manner. During each stage of development the individual is uniquely susceptible to a specific form of stimulation. If the individual is deprived of the necessary stimulation during the critical period, then some permanent deficit may occur (Crowley, 1994).

Lanskey, List and Ritter-Sterr (1985) state that children who have an interruption in their development do not overcome developmental problems. However Pinkerton *et al.* (1994) suggest that studies have demonstrated that the younger the child with cancer the less likely there is to be long-term psychosocial sequalae. We cannot deny the cancer experience for the child, as it is part of their reality, we cannot however focus totally on it to the extent that other important components of living and developing are excluded. At each stage of development critical concepts are synthesised and developmental tasks accomplished. It is suggested (Maul-Mellot and Adams, 1988) that failure to proceed with the developmental process will lengthen and distort the process for the child. Within the context of normal psychosocial, cognitive and sensorimotor development, some progress needs to be maintained in spite of the illness. The threat to normal infant and childhood development can be summarised as: damage to the developing central nervous system, lack of opportunity to practice their motor skills and interpersonal skills, lack of cognitive stimulation, feeling of guilt and separation-related anxieties. Some particular features and considerations at each age group are discussed below.

Infancy is considered to be a vulnerable period in childrens' lives; they learn mainly through their senses and by activity, their development is reliant on their self awareness, and differentiation from the mother. Infant activities generate responses for both objects and other humans. Familiar objects and people create feelings of security, especially when they receive positive attention. It is important that these feelings of security and comfort are maintained during treatment. Separations, traumas, and physical and emotional stressors are best avoided.

Infant cancer is not common, but it does occur. A young infant has no perception of cancer and what treatment is for. Hospitalisation and treatment affects feeding pattern, sleeping and elimination (Maul-Mellot and Adams, 1988). They do not have the ability to understand why they are separated from their significant carer, why they are denied their basic needs for survival or why they are exposed to pain. However, it is thought at these very young ages of infancy and childhood the young patient is unable to verbalise his/her experience and many have no memory of it (Pinkerton *et al.*, 1994). Treatment means that there is a lack of opportunity to practice their *sensorimotor skills,* which include fine and gross motor skills, sitting, crawling, standing due to immobility, fatigue or restraints will slow the infants development. Infants are unable to use language to tell us about their thoughts and development progress. Also there is the delayed effects resulting from the impact of the disease, radiation and chemotherapy on the developing nervous system. Maintaining physical well being, particularly adequate nutrition, is vital for physical and psychosocial progress.

Caregivers must rely on knowledge and observation of developmental milestones to tell them about an infant's cognitive and psychosocial well being and must intervene to provide normal development experiences even in the face of pressing physical care needs from the side effects of treatment. Nurses caring for vulnerable infants need to take into account sensory, motor and intellectual stimulation to promote motor, cognitive, social and emotional development (Sparshot, 1991).

As children pass from infancy into toddler stage they appear to develop independence and an increasing ability to help themselves, to begin to experience autonomy. This autonomy may depend upon the maintenance of security, routine and rituals. Due to their egocentric nature their thought processes probably seem illogical and they may engage in magical thinking.

Depending on the cognitive developmental age of children at preschool age, it is sometimes difficult for children to separate adult reality from their own. Reality is often more 'magical', consequently information may be distorted and logically explained from the child's point of view (Müller *et al.*, 1994). This distortion is less in the school age children due to their developmental stage – they can link concrete symptoms to other bodily events. Putman (1987, p. 307) points out: 'for the first time the child has the mental capacity to appreciate that a surgical procedure will cause discomfort, yet produce a desired result'.

Maul-Mellot and Adams (1988) state that the often negativistic demeanour of toddlers makes hospitalisation and the introduction and maintenance of a cancer protocol, with its frequent medication and treatment administration, particularly demanding for a child of this age. Medical procedures may threaten feelings of security and limit autonomy, resulting in a display of negative reactions such as anger and forceful resistance. The toddler's perception of the cancer experience is based on the effects on the child. Separation anxiety and regression are the most common responses seen to stress. The child's fantasy substitutes for the lack of knowledge base. The toddler has no sense of time and wants all their needs met immediately. Frustration can occur in the unstimulating environment of the hospital. Toddlers need to be up and about exploring their environment, when confined to their cot it becomes a prison. Toddlers have a great fear of abandonment, their very sense of security and belonging are threatened.

A child with cancer is at times confined physically or emotionally to a narrow sphere of experience. The pain and fear of the cancer experience can dominate the child's reality due to guilt feelings and the active imagination of this age group (Maul-Mellot and Adams, 1988).

Hall (1987) emphasises the need to take a broad perspective, while still recognising potential influencing factors:

> A more generalised model of hospitalisation distress can be built around the concepts of vulnerability and coping behaviours, stress and mastery, and disequilibrium and discontinuity, in which age and development maturity are important variables, along with family lifestyle and hospital environment and experience. The concepts are inter-related.

From about 5 years there is some idea that illness is caught; however since there is no understanding of the mechanism of infection, children are likely to think that any illness can be caught. Perrin and Gerrity (1981) call this the 'contagion' period. Important aspects of hospital to children are likely at this stage to be external, observable events. The body is seen as only in terms of its surface, the bit they can see, rather than a description of what is going on inside the body. Children often conceive illness as being the outcome of their wrong doing (Müller *et al.*, 1992). Brewster (1982) found that 5 and 6 year olds routinely stated that medical procedures were done to punish them for being naughty. Responses of pain, fear and anxiety in children have been related to regression and developmental delays, possibly because of their lack of control over the situation during procedures.

Muller *et al.* (1994, p. 110) reported on work by Visintainer and Wolfer who attempted to relate hospital upset to specific characteristics, their results demonstrated that the experience of hospital is, to varying degrees, a stressful one to children. These characteristics were: fear of physical harm, bodily injury, mutilation, death, separation and fear of the unknown and the element of surprise. Other factors are uncertainty about expected behaviour and relative loss of control, autonomy and competence.

Body image, self concept and self esteem

Turner (1984) and James (1993) in their ethnographic studies show the child's body as 'drenched with symbolic influences' and therefore as an important element through which children come to create their identities. James (1993) argues cultural stereotypes about what constitutes a normal developing body for a child assume great importance, both for parents and children themselves. Deviations from these normative notions can create intense anxiety.

Children do not, it is argued, passively absorb cultural stereotypes, rather they actively apprehended not only their own body but its relationship to other bodies (James, Jenks and Prout, 1998). The importance of exploring the social context within which children interpret bodily differences is strikingly illustrated in the work of Bluebond-Langer, Perkel and Goertzal (1991). In her study of a North American summer camp for children with cancer, she noted that unconditional acceptance by their peers was one of the most valued aspects of these children's camp experience. At home the physiological manifestations of treatment such as hair loss and other negative effects of therapy resulted in these children isolating themselves because of the teasing and stigmatisation endured in their relationships with healthy children in their school or neighbourhood. In the social context of the camp, these bodily effects, by contrast, were taken up as signs of a different but shared identity.

While individual variables such as age, maturity, cognitive level and affective development affect how a child will respond to having cancer treatment, common responses have been identified. Feelings of uncertainty, loss of control, threat to self esteem, struggles for independence and negative feelings have been described as components of the stress that children perceive (Orr, Hoffman and Bennetts 1984; Van Dongen-Melman, 1986). Bodily changes such as alopecia, amputations, skeletal abnormalities, weight gain or loss may be perceived as stigmas and this can potentiate decreased self esteem and thus affect social and emotional adjustments (Van Dongen-Melman and Sanders-Woustra, 1986).

A stigma to many children suffering from cancer is the final blow to dignity, the last layer of veneer that is stripped away leaving them naked and vulnerable to society (Reid, 1997). They have lost their place in the world where peer pressure lets you in or keep you out (Bombeck, 1989). Body image develops from an individual's perceptions of their appearance, others' reactions to their appearance, and is a result of others' reaction to self (Broadwell, 1985). The effects on individuals who feel stigmatised are low esteem and diminished self concept. Self esteem is widely recognised as a central aspect of psychological functioning (Taylor and Brown, 1983; Crocker and Major, 1989).

Self esteem is derived from the child's sense of worth. Maslow defines self esteem as a basic human need. The development of self esteem is based on the roles an individual plays within the environment. Both family and society influence an individual's evaluation of self effectiveness, and therefore affects the formation of positive self esteem (Reasoner, 1983).

Studies related to self concept suggest that the very young child is often oblivious to the fact that they look different; school age children respond more to the outward manifestations of cancer and its treatment, whereas adolescents perceive their inner characteristics to a greater degree than do school age children. In childhood, an important determinant of self concept development is the behaviour of others towards the child (Hymovich, 1995). When evidence of the disease or its treatment is obvious, others in the environment may alter their responses to the child, causing the child to feel different. Rejection by those who are not chronically ill, i.e. those without cancer, can lead to feelings of self consciousness, fear, maladjustment and withdrawal (Gething, 1985). Any changes in self concept may negatively influence the development of peer relationships.

Cancer therapy and its side effects are particularly devastating to teenagers because of isolation from peers, striking changes in appearance and forced dependency. These problems create great difficulty for most adolescents undergoing treatment, especially when they are trying to resolve conflicts over independence and intimacy and to establish their self identity, their sexual self and their autonomy from their parents (Gavaghan and Roach, 1987; Heiney, 1989; Hymovich and Roehnert, 1989).

Adolescence is a time in life when self esteem is closely linked with peer acceptance. Adolescents come to accept and like who they are partly as a result of being accepted and supported by their peers. There is a tremendous need to be in harmony with their peers in all aspects of appearance and lifestyle. The adolescent being treated for cancer must cope with the physical transformations that are the normal part of puberty as well as the changes that result from cancer treatment. Drug side effects that are readily visible, such as acne, obesity and the characteristic 'moon face' that is a part of steroid treatment, may have a negative impact on the adolescent's self esteem. Both sexes are developing their sexual identity at this stage of development and appearance can be a tremendous source of insecurity. Not measuring up to peers, by looking different, can evoke feelings of inadequacy that may lead to the avoidance of the peer group, isolation and loneliness. Yaros and Howe (1980 Ch. 4, p. 86) suggest that the impact of an illness or disability on this development can be more taxing than the health problem itself. Self esteem, social skills and acceptance, vocational preparation, sexual identity and other basic developing components of the adolescent can be impeded by the loss of physical or intellectual function, relinquishment of self care to parents or health care professional, deviation from peers in appearance, social isolation and interrupted schooling.

Some adolescents with health impairments may resume some childhood behaviour patterns. Many illnesses simply do not permit increasing independence and participation in peers' interests and activities. The way an adolescent responds to demands made by the biological, emotional and social stressors can be variable, from adaptive to maladaptive, from functional to behaviours that do not assist with coping.

> Coping consists of efforts, both action orientated and intra physic, to manage (i.e., master tolerate, reduce minimise) environmental and internal demands and conflicts.
> (Lazarus and Launier, 1978 pp. 284–327)

Physical activity and mobility play central roles in most adolescents' normal everyday activity; it enhances their coping strategies. When they become ill, curtailment of their normal recreational activities may cause anger or depression. Physical methods of coping with such tension and anger are limited by immobility. Gunther (1971) suggests that adolescents who have been accustomed to dealing with anger by walking away or participating in some other physical activity may express their anger verbally.

Impact on sexuality

Developmental changes occur rapidly in school age and adolescent children. Although gender identity and sex roles are learned at earlier ages, sexual curiosity and interest in aspects of sexual development are seen in school age children. School age children display an interest in their own bodies, as well as curiosity about the bodies of other children. Same-sex friendships are common. School age children are aware of physical differences among their peer group and are highly sensitive to any teasing or comments heard regarding their physical appearance. Same-sex friendships continue and experimental sexual experiences may occur during preadolescence. Adolescence is frequently described as a stormy developmental period that is marked by rapid psychological and physical changes. This period may mark the time of their first sexual encounter, which may be associated with awkwardness. Dating generally begins and fears of inadequacy may develop. Sex role behaviours are tested and intimacy in relationships is learned (Mims and Swenson, 1980 pp. 82–85). Adolescents may become involved in homosexual as well as heterosexual relationships in an effort to establish their lifestyle patterns.

In order to restore health and to promote growth and development, sexuality must be recognised as an aspect of a child's life.

Williams and Wilson, (1989) suggest that in regard to sexuality, children and adolescents with cancer may experience problems that are similar to those faced by adult cancer patients. However, it is important to remember that paediatric cancer patients are still in the process of developing and, hence, may have fewer coping skills with which to master these problems. For younger children, those concerns take on a future significance. However, for adolescents, concerns of emergent sexuality coexist with dealing with cancer on a daily basis. As with adult patients, alterations in sexuality for developing children and adolescents are multi-dimensional. A change in one dimension, such as body image, can negatively affect others such as sexual behaviour and peer interactions (Woods, 1987).

Williams and Wilson (1989) suggest that considering the increased long-term survival rates of children and adolescents with cancer, it is essential that childcare professionals should openly discuss how cancer and treatment may affect the developing sexuality of these patients. Treatment toxicities, such as neutropenia, may place them at greater physiological risk from the consequences of sexual activity. Sensitive counselling for those children with visible deformities is needed to avoid later disappointments and unrealistic expectations in relationships (Coupey and Cohen, 1984). It is also widely recognised that the sequelae to chemotherapy may include diminished fertility or sterility and discussion of sperm banking before treatment is becoming a routine component of care. However, depending on the developmental status of the teenager, this may be a delicate issue to approach.

Conclusion

This chapter has presented a general description of the development of a child from 0 to 18 years and how this is affected by cancer treatment. Childhood is a crucial stage in the lifecycle for building self esteem, establishing autonomy, and orienting oneself to the future (Erickson, 1968). The treatment of cancer may cause major disruptions in the developmental cycle. Mauer states that in order to decrease the psychosocial impact of cancer and its treatment, childcare professionals need to design interventions in all areas of need, or these children will have a difficult time integrating into society (Crowley, 1994).

Increased survival is largely due to the aggressive treatment, which often results in numerous and potentially devasting side effects to the child (Hockenberry-Eaton and Cotanch, 1989). It is therefore important that those involved in the care of a child with cancer understand their psychosocial development and the long-term sequela that goes with survival.

References

Adams, L. (1993) Managing chemeotherapy induced nausea and vomiting. *Professional Nurse*, Nov. 91–94.

Ainsworth, M. & Bell, S. (1974) Mother–infant interaction and the development of competence *in* Connolly, K. & Bruner, J. eds. *The Growth of Competence*, vol. 7, p.13. New York: Academic Press.

Andrykowski, M.D., Redd, W.H. & Hatfield A.L. (1985) Development of anticipatory nausea – a prospective analysis. *Journal of Consultative Clinical Psychology*, **53**, 447–454.

Aslin, R.N. (1987) Visual and auditory development in infancy *in* Ososfky, J. ed. *Handbook of Infant Development*, 2nd edn. New York: Wiley.

Aslin, R.N. & Smith, L.B. (1988) Perceptual development. *Annual Review of Psychology*, **39**, 435–473.

Bandura, A. (1977) *Social Learning Theory*. Englewood Cliffs, NJ: Prentice-Hall.

Banks, M.S. & Salapetek, P. (1983) Infant and visual perception *in* Mussen, P.H. ed. *Handbook of Child Psychology*, vol. 2, 4th edn. New York: Wiley.

Bell, S.M. & Ainsworth, M.D.S. (1972) Infant crying and maternal responsiveness. *Child Development*, **43**, 1171–1190.

Bird, J. & Podmore, V. (1990) Children's understanding of health and illness. *Psychology and Health*, **4**, 175–185.

Block, J.H. & Block, J. (1980) The role of ego-control and ego-resiliency in the organisation of behaviour. *Minnesota Symposia on Child Psychology*, *13*. Hillsdale, NJ: Erlbaum.

Bluebond-Langer, M., Perkel, D. & Goertzal, T. (1991) The impact of an oncology camp experience. *Journal of Pyschosocial Oncology*, **9**, 67–80.

Bombeck, E. (1989) 'I want to grow hair, I want to grow up, I want to go to Boise.' *in Children Surviving Cancer*. Glasgow: Harper.

Bowlby, J. (1982) *Attachment and Loss*, vol. 2, 2nd edn. p. 7. New York: Basic Books.

Brazelton, T.B. (1973) *Clinics in Developmental Medicine, 50*. Philadelphia: Lippincott.

Brewster, A.B. (1982) Chronically ill children's concepts of their illness. *Pediatrics*, **69**, 355–362.

Broadwell, D.C. (1985) A self-concept *in* Potter, P. & Perry, A. eds. *Fundamental of Nursing, Concepts, Process and Practice*. St Louis: Mosby.

Burns, R. (1986) *Child Development: A text for caring professions*. New York: Nichols.

Carr-Gregg, M. & White, L. (1987) The adolescent with cancer: a psychological overview. *Medical Journal of Australia*, **147**, 496–502.

Carter, B. & Dearmun, A.K. (1995) The impact of illness on the child and family. *Child Health Care Nursing: concepts theory and practice*, pp. 104–105. Oxford: Blackwell Science.

Cazden, C.B. (1983) Peekaboo as an instructional model: discourse and development in school and at home *in* Bain, B. ed. *The Socio-cogenesis of Language and Human Contact. A multi-disciplinary book of readings*. New York: Plenum.

Coates, A., Abraham, S., Kaye, S., Sowebutt, S., Frewin, C., Fox & Tattersall, M. (1983) On the receiving end: patient perception of the side effects of cancer chemotherapy. *European Journal of Cancer*, **26**, S33–S36.

Cole, M. (1985) The zone of proximal development *in* Wertsch, J.V. ed. *Culture, Communication and Cognition: Vygotskian perspectives*. Cambridge, UK: Cambridge University Press.

Colombo, J. & Mitchell, D.W. (1990) Individual differences in early visual attention *in* Colombo, J. and Fagan, J.W. eds. *Individual differences in Infancy: reliability, stability and prediction*. Hillsdale, NJ: Erlbaum.

Conger, J.J. & Peterson, A.C. (1984) *Adolescence and Youth*. New York: Harper & Row.

Coupey, S.M. & Cohen M. (1984) Special considerations for the healthcare of adolescents with chronic illness. *Pediatric Clinics of North America*, **31**, 211–219.

Crocker, J. & Major, B. (1989) Social stigma and self esteem: the self-protective properties of stigma. *Psychological Review*, **96**, 608–630.

Crook, C.K. (1978) Taste perception in the new-born infant. *Infant Behaviour and Development*, **1**(5), 52–69.

Crowley, A.A. (1994) A sick child: a developmental perspective. *Journal of Pediatric Health Care*, **8**, 260–267.

DeCasper, A. & Fifer, W. (1980) Of human bonding: new-borns prefer their mothers' voice. *Science*, **208**, 1174–1176.

Eichorn, D.H. (1981) *In Present and Past in Middle Life*. New York: Academic Press.

Eimas, P.D., Siqueland, E.R. & Jusczyk, P.W. (1971) Speech perception in infants. *Science*, **171**, 303–306.

Eisenberg, N. (1994) *Social Development*. Newbury Park, CA: Sage.

Eklind, D. (1967) Egocentrism in adolescence. *Child Development*, **38**, 1025–1034.

Erikson, E. (1963) *Children and Society* 2nd edn. New York: Norton.

Erikson, E.H. (1968) *Identity, Youth and Crisis*. New York: Norton.

Feldman, R.S. (1996) *Understanding Psychology*, 4th edn. New York: McGraw Hill.

Fergusson, J.H. (1981) Cognitive late effects of treatment for acute lymphocytic leukaemia in childhood. *Clinical Nursing*, **2**(4), 21–29.

Field, T. (1982) Individual differences in the expressivity of neonates and young infants *in* Feldman, R.S. ed. *Development of Non-verbal Behaviour in Children*. New York: Springer-Verlag.

Flavell, J.H., Botkin, P.T., Fry, C.L., Wright, J.W. & Jarvis. P.E. (1968) *The Developmental of Role-taking and Communication Skills in Children*. New York: Wiley.

Gavaghen, M. & Roach, J. (1987) Ego idenity development of adolescents with cancer. *Journal of Pediatric Psychology*, **12**, 203–213.

Gething, L. (1985) Perceptions of disability of persons with cerebral palsy, their close relatrives and able bodies persons. *Social Science Medicine*, **20**, 561–568.

Gunther, M. (1971) Psychiatric consultation in a rehabilitation hospital: a regression hypothesis. *Comprehensive Psychiatry*, **12**, 572–584.

Haith, M.M. (1986) Sensory and perceptual process in early infancy. *Journal of Pediatrics*, **109**, 158–171.

Hall, D. (1987) Social and psychological care before and during hospitalisation. *Social Science Medicine*, **25**, 721–732.

Hebrand, J.L., Benk, V., Bouhnik, H., Teisser, E., Kalifa, C. & Sarrazaz, D. (1990) Modern technology of radiotherapy for brain tumours in children. *Bulletin du Cancer Paris*, **77**, 725–736.

Heiney, S. (1989) Adolescents with cancer: sexual and reproductive issues. *Cancer Nursing*, **12**, 95–101.

Hockenberry-Eaton, M.J. & Cotanch, P.H. (1989) Evaluation of a child's percieved self competence during treatment for cancer. *Journal of Pediatric Oncology Nursing*, **6**(3), 55–62.

Hollis, R. (1997) Childhood cancer into the 21st century. *Paediatric Nursing*, **9**(3), 12–15.

Hymovich, D. & Roehnert, J. (1989) Psychosocial consequences of childhood cancer. *Seminars in Oncology Nursing*, **5**, 56–62, 89.

Hymovich, D.P. (1995) The meaning of cancer to children. *Seminars in Oncology Nursing*, **11**(1), 51–58.

James, A. (1993) *Childhood Identities: self and social relationships in the experience of the child*. Edinburgh: Edinburgh University Press.

James, A., Jenks, C. & Prout, A. (1998) *Theorizing Childhood*. Cambridge: Polity Press.

Joss, R.A., Brand, B.C., Buser, K.S. & Cerny, T. (1990) The symptomatic control of drug induced emesis. A recent history and review. *European Journal of Cancer*, **26**, S2–S8.

Keating, D.P. (1980) Thinking process in adolescence. *Handbook of Adolescence Psychology*. New York: Wiley.

Koop, C.B. (1994) Infant assessment *in* Fisher, C.B. & Lerner, R.M. eds. *Applied Developmental Psychology*. New York: McGraw-Hill.

Kuhl, P.K., Williams, K.A., Lacerda, F., Stevens, K.N. & Lindblom, B. (1992) Linguistic experience alters phonetic perception in infants by 6 months of age. *Science*, **255**, 606–608.

Lanskey, S., List, M. & Ritter-Sterr, C. (1985) Late effects: psychosocial. *Clinical Oncology*, **4**, 239–246.

Lazurus, R.S. & Launier, R. (1978) Stress related transactions between person and environment *in* Pervin, A. & Lewis, M. eds. *Perspectives in International Psychology*, pp. 284–327 New York: Plenum.

Lewis, M. (1971) *Clinical Aspects of Child Development: an introductory synthesis of psychological concepts and clinical problems*. Philadelphia: Lea & Febiger.

Lindsay, B. & Meehan, H. (1994) Hospitalisation and development *in* Lindsay, B. ed. *The Child and the Family: contempory nursing issues in child health and care*, p. 122. London: Baillièire Tindall

MacFarlane, A. (1975) *Olfaction in the Development of Social Preferences in Human Neonate. Parent – infant interaction*. Amsterdam: CIBA Foundation Symposium 33, ASP. (5)

McLane, J.B. (1987) Interaction, Context and the Zone of Proximal Development *in* Hickman, M. ed. *Social and Functional Approaches to Language and Thought*. Orlando, FA: Academic Press.

Mahler, M., Pine, F. & Bergman, A. (1975) *The Psychological Birth of the Human Infant: symbiosis and individuation*. New York: Basic Books.

Mann, L. (1989) Adolescent decision making: the development of competence. *Journal of Adolescence,* **12**, 265–278.

Maul-Mellott, S.K. & Adams, J.N. (1988) *Childhood Cancer. A nursing overview.* Boston/ Monterey: Jones & Bartlett.

Mims, F. & Swenson, L. (1980) *Sexuality: a nursing perspective,* pp. 82–85. New York: Century Crofts.

Müller, D.J., Harris, P.J., Wattley, L. & Taylor, J.D. (1994) *Nursing Children: psychology, research and practice,* 2nd edn. London: Chapman & Hall.

Muss, R. (1982) *Theories of Adolescence* 4th edn. New York: Random House.

Neisser, U. (1988) Five kinds of Self-knowledge. *Philosophical Psychology,* **1**, 35–59.

Offer, D. (1981) *The Adolescent: a psychological self portrait.* New York: Basic Books.

Orr, D., Hoffmans, M.A. & Bennetts, G. (1984) Adolescents with cancer report their psychosocial needs. *Journal of Psychosocial Oncology Nursing,* **2**, 47–59.

Ouwerkerk, J. (1994) Cancer therapy induced emesis: the nurse's perspective. *European Journal of Cancer Care,* **3**, 18–25.

Pavlov, I. (1927) *Conditioned Reflexes.* Oxford: Oxford University Press.

Perrin, E.C. & Gerrity, P.S. (1981) There's a demon in your belly: children's understanding of illness. *Pediatrics,* **67**, 841–849.

Petersen, A.C. (1988) Adolescent development. *Annual Review of Psychology,* **39**, 583–607.

Phillips, R.D., Wagner, S.H., Fells, C.A. & Lynch, M. (1990)

Do infants recognise emotion in facial expressions? Categorical and 'metaphorical' evidence. *Infant Behaviour and Development,* **13**, 71–84.

Piaget, J. (1970) Piaget's theory *in* Mussen, P.H. ed. *Carmichael's Manual of Child Psychology,* Vol. 1, 3rd edn. New York: Wiley

Piaget, J. & Inhelder, B. (1969) *The Psychology of the Child.* New York: Basic Books.

Pinkerton, C.R., Cushing, P. & Sepion, B. (1994) *Childhood Cancer management. A practical handbook.* London: Chapman and Hall Medical.

Pochedly, C. (1987) Cancer in children. *Hematology/Oncology Clinics of North America,* **1**(4), 87.

Porter, H. (1994) Mouth care in cancer. *Nursing Times,* **90** (14), 27 29.

Pretchtl, H. & Beintema, D. (1964) *Clinics in Developmental Medicine: No 12. The neurological examination of the full term new-born infant.* London: Heinemann.

Putnam, N. (1987) Seven to ten years: growth and competency *in* Dixon, S.D. & Stein, M.T. eds. *Encounters with Children: paediatric behaviour and development.* Chicago: Year Book Medical Publishers.

Reasoner, R.W. (1983) Enhancement of self esteem in children and adults. *Family Community Health,* **6**, 51–64.

Reich, P.A. (1986) *Language Development.* Englewood Cliffs, NJ: Prentice-Hall.

Reid, U. (1997) Stigma of hair loss after chemotherapy. *Paediatric Nursing,* **9**(3), 4.16–18.

Rotter, J. (1966) Generalised expectancies for internal versus locus of control of reinforcement.

Psychological Monographs: General and Applied, **80**, 1–28.

Rutter, M. (1987) Continuities and discontinuities from infancy *in* Osofsky, J. ed. *Handbook of Infant Development,* 2nd edn. New York: Wiley.

Sander, L.W. (1975) Infant and the caretaking environment *in* Anthony, E.J. ed. *Explorations in Child Psychiatry,* vol. 7, pp. 9, 11. New York: Plenum.

Sparshot, M. (1991) Creating a home for babies in hospital. *Paediatric Nursing,* **3**(80), 20–22.

Spirithall, N. & Collins, W.A. (1984) *Adolescent Psychology.* New York: Addison-Wesley.

Sroufe, L. & Cooper, R.G. (1988) *Child Development: its nature and course.* New York: McGraw-Hill.

Swanwick, M. (1990) Knowledge and Control. *Paediatric Nursing,* **2**(5), 18–20.

Taylor, S.E. & Brown, J. (1983) Illusion and well-being: some social psychological contributions to a theory of mental health. *Psychological Bulletin,* **103**, 193–210.

Teung, A. (1982) *Growth and Development: a self-mastery approach,* p. 35. East Norkwalk: Appleton-Century-Crofts.

Trehub, S.E., Schneider, B.A., Thorpe, L.A. & Judge, P. (1991) Observational measures of auditory sensitivity in early infancy. *Developmental Psychology,* **27**, 40–49.

Turner, B.S. (1984) *The Body and Society: explorations in social theory.* Oxford: Blackwell

Valiant, G.E. (1977) *Adaptation to Life.* Boston: Little, Brown, Co.

Van Dongen-Melman, J.E. (1986) Coping with childhood cancer: a conceptual view. *Journal of Psychosocial Oncology,* **2**, 47–59.

Van Dongen-Melman, J.E. & Sanders-Wondstra, J.A.R. (1986) Pscychological aspects of childhood cancer: a review of the literature. *Journal of Child Psychology and Psychiatry*, **27**, 145–180.

Van Eys, J. (1977) *The Truly Cured Child*, pp. 82–89. Baltimore: University Park Press.

Vessey, J. (1988) Comparison of teaching methods on children's knowledge of their internal bodies. *Nursing Research*, **37**, 262–267.

Vygotsky, L.S. (1978) *Mind in Society*. Cambridge, MA. MIT Press.

Vygotsky, L.S. (1986) *Thought and Language*. Cambridge, MA: MIT Press.

Watson, J. & Royle, J. (1987) *Watson's Medical-Surgical Nursing and Related Physiology*, 3rd ed. London: Baillière Tindall.

Whitehurst, G. & Vasta, R. (1977) *Child Behaviour,* p. 13. Boston: Houghton Mifflin Co.

Wickham, R. (1989) Managing the chemotherapy-related nausea and vomiting: the state of the art. *Oncology Nursing Forum*, **16**, 563–574.

Williams, H.A. & Wilson, M.E. (1989) Sexuality in children and adolescents with cancer: pediatric oncology nurses' attitudes and behaviours. *Journal of Pediatric Oncology Nursing*, **6**(4), 127–132.

Wolff, S. (1989) *Childhood and Human Nature*. London: Routledge.

Woods, N.F. (1987) Towards a holistic perspective of human sexuality: alterations in sexual health and nursing diagnosis. *Holistic Nursing Practice*, **1**, 1–16.

Yaros, P.S. & Howe, J. (1980) *Nursing Care of Adolescents*, Ch. 4, p. 86. New York: McGraw Hill.

Impact of treatment on the family

ALISON SLADE

With thanks to Katie Scanlon (RGN RSCN ONC) for her help and support during the writing of this chapter.

Introduction

This chapter aims to focus on the needs of the family of the sick child. Childhood cancer is recognised as a family disease simply because its effects reach all members of the family. It alters the relationships between family members, and thus changes the equilibrium within the family unit.

While it is accepted that all those involved with the sick child are to some degree affected, the aim will be to concentrate on those individuals who are closest to the sick child. The parents, siblings and grandparents generally suffer most acutely after the diagnosis has been made. It is their lives that will change significantly, requiring sacrifice and adaptation from everyone in order to maintain some form of normal family life, while giving optimal care to the sick child.

For every family the effect of diagnosis will be different, the stresses imposed are enormous and each family member will react in their own way. The first section examines some of the common influences that determine the way individual family members react to this enforced change in their lives. This will give some indication of the attributes to look for in families during initial assessment, and throughout treatment, highlighting issues that can cause possible difficulty, and thereby allowing early intervention, preventing possible deterioration in family relationships.

Isolation and separation, stigma, facing mortality and empowering individuals in a vast unfamiliar health care system; these are issues that affect all families with children suffering from serious illness. These areas will be discussed in turn, and the importance of being sympathetic to differing cultures highlighted. Several short case studies will be presented throughout the text demonstrating some of these issues and discussing some of the problems faced

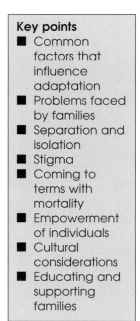

Key points
- Common factors that influence adaptation
- Problems faced by families
- Separation and isolation
- Stigma
- Coming to terms with mortality
- Empowerment of individuals
- Cultural considerations
- Educating and supporting families

by families and health care professionals. These should help the reader place the issues raised in this chapter into a practical context.

The final section discusses some of the best ways to work in partnership with families to reduce the stresses and ease some of the problems faced by both families and care workers. This will involve looking at the education of families and the various support groups available to them.

This chapter is therefore primarily aimed at increasing awareness of the problems faced by family members close to the sick child. It is hoped that readers will subsequently be able to recognise potentially stressful situations before they become too difficult to deal with, and so help families to work together for the sick child, with everyone feeling that they can play a useful part in helping the child to get well.

Common factors that influence adaptation

It is recognised by those working in the field of childhood cancer that the illness has a direct influence on all family members. Recent research into the psychological aspects of living with childhood cancer is limited, with the majority being American in origin. Faulkner, Peace and O'Keeffe (1993), reported on work by Culling (1988) and Casey (1990), who both concluded that intervention on behalf of health care professionals to support families in adjusting to the diagnosis, and an uncertain prognosis, was largely based on clinical experience, intuition and guesswork. Most of the available information concentrates on the sick child, parents and siblings. The role of grandparents and their concerns and feelings appear to be largely ignored, hence, the conclusions discussed in this chapter have been formed from observation and experience. The increasing number of families with children surviving cancer has caused interest to grow in finding ways to ensure that families remain healthy well-adjusted units, able to integrate their experience into their everyday life.

As a result of the increased success in the treatment of childhood cancer, families are having to face new challenges that extend from the time of diagnosis, through the treatment phase, and into a period where, although the child is well, there is always the underlying worry about relapse. Koocher and O'Malley have described this situation as the 'Damocles syndrome' (Culling, 1988). Many families are constantly under stress from the time when the child first becomes ill, and repeatedly have to adapt in order to cope with new problems and uncertainties.

Every family faces cancer under different circumstances, and each individual will respond differently. There are, however, some common themes that influence the way family members cope and adjust, trying to maintain a 'healthy' family unit.

Each person's knowledge of cancer will alter the way they react when the sick child is diagnosed. Cancer is a very powerful word, and evokes many fears about painful traumatic treatment and death in those old enough to have some understanding.

Past experiences influence the response of all family members. Previous contact with illness, whether their own or someone else's, and the resultant outcome can affect the way they react at the time of diagnosis, and their outlook during the treatment. Faulkner *et al.* (1993) describe a child who had seen her grandmother die of cancer. This experience had not been too upsetting because it was expected, and the grandparent had wanted to die. This was compared to the case of the child's brother being diagnosed with cancer; by contrast, this was far more distressing, being completely unexpected. A parent who has previously lost a family member or close friend from cancer may find it harder to disassociate their past experience from their present feelings when faced with a similar diagnosis in their child.

The course of events leading to the diagnosis of cancer can influence the way parents react to it and to their sick child. Faulkner *et al.* indicates that parents felt guilty if they initially failed to believe, or take seriously, their child's early complaints of pain, lethargy or nausea. Culling (1988) acknowledges that parents often express feelings of guilt that they are in some way responsible for the illness and should have sought medical help earlier. This can lead to overprotective behaviour towards their sick child.

Having trust in the health care professionals caring for their child helps parents to deal with the situation. If the path to diagnosis after medical help was first sought proved difficult, for example, with health care professionals not always taking symptoms seriously or acting quickly enough, parents can lose their faith and confidence in the medical profession and this can affect their outlook on treatment (Faulkner *et al.*, 1993).

It is important that parents talk to each other throughout their child's treatment; Mott (1990) indicates that couples previously accustomed to sharing their feelings are better able to communicate in a way that gives them greater satisfaction and mutual support.

Siblings of the sick child also face many changes in their lives, and their response to the illness will depend on several factors:

● Their age and cognitive stage of development; an understanding of the concept of illness gradually develops through childhood (Heath, 1996). The stage a child has reached affects their level of understanding of what is happening to the family and their ability to rationalise it.

- The age of the ill child: the closeness in age to the sibling. Those close in age often worry more about the same thing happening to them.
- The relationship between the well and the ill child. Is there a close sibling bond?
- If the two are close the well child will inevitably feel worried and distressed, but how does a well sibling feel when the relationship is not that devoted?
- Does this increase the feelings of jealousy when the family's attention is with the sick child? Does the well child just think 'thank goodness it's not me', and does this later leave them feeling guilty that they did not care enough?
- The reaction of the family to the diagnosis: do the siblings continually see their parents upset, stressed and irritable?
- The way the family usually deals with a crisis: have they faced previous serious problems within the family?
- The amount of disruption to their everyday life.
- How the illness is explained to them. Is it at a level they can understand? Are they able to express their feelings? Most importantly, are they told the truth? Parents often find it very difficult to explain the illness and the changes that will inevitably occur in the family to their healthy children. It is however important that parents are honest, because children are good at detecting stress and worry in their parents, and thus deception, even if well meaning, can cause confusion and anxiety. Studies have shown that siblings from families adopting an open style of communication, in which information is shared freely, emotions are expressed and appropriate psychological defences are used, cope better when faced with a crisis in their family (Gallo et al., 1992 cited in Cincotta, 1993; Ross-Alaolmolki et al., 1995).

A great deal of work has been carried out examining the effects on the children when separated from their parents during hospitalisation. John Bowlby and James Robertson both did much to stimulate discussion and promote advances within the health care environment during the late 1950s through to the early 1970s; for example, advocating that parents be able to stay with their sick child in hospital, a concept taken up in the Platt Report (Platt, 1959). The treatment of cancer involves many periods of hospitalisation, so it must be remembered that when parents stay with a sick child, the siblings may be left in the care of other family members, such as grandparents or aunts and uncles, or with close family friends. When separated from their parents, do these children suffer in a similar way to the sick children described by Bowlby and Robertson? Regular visits to the hospital may help to overcome some of the effects of separation, although travelling arrangements can be problematical. Jennings (1986), in a descriptive paper about parents caring for their sick children in parent care units, indicates that siblings benefit from being with the family in hospital because it alleviates the strain of separation and dispels some of the fantasies they may have regarding their sick brother or sister. This however must be weighed against the disruption in these healthy children's lives, especially if they are attending school and are members of sports and social groups.

It can be argued that the siblings cope better if they are cared for in their own home, which is a familiar safe environment, preferably by one parent. Provided they have regular contact with both their parents and the sick sibling, this may be the best way of meeting their needs. Doyle (1987) stresses how important it is for siblings to know that they are loved even though they may be left at home, separated from their parents. It is recognised that the serious illness of a child can cause negative outcomes for the healthy siblings, such as increased anxiety, feelings of isolation and behavioural changes. However Ross-Alaolmolki et al. (1995) indicate that sometimes positive outcomes result, such as the development of an increased ability to cope with stressful situations, improved sibling relations, increased family unity and empathy for others.

Studies indicate that the diagnosis of cancer in a child affects all family members and requires regular adjustment from all parties in order to maintain a cohesive and strong family unit. An honest communication style that allows open expression of feelings is a major factor in dealing with and adapting to this family crisis.

Problems faced by families

Every family is unique; the relationships between individual family members are continually changing in response to life events, and to the interactions that comprise family life. The diagnosis of cancer within a family changes the status of the affected member and will therefore alter the equilibrium of the family unit, creating a great deal of insecurity and worry. The occurrence of childhood cancer within the family is therefore a major and highly stressful event. It can have far-reaching effects on everyone involved with the sick child, especially those with the closest ties, and should therefore be treated as a family disease.

Separation and isolation

Parents
At the time of diagnosis parents may find they are separated

from each other for the first time since the beginning of their relationship. This occurs at a time when each is feeling overwhelmed, vulnerable, insecure, and in need of support from the person they are closest to, and who is closest to their sick child, their spouse or partner. This separation may occur because one parent, generally the father, has to continue going to work, or because one may have to stay at home to care for any other children. The frequency of occurrence of this scenario has increased as families units have become more dispersed about the country, the core family tending to become more 'nuclear', with the exended family living significant distances away. Separation generally continues throughout the treatment process because one parent regularly accompanies the sick child during periods of hospitalisation.

It is important that parents can spend some time with each other, away from their sick child. However, they may find this difficult, for fear that something will happen, or that the child will want them while they are away. If they are in an environment where they are expected to carry out parental and nursing care they may feel they need 'permission' from staff to leave. It is important that nurses are sensitive to this and form a trusting relationship with parents, so that when they are away parents can be confident that all their child's needs will be attended to. Even when these arrangements have been made, parents may find it difficult to communicate with each other at a level that satisfies both individuals' needs, each being at different stages in the process of grieving for the suffering of their previously healthy child (see 'Coming to terms with mortality', 'Parents', p. 123).

Couples who are accustomed to talking things through, and sharing their thoughts and feelings, generally find it easier to communicate in this difficult, stressful situation than those who have always avoided expressing their feelings (Mott, 1990). It is important that family members are aware that there are many different ways of reacting to, and coping with, such a huge psychological trauma; they have to try to be sensitive to, and supportive of, each others' needs. It is interesting that Lansky *et al.* (1978), in a study involving the parents of 191 children treated for cancer over a 7-year period, found a divorce rate lower than the average for that particular area in America, despite the enormous stresses these couples had faced. Lansky did not, however, conclude that the child's illness brought couples closer together, but that, although these couples had very significant problems in their marriages, they did not resort to divorce.

Each parent will obviously have different worries; these may be just alternative ways of looking at a situation or may involve a completely different understanding of the situation. Often in such a case communication becomes difficult; each parent does not fully appreciate how the other is feeling, and they become reluctant to discuss their anxieties and emotions for fear of burdening their spouse and further increasing the pressure on them. They often build a protective wall around themselves that can be difficult to penetrate. As time goes on, each parent may feel that they are carrying the greater burden. It is important that each can appreciate the role of the other in helping the family through this time of crisis.

It has previously been stated that it is generally the father who continues to go out to work while the mother, if working, stops or reduces her work commitments in order to care for their sick child. However, the situation is not always so straightforward. The decision surrounding working arrangements can cause parents a great deal of anxiety. It is common for families to be under financial pressure, many being accustomed to two income sources. It may be that the decision about which parent stops working is influenced by the necessity of keeping the largest income, which may not necessarily be the father's; this may cause resentment and frustration if both parents are not satisfied with the situation. Financial worries can cause a great deal of anger and stress in any family, and for these parents it is an extra problem that can increase any feelings of inadequacy either may have, exacerbating their feelings of isolation from one another.

From the time of diagnosis one parent will inevitably be identified as the main carer, and it is possible that they may shut out their partner, feeling that they have the major responsibility for the sick child. With the diagnosis of cancer the priorities and perspectives of parents can alter suddenly. Thoughts and concerns will obviously be with the sick child who needs a great deal of parental support, time and energy. This all limits the attention that parents can give to their other children. There can be no doubt that parents with more than one child feel torn between their feelings and responsibilities for each child, often worrying when in hospital that they are needed at home, and vice versa. They miss the child from whom they have been separated, and are conscious of the trauma that this child may be going through due to the separation. This in turn leads to feelings of guilt and inadequacy at being unavailable to comfort and care for all of their offspring all of the time.

Regular periods of hospitalisation with a sick child, and the increased stress and responsibility of caring for that child at home, affects parents' working and social lives. Many working parents are forced to take regular periods off work in order to be at the hospital and maintain home life. This all disrupts their relationships with family, friends and colleagues at a time when they need understanding and support. Barbor (1983) states that: 'It is suggested that parents who maintain and perhaps use social links fare better later'.

Some parents say that it is during this stressful period that they realise who their true friends are; they appreciate the availability and unconditional support they receive from these individuals.

Siblings

For the majority of individuals their longest relationship is with their siblings. The sibling bond develops from a complex relationship that involves friendship, love, co-operation and caring, together with the chance to experience normal feeling of competition, jealousy and rivalry (Ross-Alaolmolki *et al.*, 1995).

A child diagnosed with a serious illness, immediately becomes the focus of the parent's concern and attention, and, without deliberately doing so, the parents can view their other children's needs as less important. The well children in the family may understand the reasons why their sick sibling needs extra attention, but this does not stop them feeling hurt and neglected. Separation from one or both parents during periods of hospitalisation inevitably disrupts siblings' lives. Bryne (1994) argues that in encouraging parents to stay and participate in their sick child's care, health care professionals may be failing to meet the needs of the healthy siblings who are not only separated from their family but are unable to participate in their sibling's care. This situation fosters feelings of anxiety and isolation. Many paediatric oncology centres are able to offer family accommodation in, or close to, the hospital which means that the whole family can be close to the sick child, thus helping to alleviate the problems mentioned above. Local schools or the hospital school will often offer temporary places for the healthy siblings, but parents then have to face the dilemma of whether to disrupt these children's education and social lives. Parents often prefer siblings to remain together in the family home, with one parent, rather than with other carers, thus allowing them to care for all their children whilst minimising disruption to the lives of the healthy siblings and maintaining some normality for them during a stressful bewildering time.

Visiting the hospital is essential in maintaining and developing family relationships, and helping siblings to understand what is happening to the sick child, alleviating unwarranted fears they may have regarding the illness and treatment. However, departing at the end of a visit can be traumatic for all involved, especially if the children are young; young children may not fully understand the reason for separation from their parents who, until this crisis, have been the most stable element in their lives.

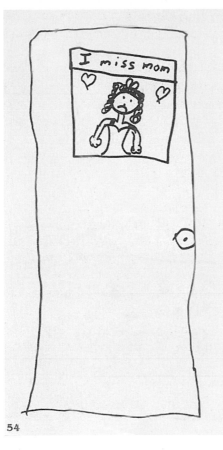

Figure 5.1 Child's drawing (reproduced with permission from The Center for Attitudinal Healing, Sausalito, CA, USA)

From the onset of the child's illness, siblings continually see their parents worried and under stress, no matter how great an effort the parents make to disguise their concerns and appear relaxed. It must be remembered that siblings have their own anxieties about many things, not solely about their sick brother or sister; for example: their own health, relationships with peers and pressures at school. The healthy siblings often complain of a reduction in the physical and emotional availability of their parents. In response to this, and with the knowledge that their parents are already under stress, these children avoid discussing their problems, not wanting to further burden their parents. This can leave them feeling isolated and confused, especially if they are not comfortable talking through their worries with anyone else.

When a healthy sibling feels unwell, or suffers any form of common childhood illness, it is important that parents, and anyone involved with the family, treat them in the same way they do the child with cancer, offering the same level of attention

Figure 5.2 Child's drawing (reproduced with permission from The Center for Attitudinal Healing, Sausalito, CA, USA)

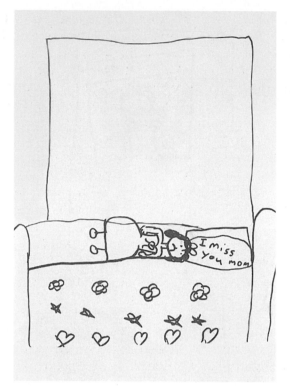

Figure 5.3 Child's drawing (reproduced with permission from The Center for Attitudinal Healing, Sausalito, CA, USA)

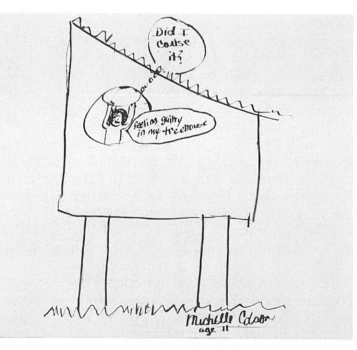

and concern. Children are always comparing themselves to their siblings, and may feel unimportant or worthless if they do not receive similar attention to their more seriously ill brother or sister.

Siblings' anxieties, and the isolation they can feel from other family members, can be very difficult for them to cope with. Many may feel that their sick brother or sister receives preferential treatment and that their parents' expectations of them are heightened, possibly to levels they regard as impossible to maintain (Harding, 1996). Parents often do indeed expect a higher level of understanding of immediate problems than the child can handle. They may also expect continuous good behaviour, and, especially with older children, acceptance of greater responsibilities in the home. These siblings are often disinclined to discuss any unequal treatment with their parents for fear that, by complaining, they may make their situation worse (Cairns *et al.*, 1979). All this can lead to increased feelings of jealousy and rivalry. Siblings are often ashamed of these negative feelings and can express guilt about being the healthy child (Kramer and Moore, 1983; Harding 1996).

Due to the combined effects of lack of attention, guilt feelings and thinking that they are less valued than the sick child, healthy siblings can have difficulty in adapting to changes in their lives. They may demonstrate many forms of behavioural change, such as problems at school, depression or withdrawal (Cornman, 1993). They may also complain of medical problems, such as increased headaches or generalised aches and pains. Being individuals, they will all have different degrees of difficulty adapting, each exhibiting different problems. It must be remembered that changes are not always negative, some children may indeed concentrate their energies into their schoolwork and show an improvement in

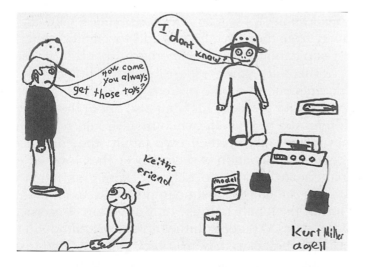

Figure 5.4 Child's drawing (reproduced with permission from The Center for Attitudinal Healing, Sausalito, CA, USA)

performance, and some enjoy the increased independence. However, this outward demonstration of coping does not necessarily mean they are 'happy' with the situation.

All the changes that occur within a family affected by childhood cancer may cause the peers of the healthy sibling to perceive the family as 'different'; (see 'Stigma' p. 118). Healthy children often find it difficult to talk to their friends about their ill brother or sister, and may fear being questioned and teased. This, together with possible restrictions on when they can see friends, due to travelling difficulties when the sick child is in hospital, or the risk of catching infections from others when the child is neutropenic at home, can leave healthy siblings feeling further isolated from their peer group.

Grandparents

Many grandparents play an important role within the family. If they live with or close to, their children and grandchildren, they are generally in regular contact with their offspring, giving advice and support to the family. Others may not have such an influential role, long distances separating them physically from their family, and personnel commitments, such as work, restricting visiting. When a child is ill grandparents are often called upon to care for the siblings, or to spend time with the sick child to give the parents a break. Conflicts can arise when grandparents are not familiar with what is happening in the children's lives. They have different expectations of the family, and may have different ideas about discipline and disagree with the parents about what is acceptable behaviour for children and adolescents within the family. This potential conflict can increase the stress for parents who, although they recognise their need and are grateful for the help of grandparents, worry about how they are coping and may resent the grandparent's interference in the running of their family. In addition, these extra responsibilities take the grandparents away from their own friends and social life, and can mean periods of separation from one another, especially if one is still working, or there are other responsibilities at home.

Grandparents often become distressed with the strain of worrying, not only about the sick child, but also about the parents, their own children. At a time of life when they should be able to relax a little, having brought up their own family, they are faced with the very distressing situation of seeing those they love suffer, often feeling inadequate, unable to help the family as much as they wish. It can be difficult for grandparents to discuss their anxieties with the rest of the family because they are often concerned about upsetting the stressed parents further. Therefore, although they are helping as best they can, they may feel quite isolated, especially if they are not kept up to date with the sick child's progress. They can also experience difficulty talking about such an upsetting subject with friends.

Case study 5.1

Samantha is 9 years old, the third of five children born to Mark and Jane. She was transferred to the ward, the regional paediatric oncology centre, from her local hospital and a diagnosis of acute myeloid leukaemia was made. This illness requires intensive treatment necessitating a long period of hospitalisation with minimal opportunity to spend time at home.

After overcoming the shock of the diagnosis, the family developed a routine in which Jane stayed at the hospital with Samantha, and Mark spent the week at home with the other children. Mark brought the siblings to visit at the weekend, staying in the family accommodation provided close to the hospital. Mark continued to go to work during the week. This situation meant that they had very little time together as a family and when they were together relationships were often strained.

Mark and Jane had virtually no time alone together to discuss their feelings and anxieties and how they were coping with the changes in their lives. As time progressed they talked less and less and began to resent each other: both feeling that their partner was having the easier time.

All members of the health care team could see the strain developing in the couple's relationship, through hearing them talk individually and seeing them together with the family. Jane was under enormous pressure, feeling unsupported by Mark and missing her other children, and all this gradually affected her relationship with Samantha, which became quite difficult at times.

Eventually after discussions with the team social worker who was very familiar with the family's situation and had discussed their problems with Mark and Jane, both together and individually, it was decided to suggest that the couple swap roles for a week. It was felt that this might improve the situation for everyone by:

- Giving Mark and Jane a better understanding of what each was having to cope with and thus reducing the resentment each had built up towards the other.
- Giving Jane some time away from the claustrophobic hospital environment, in her own home with her other children, so that she might return a little refreshed, possibly improving her relationship with Samantha.
- Giving Samantha some time with her father so that they could reaffirm their relationship. It was expected that stimulation from another adult would help her general well being. Also a short period away from her mother after such a long time together might give the relationship renewed affection when Jane returned.
- Mark and Jane's other children would probably enjoy some time with their mother, as she has not been at home for several months.

The couple agreed to the proposal and the team social worker assisted Mark to get extra time away from work. The proposal was put into practice the following week when Samantha's condition was stable and she was relatively well.

Although Samantha missed her mother at first she did enjoy this time with her father. By the end of the period both parents had a greater appreciation of what the other was coping with and were better equipped to support each other through the remaining treatment. Mark and Jane continued to swap roles occasionally, though usually for a shorter time period than this original change. The relationships between all family members appeared to improve and there was an easing of some of the tension that existed between them – a result that certainly benefited Samantha.

In general the whole family seemed to benefit from this change although the effect on the well siblings was less obvious to the health care team. This was probably because they did not all visit each weekend, taking turns and staying with friends and relatives.

Box 5.1

- Families who are accustomed to open communication, sharing their thoughts and feelings, tend to cope better when a child develops a serious illness
- Families should be encouraged to spend time together as a 'family unit', doing 'normal' things. This will help them to support each other and reduce feelings of isolation
- Siblings need regular, frequent contact with both their parents and the sick child
- It is important that healthy siblings are shown that they are as loved and as valued by their parents and other family members as the sick child

---

Box 5.1 helps to illustrate some of the needs and coping strategies of a family attempting to cope with a child who has been diagnosed with, and is being treated for cancer.

Stigma

Parents

When a child is diagnosed with cancer the family immediately undergoes a very stressful and significant change that makes them 'different' from other families. Parents face the daunting task of informing other family members and friends about their child's diagnosis, and what the future holds for them. They are often unable to do this at the onset of the illness because a full diagnosis has not been made and they are not yet aware of the treatment and prognosis. They continually have to fend off enquiries from concerned relatives and friends, at a time when they are very stressed themselves, worrying about the outcome of tests and what is going to happen next.

Once they have this information, parents need time to adjust to the situation before embarking on the task of telling others. This can be quite a burden; parents may not want to give out lots of information about their child, as they may feel that their family is going to be talked about by others, either family or friends. It is likely that they will not relish this thought, even if such discussion is well meaning. Most concerned well-wishers will not know another family with a child with cancer, and there is therefore a certain 'novelty' in discussing their concerns for the family with others.

Parents may also feel that there are certain people who, although close to the sick child, will not cope with knowing all that the sick child has to face. This could be the case with, for example, a frail elderly relative. Consequently, the parents may have the added burden of deciding how much information they should pass on. It is important to parents to be in charge of the dissemination of information about their child, as this can help them to control what is said by others about their family.

In many cases, the child is unwell prior to treatment, but there may be few, or no, visible signs indicating serious illness to observers. This may be especially true for those who are not really close to the child. However, once treatment starts this situation changes dramatically: hair loss, weight loss (often quite severe and sometimes resulting in the child having a long-term nasogastric tube) and severe mood swings, causing unpredictability and outbursts of temper, are all very visible signs that the child is unwell, or somehow 'not normal'. Parents not only have to accept these changes, but they also have to come to terms with the way others treat their child because the ill child is different. This could be just the altered way in which their friends treat the child when they meet, or may involve strangers staring at the child when they are in public.

In common with many other chronic childhood illnesses, childhood cancer is a subject which many people find hard to consider. When people know a family with a child that has cancer, it challenges their accepted notion of children being inherently healthy, with a full lifespan ahead of them. This can force them to reassess the vulnerability of their own family. Katz was reported as saying that (Gallo et al., 1991):

When people encounter sick children it creates a sense of anxiety and apprehension – they remind us of our vulnerabilities, subsequently many children with chronic illness are avoided.

Some people find it very hard to know how to approach the affected family and what to say, however close to the family they were prior to the diagnosis. Many worry about saying the right thing; for example, should they enquire about the child and family at all, or should they let the parents broach the subject of how everyone is managing?

These difficulties can sometimes lead to a situation in which the parents are ignored altogether; relatives or acquaintances may use this tactic to protect themselves from facing an encounter that could cause them emotional pain. Other people respond differently; for example, some may enquire about the sick child continuously. All this happens when the parents of the sick child just want to be treated normally, to have a listening and sympathetic ear available, and to know that they are in the thoughts of others. It is the stigma associated with the words 'childhood cancer', and the frightening thought of children suffering and dying, that leave people feeling inadequate, not knowing how to help.

Siblings

Throughout the sick child's treatment healthy siblings have to continue with their normal activities, such as schooling and sports. They regularly see their friends and classmates, many of whom will know from listening to their parents and friends that something is wrong with the ill child. Schools are often quite small communities, and news about a family travels quickly. Young children have a limited understanding of illness, although this develops as they grow older, through experience and teaching. However, the lack of understanding of cancer, and the influence of a society in which many children are inadvertently taught, at an early age, an intolerance of 'being different', can make them very wary of the sick child and the family. Siblings report that the illness puts a strain on their relationships with classmates (Kramer and Moore, 1983). Sometimes the sibling's friends fear that the illness is contagious and distance themselves. This adds to the sibling's feelings of isolation, which are exacerbated by any insensitive teasing resulting from fear and ignorance. These children also face continuous questioning about their sick brother or sister, an intrusion which they may resent, especially if they feel unable to answer because they do not think that they are fully informed themselves.

Sick children generally return to school for short periods during their treatment, and siblings at the same school can often feel responsible for the sick child, doing their best to protect them from teasing.

Changes in family finances and parental responsibilities (see 'Separation and isolation', 'Parents' p. 109) may mean that siblings are unable to continue with some of their hobbies and interests. Holidays and activities may have to be cancelled due to the therapeutic regimen, and this change in 'status' can also lead to teasing, and an alteration in the relationship with friends. This all adds to the feelings of isolation and fuels any resentment that siblings may feel towards the sick child.

Therefore there is clearly a certain stigma associated with having a sibling with cancer. It makes the family different at a time when, for many children, conformity with the appearance and behaviour of their peers is very important to them. Other children are curious and will often treat healthy siblings differently, generally out of fear and ignorance. This situation adds to the stresses that these healthy children have to face in continuing with their daily lives.

Grandparents

For grandparents the stigma situation is similar to that previously described for parents, although possibly less intense. The task of passing on information may be slightly easier if friends and relatives always go to the parents for a 'first hand' report; however, if they feel unable to do this, then grandparents are often the next best source. Those enquiring after the child may feel a little more comfortable talking to grandparents, thinking that they are not adding to the parents' stresses, and can thereby remain slightly detached from the situation. This can sometimes put grandparents in the difficult position of trying to impart information in the way that the parents would wish, without upsetting either party.

When grandparents take the sick child out, meeting other people can be as stressful for them as for the parents. They will feel protective towards their whole family, and worry about their children and grandchildren facing the possibly hurtful or ignorant comments of others.

Case study 5.2

Manjula, 16, has been diagnosed with B-cell lymphoma. She has two older sisters, aged 18 and 20, and a younger brother who is just 10. Her parents run their own newsagent shop, and Manjula's father and the children speak and understand good English, although the mother has a poor understanding of English. On the first day of treatment it transpired that Manjula and her sisters had decided not to tell their younger brother of her diagnosis, and their intention was to keep the diagnosis from him throughout treatment. Their father had apparently agreed to this, and it was also decided to keep the information given to their mother at a minimum. Their mother was obviously very distressed, and they felt it would be unfair to tell her exactly what was going on, because they felt she would be not be able to deal with it.

The family also decided to keep to an absolute minimum the number of extended family and friends they told. Nursing staff, medical staff and social workers advised Manjula and her sisters to be open and honest with their brother and their mother, but as the family felt they were doing the right thing at that time, the staff could only support them in their decision. A couple of days into treatment and after a lot of discussion between Manjula and her sister, they decided that they would tell their mother and also their brother. Their mother was extremely upset but felt that she now knew what she was dealing with. Their brother said he that he had guessed that things were a lot more serious, and was relieved that he was now to be fully included in all the conversations. It later transpired, when Manjula relapsed, that she had not told any of her friends the true diagnosis, but had led them to believe that she had had a severe chest infection requiring intensive treatment. As she had a home tutor, she did not have to go to school for any of her lessons, and since she lived some distance from the hospital, none of her friends came to visit whilst she was an inpatient.

Case study 5.2 highlights a number of factors that have to be taken into consideration when caring for the family of a child who has been diagnosed with cancer: Manjula's sisters and father felt that they were protecting her mother and brother by withholding the diagnosis from them. This created a difficult situation for the staff as the first days are crucial for developing a professional, trusting relationship between the nurse, family and patient. Providing the family with clear honest explanations helped to reduce the stigma attached to the diagnosis, and enabled the sisters to have the courage to inform their mother and brother of the situation.

As a close-knit family they did not feel it appropriate or necessary to involve others, including extended family, for support. It seemed apparent that the sisters had always made a major contribution to the parenting role and therefore it was a natural step for them to have so much input. Guiding the individual family members as to how to deal with the future requires time and patience; nurses are often those most closely involved with the family initially, and this link provides the foundations for building a trusting relationship.

Manjula's mother was unable to converse in English so she was in danger of becoming isolated from the conversations involving the health care professionals. It was difficult to assess how she was dealing with the situation as she was unable to talk directly with staff and all information had to pass through a third party. The sisters usually acted as interpreters, a situation that did not guarantee that information was translated correctly, but the family consistently preferred not to involve hospital translators. All staff were aware of the inadequacies of this situation but felt that as the family appeared to be dealing adequately, their wishes needed to be respected.

It should be remembered that as nurses we each have our own cultural background and it is dangerous to make assumptions about the way information is shared within the family and relayed to relatives and other social contacts, for example, family friends and school mates. For the family in Case study 5.2 the stigma of having cancer was a major issue and health care workers had to adapt their practice in order to respect and accommodate the family's wishes.

Box 5.2 describes some of the problems of stigma that can arise for a family when a child has been diagnosed with cancer.

Box 5.2

- Many people will label the family as 'different' once they know of the sick child's diagnosis
- The stigma associated with being 'different' means that the attitudes of others towards the family will sometimes change, putting a strain on previously healthy friendships
- It is important that all family members are kept up to date with the sick child's progress so that they feel confident in answering the inevitable questioning from friends and acquaintances

---

Coming to terms with mortality

Parents

In western society parents understandably expect that their children will outlive them. Furthermore, people assume that children will naturally be healthy. Having a child diagnosed with cancer directly challenges these two fundamental premises in a brutal way, and many parents perceive it as a death sentence for their child. Great care is required by health care professionals in explaining the prognosis in a balanced way so that expectations are realistic, and any incorrect assumptions dealt with.

From the time of diagnosis parents enter a type of grieving process over the potential loss of their healthy child (Culling, 1988). Barbor (1983) describes this grieving as 'anticipatory grief', and indicates that, although in many cases the child will recover, the threat of death is always present. This anticipatory grief will involve many emotions: shock at the diagnosis, fear, disbelief, anger, guilt and finally some form of acceptance of the situation (Figure 5.5).

Each person goes through this process in an individual way with feelings varying in intensity and duration. Furthermore, an individual may experience one stage only to return to it later. Parents will often be at different stages in the grieving process at

Figure 5.5 Some of the feelings that parents may experience (reproduced from *Emotional Aspects of Malignant Disease in Children* by Barbor (1983 p. 323) with kind permission from Medpress Ltd.)

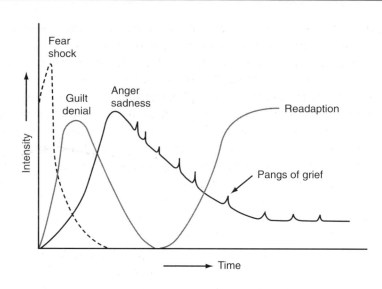

different times. This situation can increase any difficulty they have supporting each other.

At some stage during treatment parents can experience feelings of bitterness and anger at the unfairness of the situation, often at diagnosis, or when things are not going as well as planned. They express these feelings by asking 'Why me?' or 'Why us?'. They witness their whole family suffering in different ways, and miss the life they had before their child's illness. Most parents feel a sense of inadequacy that they cannot improve the situation for everyone involved, not only for the sick child.

Parents see their sick child as very vulnerable, and they can become overprotective if faced with anything they perceive as a potential threat to the child. We know that when neutropenic children are at increased risk from bacterial infections which they have no ability to fight. Fear of losing their child to a serious infection can make some parents overcompensate for the risks, thereby severely restricting their activities and reducing social interactions. It is important to preserve a balance which protects the child, while still allowing the child to develop normally and enjoy life. All parents, whether they have a sick child or not, naturally want to protect their offspring, but having their own life can be very difficult for sick children. This is especially true for adolescents who often complain of feeling 'smothered' when they simply want to get out and experience life.

The desire of parents to see their child recover is balanced against the importance of limiting suffering. Difficult decisions sometimes have to be made, and although these are made together with the health care professionals, parents bear the greater part of this responsibility. Hinds *et al.* (1996) carried out a study of parents' responses to a first recurrence of cancer in their child, recurrence being defined as any reappearance of cancer at any time, even during initial treatment. They found that parents have to overcome their immediate emotional response in order to try to make wise decisions about treatment, while accepting that the eventual outcome would be beyond their control. They strove for the best chance of cure, at the same time preparing themselves for the child's possible death. As time progresses, parents consider the limitations of the treatment, balancing their child's response to, and tolerance of, the regimen, against the suffering involved. These considerations add to the emotional turmoil that parents experience when their child has life-threatening disease.

The hospital environment forces parents to contemplate the possibility of the death of their child. In hospital, especially in the major paediatric cancer centres, they meet other children with cancer and their families, and will inevitably get to know children who subsequently die. This acts as a constant powerful reminder of what could happen to them, making them consider the possibility even when treatment is going well for their child. Parents are never able to dismiss the possibility of the death of their child; they have to learn to live with this constant threat in their lives.

Questions from others, especially other children, including the sick child's siblings, can also force parents to consider their child's possible death. Children, irrespective of their age or understanding of illness and death, will inevitably ask if the sick child is going to die. The reassuring answers that parents give may not accurately reflect the worries they have, and the fear of the possible death of their child that they carry with them.

Once a child has been diagnosed with cancer the threat of recurrence never goes away. Many parents find this as stressful to cope with as the treatment itself. It is always in their minds, becoming even more worrying at the time of check-ups. We can assume that the fear never goes away for a lot of families, even after years out of treatment, and their lives are always shadowed by this enormous life event (this has been referred to as the Damocles syndrome, mentioned in 'Common factors that influence adaptation' p. 106).

Siblings

A child's understanding of mortality is dependent on age, stage of development, intellectual ability, religious and cultural beliefs and, to some extent, past experience (Culling, 1988). Lindsay (1995) indicates that many adults including health care professionals find the idea of discussing death with children, even healthy children, difficult, feeling that they will not understand and regarding it as a subject not fitting for discussion with children.

Young siblings will have very little appreciation of the vulnerability of the sick child and the potentially fatal threat that the cancer poses. Older children have a greater understanding of the problems associated with having a seriously ill brother or sister. Bendor (1990 p. 26), when studying a group of siblings of cancer patients aged 8–14 years, concluded that: 'A sense of danger, damage and possible death was ever present in the well siblings' lives.'

This group had some understanding of the risks of treatment, picked up from hearing their parents talking, and from their education. Adolescents, also studied by Bendor, were even more worried about their sibling's possible failure to respond to treatment and the complications resulting from therapy. They recognised the sick child's vulnerability, showing concern about the possibility that they might pass on an infection that could be fatal.

Most siblings consider their own vulnerability to some degree, worrying that they might develop cancer themselves. The level of concern varies with age, older children generally have a better understanding of illness, knowing that cancer cannot be 'caught'. Genetic causes of cancer are often mentioned in the popular media, but these are mostly adult cancers; paediatric malignancies are very rarely passed on through genetics. Personnel working within paediatric oncology may need to explore this area with some individual family members and provide information and reassurance. Younger children, lacking understanding of the disease process, may see many similarities between themselves and the sick child, especially if they are the same sex or close in age. They will have had many similar life experiences, causing them to worry that they too could become ill. Indeed some children actually expect to develop cancer, especially if there is a family history of children being ill; well siblings can simply expect to be next. While adults accept that the cause of paediatric cancer is at present largely unknown, it is difficult for children to understand how something that causes such major changes in their lives can have no apparent cause or reason. This can lead them to fantasise about the possible reasons for the illness, and enhances the idea that it could also happen to them.

It is important to allow siblings to express their fears about the cancer. These may be difficult to understand, especially if the children are young and have difficulty vocalising their feelings. It may be necessary to use other means of expression in order to understand the child's perception of the illness, such as art or play therapy. It is important to recognise the need to try to uncover and alleviate fears in a way the child can comprehend.

Younger children tend to carry on with daily activities without much questioning, however much their life is disrupted. Adoles-

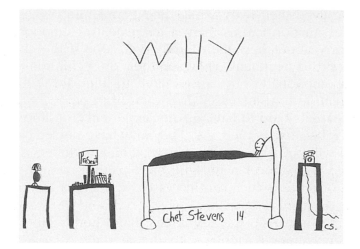

Figure 5.6 Child's drawing (reproduced with permission from The Center for Attitudinal Healing, Sausalito, CA, USA)

cents, however, express much more conflict in getting on with their daily lives and planning for the future while wanting to be available for their parents and sick sibling (Bendor, 1990). They can appreciate what the sick child is missing through illness, and often feel guilty for thinking about their own future when their brother's or sister's is so dominated by illness, and thus uncertain.

Grandparents

Grandparents, like parents, experience anticipatory grief, and they can find it particularly difficult to come to terms with the possibility of losing a grandchild. They will naturally expect to die before their own children, and certainly before their grandchildren. Most express feelings of the unfairness of the situation; if anyone in the family should be so ill it should be them, because

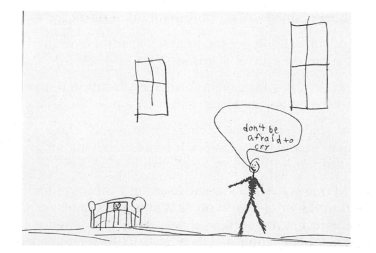

Figure 5.7 Child's drawing (reproduced with permission from The Center for Attitudinal Healing, Sausalito, CA, USA)

they have lived their lives, while their grandchild's is just beginning. The situation causes them a great deal of emotional pain. Many worry about how their family will cope if the child does not respond to treatment. They see their own children suffering so much emotionally but can do little to alleviate the pain for them, which in turn increases their own distress.

Grandparents tend to have greater experience of illness within the family, because of their age. They may have nursed close relatives and will probably have lost close family members. Having a grandchild with cancer may bring back painful memories of the suffering of others which can increase the stress of this traumatic experience.

Box 5.3 summarises the key issues that a family have to cope with when coming to terms with the mortality of one of their family members.

Box 5.3

- Family members experience anticipatory grief over the potential loss of their once healthy child. Although the feelings and emotions are similar for all those involved, everyone follows an individual path through their grief
- Children's understanding of illness and mortality is influenced by many things. Not all children of the same age will have the same insight
- Once a child has been diagnosed with cancer, however successful the subsequent treatment, family members' worries about recurrence never diminish

---

Empowerment of individuals

Empowerment is a complex and multidimensional concept, which is difficult to define but can be broadly described as:

> a process of helping people to assert control over the factors which affect their lives. (Gibson, 1991 p. 354)

Stewart (1994 p. 248) gave a further explanation demonstrating some of the qualities involved:

> Empowerment is about giving control and choice; about participation and consultation. It requires having information to work on and the ability to respond.

Empowerment has a different form and meaning for different people in different circumstances. Within the context of the child with cancer it can be seen as a way in which families can take back some of the control which is usually relinquished when the sick child is taken to hospital. Robinson (1985) indicates that some degree of relinquishment of control is implicit in a parent's decision to go to hospital with their child. Barbor (1983) agrees, suggesting that, once involved in hospital treatment, parents are no longer in complete control of what happens in the family.

Empowerment is a two-way interaction in which power is both given and taken away. Gibson (1991) notes the importance of examining this process, considering both the way the 'powerless' attempt to take power, and the way the 'powerful' release power. Within the hospital setting it is the health care professionals who are in a powerful position, being both knowledgeable and in a familiar environment, whereas families are admitted into an alien environment where they feel particularly insecure.

Parents

When parents have a child diagnosed with a serious illness they have to face the reality that they no longer have complete control of that child's destiny. Their role as protector and provider is challenged by the illness experience (Cincotta, 1993).

In their own home parents have control over their family. Home is a place where they feel secure, can have some privacy and are able to relax. Hospital is a place where they feel exposed and vulnerable, where there is no privacy, nowhere to express their emotions unobserved, and nowhere to spend time with their partner without intrusions. The importance of encouraging parents to spend time together away from the hospital so that they can express their feelings privately has already been discussed (see 'Separation and isolation', 'Parents' p. 109).

When in the hospital many parents feel that their parenting skills are under scrutiny from nurses and doctors. They feel that the way they relate to and interact with their child is being observed. This can leave them feeling inadequate at a time when they are already under immense stress. It is important that parents have some uninterrupted time with their child, allowing them all to behave in as natural a way as is possible within the bounds of the hospital environment and the child's illness.

Darbyshire has discussed the fact that the live-in parent, or indeed any parent of a hospitalised child, loses control over the passage of time, becoming dependent on the timetable of others (Taylor, 1996). This concept has been demonstrated by Taylor, suggesting that control over the child's bedtime moves from the domain of the parent to that of the nurse. Nurses also have control over the time they spend with families; even nurse–client inter-actions initiated by family members tend to be terminated by the nurse (Taylor, 1996). This demonstrates the power that health care professionals have over their own time: they prioritise their daily workload, often having to limit the time they spend with families because of the pressure of work.

Parents are unsure of what is expected of them when they bring their child to hospital. For example, how much of their child's daily care should they carry out, and what will be performed by the nurses? It is important that nurses discuss with parents what is expected of them, and also what activities or procedures the parents wish to be involved with. Knafl and Dixon, discussed in Callery and Smith (1991), analysed fathers' participation in their child's hospitalisation and argued for negotiation between nurses and parents, to determine their respective roles. Often, as the child's treatment progresses, so does their parents' understanding and confidence. They may wish to take on extra care activities which were previously the responsibility of the nurse. These might be the flushing of central intravenous lines, taking of blood, or administration of intravenous antibiotics. Learning these skills may reduce the child's visits to hospital, thus raising the ill child's quality of life through spending more time at home. These new skills also give parents greater control over their family's life, allowing them to be at home more, with less disruption to family activities. Inherent in the idea that parents may take on these roles is the realisation that nurses will have to relinquish some of the control they traditionally have over these activities. For parents to be empowered in this way it is essential that nurses promote a trusting relationship and have effective communication skills, enhancing parents' confidence both in their abilities as a parent and in their nursing role.

When considering the involvement of parents in their child's care it is important that nurses ensure that the parents are willing to take on extra activities other than normal parenting roles. Parents can sometimes feel pressurised into carrying out care that they do not feel confident to do. This may arise because of the pressure on nurses' time, due to their workload, leading to them expecting parents to carry out some nursing activities for them. Alternatively it may come from knowing that other parents carry out these nursing tasks for their children, making them feel they should be able to do the same. It is important that nurses remain sensitive to parents' knowledge and experience, encouraging their involvement in their child's care without pressurising them or making them feel that they are 'allowing' them to be involved.

Effective communication between parents and all members of the health care team is essential in giving them the information and skills they need to care for their child. It is important that this communication is on-going, as parents' needs and understanding will alter as their child progresses through treatment. Accurate and up-to-date information will help parents to make decisions that are in the best interests of their child and family. Understanding each phase of the treatment programme, together with its possibilities and pitfalls, will assist parents in retaining control over the dissemination of information about their child among relatives and friends.

Empowerment of parents is essential in redressing the balance between everyone involved in the sick child's care. Gibson (1991 p. 357) indicates that the less powerful party must have a desire to take this on for it to be successful:

> Healthcare professionals cannot empower people; people can only empower themselves. However, nurses can help them develop, secure and use resources that will promote or foster a sense of control and self-efficacy.

Siblings

Healthy siblings are very vulnerable when their family is under the immense stress of caring for a child with cancer. They tend to occupy a position which allows them very little control over their own environment. Children need to feel secure within their family environment in order to confront their parents about any injustice they feel is occurring due to their sibling's illness (see 'Separation and isolation', 'Siblings' p. 112). Explanations of, and involvement in, the sick child's care may help them to feel an important member of the family, giving them the confidence to take issue with their parents and gain a little control over their own situation.

Healthy siblings need to be kept up to date with their sick brother or sister's progress. They need to have things explained to them in a way they will understand. This knowledge will help them to answer the inevitable questions from their peers. Understanding what is going on will help to increase their sense of security within their peer relationships. Adolescents, with their greater understanding and ability to examine information, will be able to have more control over how much they pass on to their friends. In this way siblings will feel more empowered.

Grandparents

Grandparents generally spend far less time in the hospital ward than parents, but they may come to visit the family, or look after the sick child when parents have a break. They are often quite intimidated by the ward environment, with so many machines and nurses who always appear busy. It is important that parents keep them updated on the child's progress so that they know what to expect when they visit their grandchild.

Grandparents who spend time alone with the sick child are often very unsure of what is expected of them by both the parents and nurses. It is important that the parents let them know what to expect during the time they are away; this will make them feel more confident about staying with the child. Nurses must not expect the general child care or nursing activities that had been carried out by parents to be continued by grandparents, so should find out to what extent the grandparents are confident to participate in the child's care, and should offer support throughout their stay.

When grandparents care for healthy siblings they often feel very insecure, especially if they are not closely involved with the family's usual activities. Conflicts may arise between parents and grandparents which will only be resolved through discussion and negotiation between both parties (see 'Separation and isolation', 'Grandparents' p. 116). Hospital staff should encourage this communication as it will give everyone an understanding of each other's expectations and let them all have some degree of control over the family. This will help to alleviate the stress felt by everyone involved. These steps should enable the grandparents to feel that they too are empowered individuals.

Case study 5.3 aims to demonstrate empowerment and the importance of partnership between the family carers and health care professionals. As Casey stated:

> The care of children, well or sick, is best carried out by their families, with varying degree of assistance from members of a suitable qualified healthcare team whenever necessary. (Casey, 1988 p. 8)

Case study 5.3

Noah, 4½ years old, was diagnosed with a solid tumour and required intensive chemotherapy which culminated in numerous neutropenic episodes. Consequently, Noah spent a lot of time in hospital. Noah and his sister Lucy, 2, live with their parents Joanne and Owen, 12 miles from the hospital.

It was very important for Joanne to maintain as normal a routine as possible throughout Noah's hospital admissions. In collaboration with the nursing staff and play specialist, she devised a routine for each day. This enabled her to maintain control and play an active part in all aspects of Noah's care. As Owen worked away from home he was able to organise to take over in the evening and do the night shift, with Joanne returning in the morning. Lucy spent all or part of the day on the ward or with her childminder who lived locally to Joanne and Owen. Unfortunately, this meant that Joanne and Owen spent very little time together during the week, though the weekends did give them some opportunities to spend time together. If possible all chemotherapy was scheduled for weekdays.

Joanne felt strongly that Noah should continue with learning his basic numeracy and literacy skills already started at nursery. She also devised various art and craft projects and involved Lucy in all these activities. She ensured Noah had his meals at the same time as herself and Lucy. Even when he was anorexic she acknowledged meal times by offering him a high calorie drink or a snack. In the afternoon, a nurse or the play specialist would arrange to spend a period of time with Noah, allowing Joanne to go out with Lucy or merely have some time out to herself. Medical staff respected Joanne and Owen's wishes and if possible avoided visiting Noah on their daily round between 10.00 and 10.30 so that the children could watch *Playdays* uninterrupted.

Joanne and Owen were taught how to correctly take and record Noah's temperature and to care for his Hickman line. As is normal practice on the ward, they had full access to his nursing records throughout each admission.

Joanne and Owen developed an open and trusting relationship with the nursing staff. Lucy remained a well-adjusted toddler and Noah a bright and lovable little boy who adapted to school life extremely well.

Joanne and Owen felt strongly from the outset that they wanted to maintain as much control and choice as possible in all aspects of Noah's care, and were able to adjust their lifestyles accordingly. Not all families have the desire or resources to exercise this level of independence or autonomy from the first admission, but as empowerment requires ongoing negotiation it should be re-assessed at each admission. Noah and Lucy benefited from having a routine that was similar to home. Meal times, activity times, quiet times and bedtimes were maintained appropriately, enabling the whole family to have some semblance of normality.

It can be intimidating for health care workers when parents or carers express their needs objectively and openly but all families should be given this opportunity. Empowerment is necessary and will only benefit the child and family if all involved are prepared to be flexible. Box 5.4 summarises the factors involved in empowerment.

Box 5.4

- When a child is diagnosed with cancer parents have to recognise that they are no longer in complete control of their child's destiny, or indeed the everyday life of their family
- Effective communication between the family and all members of the healthcare team is essential if parents are to be 'empowered' individuals, involved in the care of their child
- Everyone involved in assisting the family care for the sick child should discuss their expectations of one another in order to help avoid areas of conflict arising

Cultural considerations

Childhood cancer is an indiscriminate illness that affects all races and social classes. Modern societies are made up of diverse multi-cultural communities, individuals and groups having widely differing beliefs and customs which can influence the way they view illness and disease. This in turn affects the manner in which they seek and view the advice and treatment given by health care workers. Fuller and Toon (1988, p. 56) describe health beliefs as:

> an accumulation of notions, ideas and experiences, which provide explanations for illness and good health, as well as recommendations for action in illness or for continued health.

Health care workers are involved with families who are suffering both psychologically, socially and physically. Under these circumstances, many turn to their religious or cultural beliefs more intently than ever before in a search for explanations, strength, guidance and support to help them through the crisis of their child's illness. The importance of understanding and respecting these beliefs and customs forms an integral part in developing a trusting relationship with families; Rajan (1995 p. 452) states:

> To be culturally sensitive is to show respect. To show respect is the first step in the development of a trusting and therapeutic relationship.

Knowledge of the religious and cultural beliefs of the family will enable health care professionals to tailor advice and treatment so as not to conflict with these beliefs, wherever possible. This will promote understanding and acceptance of treatment, and reduce areas of conflict both within the family, especially where a large extended family is involved, and between the family and those responsible for the treatment of the sick child.

The importance of effective communication between the family and the health care team caring for the sick child has been discussed throughout this chapter. In some cultures it is the case that the head of the family makes the decisions regarding family members, so communication regarding the sick child should be made through them. It is usually the father who occupies this position; once he has the relevant information he will usually discuss the available options with other family members before making any decisions. However the father may not be involved in the physical care the other family members give the child, and may, like other male family members, leave when nurses are carrying out certain activities. This behaviour must be appreciated as normal for that family, and normal within that culture.

There are many situations when, once a family becomes involved in the health care system, they react differently depending on their religious and cultural beliefs. Families express different priorities and expect different things from the hospital, so some understanding of their cultural requirements will help nurses to offer care that is sensitive to their needs; for example, offering the correct diet, appreciating their need for uninterrupted time for prayer or special considerations associated with certain religious festivals.

For many families their cultural identity remains a very important feature of their life throughout all their experiences, both good and bad, and therefore should never be overlooked. Rajan (1995) suggests that by allowing individuals to express their cultural differences and providing care which is suited to their particular culture, health care professionals encourage compliance with, and understanding of, the treatment they prescribe.

Educating and supporting families

Health care professionals play a vital role in the support and education of families whose lives are suddenly thrown into turmoil by the diagnosis of childhood cancer. It is important from the outset to foster an honest trusting relationship with the family, which will in turn increase their confidence in those caring for their child. Having this kind of relationship with families will help communication, making them feel more able to discuss their concerns and leaving them more open to suggestions when help is needed. Casey's Partnership model, as discussed in Chapter 1, involves a process by which nurses who initially perform the majority of care for the sick child, gradually facilitate parents to take over more care themselves. It is a transition that requires negotiation between all parties, each requiring confidence in the other's abilities, and aims to establish a relationship where parents and professionals have equality in a partnership aimed at providing the optimum care to the sick child.

From the time of admission families are continually searching for information. They start from a point of minimal knowledge and will want to know all about the tests and possible outcomes. At this time it can be difficult for health care workers to satisfy this need, being aware of the dangers of giving information that may be inaccurate because the full picture is unavailable, but it is important to keep parents updated, giving them accurate information as it becomes available, thus ensuring that they feel they have some control during this very difficult time.

Educating parents and other family members is an important

part of the role of health care workers in both the hospital and community setting from the time of initial contact. This can take many forms such as verbal communication, practical demonstration, performing care together and providing written information. Paediatric cancer centres have many booklets, some explaining cancer and the treatment in general terms, and others specific to certain conditions. This written information given at the time of diagnosis is invaluable to families, as it gives them something to refer to at a time when it is very difficult to remember everything that is said to them about the sick child by doctors, nurses and other members of the team. There is also information available for parents to help them explain the illness to siblings – a problem that often causes them much anxiety and distress.

Communication is a two-way process: the time of diagnosis is an important time for health care workers to learn about the whole family. It is important that they take time to listen to the family and try to develop some understanding of the family dynamics, as this may provide a guide to the way the family will cope with this very stressful experience and how information can be most helpfully given and support offered.

It is important to ensure that communication between families and professionals is effective. This means always allowing time to listen to family members and trying to ensure that they have understood the information they have been given. Initially this may mean explaining issues several times, as everything will be unfamiliar and they will be in a highly stressed state; however as parents become more accustomed to the terminology and treatment they may need less explanation. It is important however to remember that during times of stress even parents who are very familiar with the hospital environment and their child's treatment may need extra time and explanation from staff with whom they have already built up a trusting relationship.

Throughout the child's treatment parents and families gradually build up their knowledge base and increase their skills in caring for a child with a life-threatening illness. As previously discussed under the section on 'Empowerment of individuals' (p. 128), knowledge and information helps parents take some control over their family's situation. With this increase in knowledge and skill developed through experience and gathering information they often become the 'experts' in many aspects of their child's condition and it is important that health care professionals recognise and value this expertise.

Individual family members generally give support to one another, however it must be remembered that each is going through a very stressful experience that challenges their ability to adapt and cope. It may sometimes be difficult for family members to gain all the support they require from within the family unit, or from friends or community groups of which they might be members. Thus many look to individuals or groups who have some knowledge or experience of what they are going through to provide much needed support. They may rely on health care workers for support, but many use peer support from others undergoing a similar experience. Carpenter *et al.* (1992 p. 27) acknowledge that:

> The provision of peer support by individuals who have had personal experience with a particular crisis can be a vital component in facilitating the adjustment process of others who are confronted with the same crisis.

Parents often gain this support from other parents they meet on the ward, they have an empathy towards each other and form friendships that give each support throughout treatment and the difficult time when close contact with the hospital diminishes.

Many paediatric oncology centres run support groups for parents. These are very individual and aimed at meeting the particular needs of participants. Some are organised entirely by parents and others have some professional input, but they are continually evolving as the membership changes. Obviously the parents will have children at different stages of treatment and thus those farther into treatment will often be able to offer support to those at an earlier stage of the treatment regimen. Difficulties may arise when a child dies. Is there a separate support group for bereaved parents? If so, should they be expected to leave the group that has been a major support to them to join a new group at a time when they are facing such an enormous loss, or should the group accommodate parents of children in and out of treatment as well as bereaved parents? These are issues that each group must resolve.

Many centres also offer siblings a support group and arrange special days for siblings to meet socially and ask questions they do not feel they can trouble their parents with. They also offer the opportunity to be with other children facing similar situations to themselves and experiencing similar feelings and emotions. Many health care professionals recognise the need to provide this facility, but encouraging such a group requires consideration of many issues such as confidentiality, providing a 'safe' place for them to express themselves, the ages of the children involved and who should be in the group. The same considerations have to be given to the issue of bereavement as with the parent groups. The group should develop to meet the needs of those participating without a set agenda, as different groups may have different priorities and concerns.

Although professionals recognise the need for these sibling groups, Woodhouse (1996) indicated that sibling days organised by one centre to provide education and peer support for these children were poorly attended. Other centres reported a similar picture. Woodhouse questions whether this is due to parents being too concerned with the sick child to recognise the needs of their other children, or possibly that they do not want to visit the hospital on a day when they could be at home. Finally she asks whether these children, despite the research evidence, have the need for professional and peer group support.

It must be remembered that many families do not live close to the paediatric oncology centres providing specific support groups and thus have very limited access to these facilities. These families often rely on the network of families they meet through the hospital, especially those whose children share the same condition, or local hospital and thus live in the same area for peer support.

There are national disease specific groups that parents can access for information and support and all centres should carry information of what is available and how to contact these groups and organisations.

Conclusion

The idea that childhood cancer affects the whole family has been borne out by the literature researched for this chapter. The effect on every family member is individual, however there is a common pathway of feelings and emotions that many experience. Each person experiences these at different times and to different intensities, and it is the stage that a person is in at a particular time that can affect the way they are coping, their need for support from others and their ability to offer support themselves.

As health care workers we must remember that every family member is affected and try to remain sensitive to the feelings of everyone involved. Everyone will face to some extent the problems highlighted throughout this chapter. Effective communication, education and the support of other families helps the family members manage these issues and feel less isolated. It is important to remain observant and listen to all members of the family – this will help build a picture of how everyone is managing, and if and where any professional intervention might be helpful.

We must remember that the family will always be affected by the consequences of the treatment of childhood cancer, whatever the outcome for the sick child. The feelings that they have experienced will affect the way they develop as individuals and adapt to other major changes in their lives, so it is important that health care workers and support organisations try to help them adapt to this crisis in as positive a way as possible.

References

Barbor, P. (1983) Emotional aspects of malignant disease in children. *Maternal and Child Health*, **8**, 320–327.

Bendor, S.J. (1990) Anxiety and isolation in siblings of pediatric cancer patients: the need for prevention. *Social Work in Health Care*, **14**(3), 17–35.

Bryne, D. (1994) Out in the cold. *Nursing Times*, **90**(11), 38–40.

Cairns, N.U., Clark, G.M., Smith, S.D. & Lansky, S.B. (1979) Adaptation of siblings to childhood malignancy. *Journal of Pediatrics*, **95**, 484–487.

Callery, P. & Smith, L. (1991) A study of role negotiation between nurses and the parents of hospitalized children. *Journal of Advanced Nursing*, **16**, 772–781.

Carpenter, P.J., Vattimo, C.J., Messbauer, L.J., Stolnitz, C., Bell Isle, J., Stutzman, H. & Cohen, H.J. (1992) Development of a parent advocate program as part of a pediatric hematology oncology service. *Journal of Psychosocial Oncology*, **10**(2), 27–38.

Casey, A. (1988) A partnership with child and family. *Senior Nurse*, **8**(4), 8–9.

Cincotta, N. (1993) Psychosocial issues in the world of children with cancer. *Cancer Supplement*, **71**, 3251–3259.

Cornman, J.B. (1993) Childhood cancer: differential effects on the family members. *Oncology Nursing Forum*, **20**(10), 1559–1566.

Culling, J.A. (1988) The psychological problems of families of children with cancer *in* Oakhill, A. ed. *The Supportive Care of the Child with Cancer*, pp. 204–237. London: Butterworth.

Doyle, B. (1987) 'I wish you were dead'. *Nursing Times*, **83**(45), 44–46.

Faulkner, A., Peace, G. & O'Keeffe, C. (1993) Future imperfect. *Nursing Times*, **89**(51), 40–42.

Fuller, J.H.S. & Toon, P.D. (1988) *Medical Practice in a Multicultural Society*. Oxford: Heinemann Professional.

Gallo, A.M., Breitmayer, B.J., Knafl, K.A. & Zoeller, L.H. (1991) Stigma in childhood chronic illness: a well Sibling perspective. *Pediatric Nursing*, **17**(1), 21–25.

Gibson, C.H. (1991) A concept analysis of empowerment. *Journal of Advanced Nursing*, **16**, 354–361.

Harding, R. (1996) Children with cancer: the needs of siblings. *Professional Nurse*, **11**(9), 558–590.

Heath, S. (1996) Childhood cancer – a family crisis 1: the impact of diagnosis. *British Journal of Nursing*, **5**(12), 744–748.

Hinds, P.S., Birenbaum, L.K., Clarke-Steffen, L., Quargnenti, A., Kreissman, S., Kazak, A., Meyer, W., Mulhern, R., Pratt, C. & Wilimas, J. (1996) Coming to terms: parents' response to a first cancer recurrence in their child. *Nursing Research*, **45**(3), 148–153.

Jennings, K. (1986) Helping them face tomorrow. *Nursing Times*, **82**(4), 33–35.

Kramer, R.F. & Moore, I.M. (1983) Childhood cancer: meeting the special needs of healthy siblings. *Cancer Nursing*, June, 213–217.

Lansky, S.B., Cairns, N.U., Hassanein, R., Wehr, J. &

Lowman, J.T. (1978) Childhood cancer: parental discord and divorce. *Pediatrics*, **62**(2), 184–188.

Lindsay, B. (1995) Like skeletons or ghosts: developing a concept of death and dying. *Child Health*, **2**(4), 142–146.

Mott, M.G. (1990) A child with cancer: a family in crisis. *British Medical Journal*, **301**, 133–134.

Murray, G.G. & Jampolsky, M.D. (1982) *Straight from the Siblings. Another look at the rainbow*. Berkeley, CA: Celestial Arts.

Platt, H. (1959) *The Welfare of Children in Hospital. Report of the commission, Department of Health, Central Health Service Council*. London: HMSO.

Rajan, M.J. (1995) Transcultural nursing: a perspective derived from Jean-Paul Sartre. *Journal of Advanced Nursing*, **22**, 450–455.

Robinson, C. (1985) Parents of hospitalised chronically ill children: competency in question. *Nursing Papers*, **17**(2), 59–67.

Ross-Alaolmolki, K., Heinzer, M.M., Howard, R. & Marszal, S. (1995) Impact of childhood cancer on siblings and family: family strategies for primary health care. *Holistic Nursing Practice*, **9**(4), 66–75.

Stewart, A. (1994) Empowerment and enablement: occupational therapy 2001. *British Journal of Occupational Therapy*, **57**(7), 248–254.

Taylor, B. (1996) Parents as partners in care. *Paediatric Nursing*, **8**(4), 24–27.

Woodhouse, S. (1996) Do siblings need a special day? *Paediatric Nursing*, **8**(3), 8–9.

Impact of treatment on the nursing team

SUSAN BULLEY

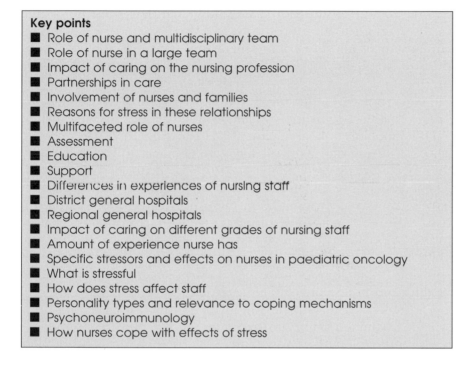

Key points
- Role of nurse and multidisciplinary team
- Role of nurse in a large team
- Impact of caring on the nursing profession
- Partnerships in care
- Involvement of nurses and families
- Reasons for stress in these relationships
- Multifaceted role of nurses
- Assessment
- Education
- Support
- Differences in experiences of nursing staff
- District general hospitals
- Regional general hospitals
- Impact of caring on different grades of nursing staff
- Amount of experience nurse has
- Specific stressors and effects on nurses in paediatric oncology
- What is stressful
- How does stress affect staff
- Personality types and relevance to coping mechanisms
- Psychoneuroimmunology
- How nurses cope with effects of stress

Introduction

This chapter is an eclectic view of stress using research, anecdotal evidence, personal experience and reflection to illustrate the impact of caring for children with cancer and leukaemia, primarily on nursing staff.

When addressing the topic of stress it is widely accepted that nurses are a particularly high risk group primarily because of the 'hands-on' nature of the work (Kunkler and Whittick, 1991). This chapter focuses on the experiences of nursing staff, in particular the effect that stress plays in the day-to-day work of tending to the needs of children and their families. The subject of occupational stress has yielded a large body of research and literature and yet the nursing profession tends to view stress as an individual problem and the alleviation of it as a personal responsibility (Harris, 1989). The consequences of stress have financial implications affecting patient care and nurse relations (Kennedy and Gray, 1997). More worrying, however, are the high rates of suicide among nurses related to issues of stress (Wheeler, 1997).

Selye (1980) describes stress as the non-specific response of the body to any demand made upon it. Mast *et al.* (1987) puts forward the idea that human beings are constantly faced with potentially stressful situations that require physical, emotional and/or behavioural adjustments. No two people respond in exactly the same manner to a given situation. Each individual perceives the degree of threat in a situation on the basis of past experiences, present circumstances and the coping mechanisms available to deal with the stressor. Bailey (1985) summarises that stress emanates from the meaning given to the demands placed upon the nurses and the value nurses put on the importance of caring for others.

The chapter begins by focusing on the role of the nurse within a large multidisciplinary team (MDT), caring for children with cancer. Nursing staff work closely with families, and to ensure that their needs are met rely on the MDT to provide a holistic approach to meeting those needs. Therefore not only are nursing staff exposed to stress brought about by cancer care, but this unfortunately can be compounded by interdisciplinary conflicts creating further stress. Research suggests that a greater understanding of one another's roles can help promote cohesiveness in working relationships and ultimately provide better care. Recent moves to bring health care professionals together in education will be discussed.

The recent Calman–Hine report (Department of Health, 1995) will be examined with particular reference to the recommendations for the role nurses now play in referring patients to members of the multidisciplinary team. This report has also promoted the centralising of cancer services to create centres of specialist care. The present paediatric oncology model is that of shared care between regional and district general hospitals. My own experiences as a staff nurse on a general paediatric ward in a district general hospital, and as a student in a regional centre (whilst on the ENB 240 paediatric oncology course), will be used to illustrate how this model works. It is of relevance to families and health care professionals who observe a break in partnerships at some point when families attend one of the two hospitals. The chapter will focus directly on the experiences of nurses in regional centres and district general hospitals, exploring specific causes of stress pertinent to these different care settings. The discussion points at the end of the chapter will provide useful exercises to help you to contrast the evidence of stress, the effects and coping mechanisms and will be referred to throughout the chapter. The reader should remember that comments from the surveys are relevant only to the time and areas they were conducted in. However they are easy to recreate and could be applicable to other areas of paediatric oncology.

As mentioned above, nurses and other members of the MDT work very closely with children and their families, therefore it is of significance that partnerships in care are discussed, in particular how these partnerships relate to the ward environment and how they play a part in creating stress for all involved. In the beginning families can immediately lose control in the face of bad news, and become overburdened by the information given by so many different members of the MDT. It is at this point the nurse plays such an important role, placed into an often difficult situation when trying to form a relationship, which may prove to last some time. This first meeting takes sensitivity and skill to ensure the child and family feel they have someone who will help them and be someone they trust and like. This encounter is also the point at which the nurse is exposed to a family thrown into turmoil and, as the literature suggests, is a stressful time for the nurse who has to help the family through a variety of emotions.

Anne Casey's (1988) model of partnerships in care will be used to depict the many relationships a child and family become involved in. The model, although not exclusive, does provide a structure which allows the nurse and family flexibility when planning care suitable for the ward and home environment. Again the nurse is pivotal in providing the family with the necessary skills to use partnerships effectively, empowering them to ensure their needs are met and the child achieves optimum health. Darbyshire (1994) found that one cause of stress to parents was the lack of control they had in their child's care. It is therefore reasonable to assume that if parents and children are stressed it makes the role of caring that much more difficult for all staff who may not be fully aware of how parents feel.

Evidence shows the impact of caring for children with cancer and leukaemia affects nurses in different ways depending on their experience and level of skill. Work by Benner (1984) will be used to illustrate the nurses' journey from novice to expert and how stress is dealt with at each level. To understand evolving skill it is necessary to try and grasp how the nursing profession conceptualises hands-on care. By discussing reflection on nursing practice using Carper's fundamental ways of knowing (Carper, 1978), it is hoped to show how nurses describe what they do in concrete terms, and therefore how they are able to learn and share knowledge to combat the effects of stress brought about by caring for children with cancer. Many of the problems nurses face from cancer care may be lessened through guidance and support from 'expert' nurses who have faced and used stress to help them through difficult situations. Peplau's (1988) descriptions of the different roles a nurse fulfils will be explored in relation to helping others deal with stress.

The chapter concludes with a short examination of the coping mechanisms nurses employ when faced with prolonged stress. It is also at this point in the chapter that personality will be analysed, in particular the increasing body of evidence that suggests there may be a link between behaviour and cancer. The reason for including this came from the idea that stress may play a part in causing cancer as argued in various research studies, and the relevance to nurses' own behaviour when caring for patients with cancer. It is not to make any particular point but for the reader to draw their own conclusions.

The role of the nurse and the multidisciplinary team

Kerstetter (1990) describes cancer care as a good example of health care organised and carried out by a number of health care professionals. However, it appears that team members know very little about overall treatment and goals for patients with cancer (Kerstetter, 1990). It would be fair to suggest that the nurse provides an important role in communicating care between professionals, nurses are after all the one member of the team in closest contact with patients and their families. It is important for nurses to recognise this and act in a collaborative manner, as directed in the United Kingdom Central Council (UKCC) Code of Conduct for Nurses, Health Visitors and Midwives (UKCC, 1992a), to achieve optimal care for their patients.

As a child's treatment proceeds, it is important that relevant referrals are made at appropriate times. The nurse is well placed to make the referrals or suggest to medical staff that another service is required. Stutzer (1989) recognised that paediatric oncology nurses believed they were close enough to situations to know what the child wanted and needed and yet they were seldom, if ever, included in decisions concerning their patients. It would be unfair to suggest this is a problem for all nurses as many oncology units have regular MDT meetings to discuss individual patient care and is a chance for all members involved to make their comments. If however communication is an issue, Tyler and Ellison (1994) suggests the idea of nurses attending business courses and stress management programmes. Kerstetter (1990) believes effective communication is a key factor in bringing together all services to provide effective holistic care. This is further endorsed by the recent Calman–Hine report (Department of Health, 1995), which states that services should take account of patient needs and in particular good communication between client and professional. An earlier report by the World Health Organization (WHO) in 1988 also stressed the need for collaboration and good relations between allied professionals. The report went on to suggest that health care professionals could become more aware of one another's role by attending courses together. Many advantages can come from health care professionals training together, perhaps one advantage being that members of a MDT are aware of their role and that of others, therefore not confusing professional boundaries. That is to say one professional trying to take on all roles for their patient. If this happens it is arguable that the patient is not receiving the best care and can create further problems for the patient and the professional brought in at a later time. This can perhaps be illustrated by a piece of personal reflection exercised after another member of the MDT was upset and stressed by a referral made to her (Case study 6.1).

The situation illustrated in Case study 6.1 shows how one fairly common problem like oral thrush can lead to another potentially long-term problem of weight loss and anorexia. Nursing staff had acknowledged that Ruby was losing weight, and with the best of intentions, had given advice. On reflection it would have been better if a dietician had been contacted at the earliest possible

Case study 6.1

A number of staff had noted how Ruby, a 9-year-old child, had been losing weight over the last 6 months during her treatment for leukaemia. Staff had offered suggestions about diet to Ruby's mother. On seeing just how much weight Ruby had lost and that she had little or no appetite, I asked her consultant if we could bring in a dietician to help Ruby. Pam, Ruby's mother, was grateful for the dietician's help and explained how she felt that Ruby's appetite had diminished since experiencing a particularly painful episode of oral thrush some months back. Pam felt guilty at letting the problem go on for so long but was aware that forcing Ruby to eat would not help matters. After a long chat with Pam and Ruby, the dietician offered a variety of nutritional supplements, tasted and accepted by Ruby. A short-term plan was developed and reviewed on a regular basis while Ruby was an inpatient. The dietician then came to me and explained how she felt she could have achieved more through being contacted sooner or perhaps avoided Ruby losing so much weight if brought in at the beginning of treatment. She pointed out how sad she felt that as well as the leukaemia Ruby and her mother had yet another significant problem to deal with. She also described her feelings of frustration at believing she had not achieved a great deal for the family and would take some time to make progress.

Can you think of a common problem, which you have encountered in a patient, that has led to a more potentially serious problem?

point to help Ruby. The case study shows how nurses felt it was reasonable to give dietary advice despite having another professional who deals exclusively with this area of care. It might be suggested that professional boundaries were misjudged and an appropriately timed referral was not made. The case study also illustrates how as professionals we can create stress for one another through ineffective decision making and planning. The dietician was brought in at a point that could almost be described as 'crisis management', which upset her. It is important therefore that we acknowledge that other members of the MDT are also stressed by caring for children with cancer and leukaemia and should be part of the child's care from an early point; it would also be helpful if staff understood each other's role so that referrals can be made appropriately. The problem in the above situation is trying to be rectified by involving dietetic services at diagnosis and ensuring parents know the service is there for them to use as they feel is necessary. On a broader issue Plymouth now offer an MSc in Cancer Studies for professionals from various disciplines to study together (including nurses).

There is of course the other extreme where, as Geen (1986) recognises, the family and child are visited by many professionals. The temptation may be to ensure the child has all the relevant professionals involved in their care at the same time. The problems caused by this are obvious, resulting in the child and family being overburdened by information and perhaps then unable to use any of the information effectively. Kerstetter (1990) warns against the fragmentation of care through a MDT approach, therefore a continual communication between members is of importance to avoid this. The answer may be a gradual introduction to the MDT during the first few hospital admissions and for the named nurse to ensure the family understands the relevance of each team member to their child's care and how to use their expertise. Fradd (1994) is an exponent of empowering patients and believes nurses have an influence to empower patients in their care. Davidson and Lucas (1995) believe that cancer care can be enhanced by including the patient's voice. With guidance from experienced nurses and medical staff problems may be prevented, saving members of the MDT from having to 'crisis manage' and encourage parents and children to have some control over their lives before they also reach crisis.

Partnerships in care

Parent participation and family-centred care has been advocated in paediatric services for many years. The Platt Report published in 1959 supported parental involvement in the care of their own hospitalised child (Platt, 1959). An increasing body of literature since that time reveals the benefits for children and their families being together in hospital. Early studies have shown the potential damaging effects on children when separated from their parents (Robertson, 1958; Bowlby, 1973). Other studies focusing on parental anxiety of their hospitalised child found parents worried about the emotional and physical well being of their child (Casey, 1988; Coyne, 1995). Work examining the needs of children in hospital have helped nursing staff to accept parents participating in the care of their child and have led nurses to expand on the philosophy of partnerships in care. This process however has been further forged through governmental endeavours to bring choice to the consumers of health. Initiatives such as the Patient's Charter (Department of Health, 1991) and the Children Act (1989) have brought partnerships in care to the forefront, in order to keep consumers informed of their care and to have some control over their lives while patients.

Nurses are attempting to use holistic care to empower their clients, thus adopting initiatives from reorganisations within the health service to give choice and power of decision making to users, and perhaps moving patients away from the image of the doctor always making the decisions about care. However, as Fradd (1994) suggests, nurses must first believe they have some power before they can empower patients in their care. The introduction of the 'Named Nurse' initiative as part of the Patient's Charter (Department of Health, 1991) should place the nurse closer to knowing the needs of their patients. Individual nurses are able with their patients and carers to prescribe care that often extends beyond the hospital setting, enabling parents to give care in hospital that continues at home. All this considered, nurses are arguably now much closer to the children, their families and the stress that cancer can bring. Nurses are expected to adapt to the ever-changing treatments for childhood cancer and assess the abilities of parents to take on specific care in their child's treatment. As Fradd (1994) recognises, nurses must first believe in their own abilities and feel confident in the care they give. Various studies have shown that nurses feel stressed by their lack of knowledge in such a specialist field and therefore may have difficulty in helping parents to achieve some control over their child's care (Lansdown, Pike and Smith, 1990; Hinds, Quargnent and Hickey, 1994); this must also create problems in communication between the nurse, child and carers.

Evans (1994) believes in the philosophy of care by parents but suggests that in all probability it finally came as a result of reducing staff numbers in newly formed trusts. Therefore there is a need for nurses to be more sensitive to parents who feel further stressed by taking on more technical roles in caring for their children while in hospital, especially when trying to form new working relationships with those families (Cleary, 1992). Anne Casey's model describing partnerships in care allows a flexibility of roles. The model is defined as not having a rigid structure so it may be adapted to any speciality in paediatric care (Casey, 1988). Negotiation of care must be realistic and consistent, with parents involved as much as they feel able with the support of nursing staff. Robinson (1985) describes how parents are expected to be clinical experts in the home yet relinquish these skills in the presence of nurses and doctors. In paediatric oncology care where parents are required to take on new skills in caring for their child, a supportive and educational partnership is needed, allowing the child to reach its full potential and keeping the parents' role consistent. Casey's model recognises this need and believes the ability for the family to function socially, emotionally and physically is important for the sick child to grow and develop (Casey, 1988). Parents are active in the care of their child, and this can often span years of intensive treatment, remissions and relapses – it is this element of cancer care that creates differing dependence on professionals through the years. Often partnerships change with parents taking the lead in their child's care, and relinquishing it for a time in the light of a relapse or the beginning of palliative care, creating a heavy reliance on nursing staff and other members of the health care team both on the ward and in the community.

The recent Calman–Hine report (Department of Health, 1995) favours collaboration in care for patients with cancer to provide a holistic approach to their management. As the person often closest to the patient, the report places a greater emphasis on nursing staff to refer patients to the appropriate members of the health care team. This may be a source of potential conflict on the wards, as historically doctors have made referrals when they feel it necessary to do so. Casey (1995) suggests that individuals have a problem with professional identity and believe they can take care of all aspects of a patient's care, resulting in the child and the family not receiving specialist help from the appropriate member of the MDT. The report and similar initiatives may be an opportunity for nurses to recognise their skills and present them to doctors when addressing patient's need for other professionals to become involved.

As the treatment for cancer and leukaemia can potentially affect an individual's physical and psychosocial well being, there is the opportunity for patients to come into contact with many members of the MDT. It is important that the nurse has some concept of

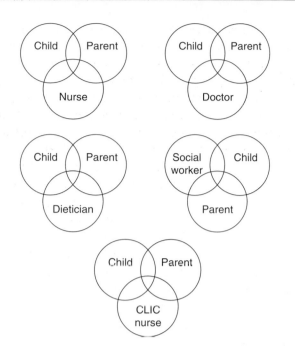

Figure 6.1 Examples of some of the partnerships a child and family are involved in during and beyond treatment.

the vast array of health care professionals involved in cancer care, and Figure 6.1 depicts some of the many partnerships that a child and family are involved in during and beyond treatment.

The named nurse can help the child and family to form the many partnerships and use them effectively when perhaps other members of the MDT do not recognise their encounters as a partnership. The nurse must also be able to use skills and experience to refer children at a time that is right, keeping numbers of professionals involved at any one time to a minimum.

It is obviously important for nurses to ensure continuity of care is maintained for the child and family; however this may prove difficult for hospitals that share care with regional centres. Recent moves to centralise services for oncology patients often mean shared care, such as that between Plymouth and Bristol for children with cancer and leukaemia. In Plymouth children with a malignancy often present on one of the general paediatric wards with symptoms of their disease. Once a provisional diagnosis of cancer is made the child is transferred to the Bristol Royal Hospital for Sick Children (BRHSC). At present, a number of children when diagnosed spend some time in the BRHSC. Visits include commencement of treatment once diagnosis and staging is completed, bone marrow transplantation, stem cell transplantation, administration of high does methotrexate and times when children become so unwell they may require treatment and specialist help not available in Plymouth. Plymouth does however offer a wide range of treatment, which means children and their families can return home quicker with subsequent care provided. With advances in oncology care district general hospitals (DGHs) like Plymouth can offer more to children and families, which means less time spent in regional centres like Bristol but ensuring a high standard of care is still achieved. However as children and their families do go to Bristol it does mean that partnerships formed in Plymouth are broken and new ones have to be established. At a time of anguish for families this can be yet another cause of stress, and nurses need to be sympathetic to this. It does mean that on subsequent visits the partnerships are hopefully still in place and this makes the overall experience of moving from one hospital to another a little easier for families and staff.

From a nursing perspective in a DGH it can be difficult forming effective partnerships if the child has been transferred to a regional centre quickly after initial diagnosis. Nurses have limited time to talk to the child and parents, making preparation for the transfer and subsequent treatment difficult. From experience families have often said they felt 'safe' in Bristol because of the specialist knowledge there, and so feel apprehensive when returning to Plymouth where the ward caring for children with cancer does not cater solely for paediatric oncology. In these circumstances partnerships in care can be difficult to form without time and understanding from both parties. When a child and family are facing a life-threatening illness it is part of the nurses' role to build confidence in the care received in a DGH, and ensuring a child has consistency in their care, feeling able to trust those responsible for meeting their needs (Casey, 1988). To help this situation nurses from the ward in Plymouth caring for these children are encouraged to visit the BRHSC to see the work carried out there and to have some understanding of the parents' anxieties. This visit takes the form of a 2-week course introducing staff to paediatric oncology from an educational and practical basis. Nurses in Plymouth find this helpful as it gives them an idea of what will happen to the child once in Bristol and are able to inform the child and their carers before they leave Plymouth. It also provides a link for nursing staff in both hospitals, making future contact easier. This contact also provides an opportunity for staff to share ideas of nursing care, which provides a consistency of nursing practice between the two centres.

In the regional centres nursing staff also experience a break in partnerships and often lose contact with a child and family once they return to their own DGH. As mentioned previously, DGHs are able to take on more and more of a child's care with direction from regional centres. This allows the regional hospitals to discharge patients quicker and take on more children for treatment. However, as Harding (1994) points out in a study conducted at the BRHSC, more of the rarer forms of cancer are being seen in regional centres often with a poorer outcome exposing staff to more deaths. The fact that more rarer cancers are getting to the stage of being treated may have something to do with recent advances in the way in which cancer and leukaemia is managed (Pinkerton, Cushing and Sepion, 1994). Treatments have become more aggressive and complex, which has an overall effect on the numbers of children surviving longer, creating a demand for beds in regional centres (Pinkerton *et al.*, 1994). This of course impacts on the nursing experience in both DGHs and regional centres, and this will be examined later in the chapter.

From experience, partnerships and relationships can create stress but can also be very productive for nurses and families if both parties are realistic in what they want from the relationship. For families this is difficult when dealing with a child with cancer, therefore nurses should set boundaries for the relationship in the beginning. This gives the child and family an idea of what to expect from the nurse. Personal beliefs are that the nurse in being so close to the family for some time, also needs to be protected from stress while caring for the child and family. It is inevitable that the family and nurse get to know one another well during treatment and it is not to say that the nurse should distance any personal feelings. However as the chapter shows, nursing staff have a great deal to cope with as the child's advocate and 'secondary' carer, and to continue in paediatric oncology, need to think of self preservation, therefore the nurse needs to be aware of professional boundaries.

Can you think of a family you have dealt with when perhaps the level of stress you felt at the time was difficult for you to deal with

The nurse's role in assessment, education and support

As already identified paediatric oncology nurses as with other paediatric nurses are encouraged to use a partnership in care philosophy. This partnership is between many members of the MDT, parents and child. With so many professionals involved, parents may well feel they lack any sort of control over their child's care. Darbyshire (1994) uses parents' feeling and experiences while in hospital with their child to illustrate this point. He found that their perceived lack of power was due to their position as primary carer being taken over by the many members of the MDT. He further explains how children feel powerless to ask their parents to make them better. To overcome parents' and children's lack of control, it can be argued that steps must be taken to empower them. This is especially so in paediatric oncology, where parents have traditionally taken on so much information and care relating to their child's disease and treatment. Parents are expected to know when their child needs hospitalisation to prevent potentially life-threatening situations like the child being febrile and neutropenic. To understand the implications of this takes knowledge and skills on the part of the parents. Negotiation of care between child, family and the nurse promotes an environment in which nurses are able to empower those in their care not only on the ward but also at home (Norris, 1995).

The process of negotiation in care begins with the child's admission to hospital. Assessment of care at this time involving the parents gives the nurse the opportunity to plan care using vital information relating to the child's normal activities and routines. Casey's model suggests parents are given the chance to discuss what they feel able to do for their child at admission and throughout the child's stay in hospital. The recent Scope of Professional Practice document (1992) now provides nursing staff with the choice of expanding and developing their roles at a ward level. This arguably brings choice to parents and children who with supervision may also want to take on more technical roles. Nurses are able to carry out tasks traditionally done by doctors, therefore giving a more holistic approach to care (Wilson, 1996). Training and assessment ensures nurses are competent to undertake new skills and can pass on these skills at the request of parents. Casey (1995) believes that when a parent is taught a skill there should be evidence that teaching has taken place and what it involved, it then becomes the nurses responsibility to judge the parent's or child's ability to carry out the task. However nurses should also ensure parents do not take on too much, as parents may feel obligated to do so if they see other parents carry out nursing tasks. As nursing staff know, on a busy shift it is often tempting to let parents do as much of their child's care as possible, thus allowing staff to continue with other work, or not take time to teach parents and therefore carry out tasks without including the parents or child. It should also be considered that parents need to take time for themselves or just to sit with their child and engage in the 'normal' routines like reading stories and talking about life away from hospital. As many studies show, parents have their own unique stresses to deal with when their child is ill and routines are upset through hospitalisation, nurses therefore have to be receptive to help parents balance being a parent and a skilled carer.

Perhaps one of the most stressful times for parents is at initial diagnosis. Often time has been spent awaiting tests results and, as Geen (1986) suggests, the child and family may have been seen by many individuals who have given advice or information. In the light of bad news parents may often have difficulty in assimilating and understanding information. This is endorsed by Dear (1995), who believes parents on receiving bad news only hear the worst and little else. Geen (1986) advocates the paediatric oncology nurse as being a constant figure in the child's care, facilitating the understanding of information by removing jargon and taking time for parents to ask questions. Although stressful also for nursing staff involved in the breaking of bad news, it could be considered an important time for initially forging a relationship which may last some years. Recent changes in nursing styles help to shape relationships between nurses, children and families. Primary nursing and family-centred care encourages the nurse to become more involved with the family, giving more that just hands-on care (Sepion, 1990). These changes, combined with advances in the treatment of cancer and leukaemia, create long partnerships perhaps spanning years (Emery, 1993), the benefits of which include continuity of care during periods of hospitalisation. The child and family may feel a little less stressed before repeated admissions, knowing there will be a familiar face who knows not only them but is well practised in the care they want to receive.

As with most relationships there can be problems. Emery (1993) recognises working with sick children can be difficult, but working with children who face a life-threatening disease requiring long intensive treatments can be stressful especially when the outcome can never be predicted or guaranteed. As a named nurse, being so closely involved with families from the time of diagnosis, remission, relapse, periods of being unwell and death brings a multitude of emotions and ultimately stress for nursing staff (Harding, 1994). Unfortunately there are also many other sources of stress that nurses have to deal with on a daily basis connected with work or perhaps of a more personal nature (this will be discussed more fully later in the chapter). All of these stresses can create difficulties when caring for children with cancer and leukaemia. Not only do nurses have to deal with their own stress but they also need to be a source of support for parents and children. Hanson (1994) suggests oncology nurses possess an inherent working knowledge about stress among persons and families with cancer. It is believed to come from the close relationships which are formed through caring, protecting and promoting the rights of the patient. In giving psychological support nurses need to acknowledge their everyday experiences, encompassing both professional practice and educational experience, which provide them with 'common sense knowledge and value' (Hanson, 1994). Therefore when discussing and planning care it is important for the nurse to draw on past experience to provide practised

take a difficult situation and make it interpretable and approachable. This skill is a valuable asset, especially if applied to new or junior staff in helping them to adjust and build upon their practice with confidence. The role of the paediatric oncology nurse is of course not in existence exclusively for the mentorship of staff. However in light of an ever-expanding speciality it is vital staff are supported, helping them to adjust and, importantly, remaining long enough in cancer care to develop advanced clinical practical skills and ultimately effective coping mechanisms.

Skills possessed by this group of nurses come from experience and/or undertaking further study like the ENB 240 Paediatric Oncology Course. Experience and further education can help paediatric oncology nurses to have the necessary expertise and up-to-date knowledge to equip them for this multifaceted role. Hanson (1994) believes that cancer nurses generally have a rich body of knowledge and ability in relation to psychosocial care and they should be given the opportunity to use these skills to meet the everyday needs of their patients. These skills are what Benner (1984) relates to in creating the theory of an expert coach; a nurse being able to talk to patients discussing their illness and making it relative to their present state and daily life. Benner and Wrubel (1989) believe that often nurses and members of the patient's family find this difficult to do, especially when the subject matter is deemed to be inappropriate. If psychological matters are not discussed it can lead to the patient feeling their problem is much worse and possibly increase their levels of stress (Hanson, 1994).

Knowledge of disease processes, treatment and outcomes must be considered as an important part of the paediatric oncology nurse's repertoire. As already mentioned, nurses become involved in very close relationships with the child and family. From personal experience a quiet time on the ward spent chatting is often an opportunity for parents and children to ask questions. To be able to give them up-to-date knowledge may give the family confidence in 'their' nurse and creates another dimension to the relationship. Reviews of literature find a lack of knowledge displayed by patients and families in, for example, overestimating the number of cancer deaths. Perhaps more alarming is that the same reviews discovered nurses caring for these patients shared the same level of knowledge (Corner, 1988). Not only does this not help the patient, it may also go some way to shattering any hope they and their family may have. Therefore it is up to nurses to ensure knowledge is research and evidence based and given at an understandable level to help families to see the overall picture of cancer and is not potentially harming them through a lack of knowledge. It is also important that nurses see a positive side to their work and consider the advances being made in oncology in bringing about a better outcome for many children.

Differences in experience of nursing staff in regional and district general hospitals

Working on a general paediatric ward within a DGH staff frequently express their feelings of stress when caring for children with cancer and leukaemia. While on secondment to do the ENB 240 Paediatric Oncology course at BRHSC, it was evident that the causes of stress for nursing staff might be somewhat different to the experience of nurses in a DGH. As part of the ENB 240 course I undertook a survey gathering the thoughts and feelings of staff detailing what they felt stressed them, how this stress manifested itself and how they coped with the feelings and other effects. This information was then compared to current research and literature as part of an assignment for the course. With the information discovered I decided to carry out the same survey in Plymouth to contrast the results, identifying any differences and possible reasons for them. This section will explore the results of the survey to give the reader an idea of the differences found. Findings discussed are by no means intended to be a generalisation of experiences around the country and apply to Bristol and Plymouth in 1995/6. Following this section a literature review will provide evidence of occupational stress taken from research carried out in Europe and America.

In Plymouth children with cancer and leukaemia are cared for on one of the general paediatric wards. Approximately 10–11 children are diagnosed in Plymouth and the catchment area each year, however these figures can vary as in any DGH. This means that compared with regional centres, staff see relatively small numbers of children with cancer at any one time in the hospital. However again this fluctuates from having no children to perhaps four or five on the ward together. A percentage of children diagnosed in Plymouth are transferred to BRHSC to commence some treatments. Despite having a shared care system with Bristol, a substantial amount of treatment is administered in Plymouth, either on the ward or in the outpatient department next to the ward. At present there are three nurses with the ENB 240 certificate, and the ward relies upon these nurses' help to teach and guide staff, both new and experienced. One nurse wrote the following account of her feelings on first encountering a child with cancer:

> I knew nothing at all about any childhood cancers or leukaemia and was not altogether happy to nurse these children.

However with help from oncology experienced nurses I learned a lot. Now three years down the line I feel more confident and can give medications, chemotherapy and blood products via Hickman lines, prior to this I had never even seen a Hickman line and so felt fairly stressed knowing I would have to use them.

The presence of nurses with the ENB 240 certificate can help to give confidence to other nurses who feel apprehensive about caring for this client group. From personal experience in providing regular teaching sessions on all aspects of cancer care in paediatrics, given either informally or more formally, this not only helps staff to learn but also lessens the workload of nurses who have the ENB 240 certificate. Not sharing information only increases the workload of specialist nurses who are ward based, and may lead to standards of care being poorer when these nurses are not on duty. It could also be suggested that an overdependence by families on specialist nurses may occur through other members of staff being excluded from vital knowledge and the benefit of experience. This overdependence is arguably counter productive and creates further stress for the nurse, who then finds it difficult to extract themselves from the needs of the child and family. Taking time away is important for nurses, especially during difficult times, for example when a child is dying, and by doing so helps to empower the family and other nurses to deal with the situation.

As previously established, empowerment of parents and child is also important to help them continue care at home with support from community nurses. Parents very quickly become conversant in most areas of their child's care, for example they come to know the norms and deficits in blood counts. This is a process which Peplau (1988) believes comes from nurses being seen as teachers using subject matter that the patient or carer finds of interest, and then building upon it using additional medical information. However other nursing members can become intimidated by a parent's knowledge; a nurse from the survey conducted in Plymouth wrote:

I do feel inadequate because of my lack of knowledge regarding blood counts and chemo, most of the parents know considerably more than me.

Another nurse stated similar feelings in writing the following statement:

Its [sic] not until I talk to the parents that I realise I don't know as much about cancer, it can be embarrassing not being able to spend time discussing their child's disease.

A different nurse's comments focus directly on working on a general paediatric ward:

> I know my oncology knowledge is not what it should be, but with eight other specialities on the ward it is difficult to know a lot about all of them.

Other comments dealing with issues of stress emanating from such a wide variety of specialities included dealing with children suffering from eating disorders and then caring for a child in the terminal stages of cancer. From personal experience it can be difficult when teenagers with cancer become upset on seeing another teenager on the ward being cared for with an eating disorder such as anorexia nervosa. However there are positive aspects to caring for children with cancer on a general paediatric ward, one nurse made the following observation:

> When I am upset caring for a child with cancer I know I can escape or gather my thoughts by caring for another child who may have a broken arm and is being discharged home very soon after their accident.

Another nurse not only felt working on a general ward helped her cope with stress, but also believed it helped parents of children with cancer. Her rationale for this was:

> Whilst there are no 'normal' situations on a paediatric ward it may be beneficial for a parent to spend time with another parent whose conversations do not include chemotherapy, blood counts and cancer.

The nurse also recognised a need for the child with cancer to perhaps integrate with the other children, but those with cancer and leukaemia are almost always accommodated in a cubicle because of the risk of infection on a ward that caters for so many specialities. The same nurse also acknowledged the tremendous support that families of children with malignancies get from one another.

Another area of stress mentioned that related more to the Plymouth experience was being present when bad news was given to families. Fortunately due to the relatively fewer cases dealt with in Plymouth this scenario is not encountered on a regular basis, but this may account for the nurses' perceived lack of communication skills in this area of care. A nurse wrote the following account:

> The first time I sat with a family while doctors explained that their child had cancer was awful. I cried almost as much as they did and felt totally useless and should have been stronger for them all.

It is fair to say that breaking bad news or being involved is never easy, and perhaps nurses judge themselves unfairly in these situations. However it may be beneficial to reflect on experiences such as breaking bad news to explore reactions and feelings to prepare for a similar experience. Nurses from both areas remarked on events such as relapse of disease, death and heavy workloads as causing stress; these issues will be explored later.

The survey carried out in Bristol included a non-random sample of 12 nurses all working on two paediatric oncology wards and the bone marrow transplant unit. The survey was chosen to establish the attitudes, opinions and beliefs of paediatric nurses caring for children with cancer and leukaemia in relation to how stress affected them personally. The same three open-ended questions were put forward encouraging the nurse to write as much or as little as was felt necessary. A total of 20 questionnaires were distributed, staff were asked only to state their grade and not their names. Grades D, E, F and G were represented in the survey. Twelve questionnaires were completed detailing causes of stress, effects and coping mechanisms used.

Nurses from Bristol believed that because the hospital was a regional centre they saw the rarer types of cancer, and because of this a poorer prognosis for the children affected. This was mentioned in a study by Harding (1994) (also conducted at the BRHSC), where nurses felt they did not see the 'successes', children tended to be admitted at diagnosis, times of relapse, intensification of treatment, when the child becomes unwell or in the terminal stages of their disease, with a great deal of the children returning to their own hospitals around the South West. Nurses also linked this to workload, remarking that they felt they had more work from children coming from all over the South West and their own catchment area of Bristol, which resulted in a high demand for beds. This workload for some had repercussions in trying to care for patients. No nurse in the Bristol survey commented on lacking communication skills, however what they did say was that they just did not have the time to sit and discuss patient care with children and their families. One nurse recognised parental distress on the ward, but felt usually she was too overloaded with work to be able to attend adequately to their needs; she wrote:

> I have feelings of inadequacy at times. I can't do everything,
> I need to support staff and feel frustrated that the patients
> and families are not getting the quality time they need.

None of the nurses in the survey commented on nursing other specialities (there were a few beds for one or two other specialities on each ward) as being a source of stress or, as the nurses in Plymouth felt, a way of dealing with stress through being able to do more than just cancer care. Harding (1994) did find that staff mentioned caring for children with non-accidental injuries on the same ward as children with cancer created difficulties for them in how they coped.

Coping mechanisms mentioned in both areas were similar, with talking to colleagues as the most quoted way of helping with stress. Nursing staff in Plymouth did consistently mention feelings of inadequacy, however this was not the same for staff in Bristol. It may be that the coping mechanisms used in Bristol are all well practiced because it is a regional centre catering for more children, compared to fewer cases in district centres where stress linked to cancer care is not a consistent feature of nursing practice. Nurses in Bristol commented on being able to see children who were 'doing well', as they felt they frequently only saw very sick children or often the worst cases. One nurse remarked that being able to rotate to the outpatient department for 3–6 months may allow nurses to see greater numbers of 'healthier' children being followed up for cancer. This was not mentioned by Plymouth staff, possibly because the outpatient department is situated next door to the ward and children attending oncology clinics almost always paid the ward a visit to chat to the staff. Again the number of children with cancer in Plymouth may be a contributing factor for staff not feeling the need to rotate to other areas.

In Bristol lack of time to care featured significantly as a cause of stress, whereas nurses in Plymouth felt lack of knowledge was a particular source of stress. Nurses in Plymouth do not have the same opportunity to continually practice skills in cancer care and therefore their progression in learning about paediatric oncology may be slower. However with advances in treatments children are living longer and requiring close follow-up for the late effects of treatment (Pinkerton *et al.*, 1994), and it may be that nursing staff in DGHs find they are caring for children with cancer and leukaemia on a more regular basis in the future. At present in Plymouth, to help nursing staff feel a little more confident, they are offered a 2-week introduction to paediatric oncology. This short course is based in Bristol at the BRHSC. Staff who have completed the course have said they feel equipped to continue learning about cancer care and believe it helps their practice. Currently the 6-month ENB 240 course is taught in Bristol, the closest centre to Plymouth, but for many nurses it is difficult to move away to attend the course due to personal commitments in Plymouth. For that reason it was not surprising to find a higher proportion of ENB 240 trained nurses in Bristol.

Although differences exist, the shared care initiative works well, with children in Plymouth and the surrounding South West receiving expert care from a multidisciplinary team in Bristol. A consultant from the BRHSC visits Plymouth once a month to discuss patient care with staff. With nurses attending the study weeks and the ENB 240 course, links are also forged with nursing staff in Bristol, which proves to be valuable in helping to increase expertise and provide support when needed.

Impact of caring on different grades of nursing staff

Research suggests that nurses with varying degrees of experience are affected by stress in a variety of different ways (Wilkinson, 1994). From personal experience it is evident that newly qualified nurses encounter different causes of stress compared to more experienced staff. Therefore it may be helpful to first illustrate levels of experience and expertise in the clinical setting. Theories from Benner (1984) will be explored to understand the journey a nurse makes from a beginner to expert. There are of course different theories and the reader is reminded to remain open to other opinions. However, to understand the difficulties a nurse faces when new to the profession and to paediatric oncology, Benner's ideas provide a framework with which to facilitate this understanding. This section will also focus on the impact of care on experienced nurses and those with the ENB 240 Paediatric Oncology certificate. The merits of reflective practice will be discussed in an attempt to show how nursing experience can be conceptualised using Carper's framework for reflection (Carper, 1978). Research has demonstrated a connection between higher levels of stress and newly qualified staff in oncology (Hinds *et al.*, 1994; Wilkinson, 1994). Lansdown *et al.* (1990) found nurses new to paediatric oncology may have taken on the work with high ideals and unrealistic expectations. Emery (1993) reported that new staff nurses felt they had to allocate themselves tasks in order to deliver nursing care and were aware of the possibility of making mistakes. Task-orientated work is reinforced in the study by Hinds *et al.* (1994), in which nurses felt a sense of urgency in trying to complete treatments and administer drugs even when time was against them. As well as the usual ward routines, newly qualified staff are in a position of caring for dying children with little practical educational preparation to help them cope for these situations (Saunders and Valente, 1994). Hinds *et al.* (1990) believes that inexperienced nurses may have their initial feelings of inadequacy reinforced by the constant confrontation with death and the inability to deal with the resulting emotional stress. If new staff are left to deal with these feelings alone, the outcome is often that they leave the speciality (Hinds *et al.*, 1994).

Benner describes newly qualified staff as being 'advanced beginners', often aware of situations on the ward, but unable to adopt a holistic approach to cope with them. At this stage nurses are still functioning at a level which encourages them to nurse by rules they have been taught in school, therefore being unable to prioritise work (Benner, 1984). This evaluation reflects the findings of research describing junior nurses as setting themselves tasks to complete delivery of care.

For newly qualified staff to negotiate difficulties and subsequent emotions, an external source of help is required (Hooton, 1994). The UKCC (1992b) proposed the role of a Preceptor to support and supervise newly qualified staff aiding the transition from student to staff nurse. However, successful transition depends firstly on the presence of a preceptor and the methods they employ to support the nurse. Benner (1984) advocates that the mentor provides guidelines to give new staff nurses cues to attend to patient needs in a holistic manner. Benner continues by stating that before this takes place, the nurse must first recognise the need to prioritise workload and time management. Peplau (1988) believes that effective learning can take place through experiences in which a person is involved and then develops around the interest the person has regarding the particular experience. Reflective practice is one way in which a nurse can learn from a pertinent experience, that is of course if the nurse is aware that learning is taking place (Boud, Keogh and Walker, 1985). Reflection often originates from practice which may have triggered uncomfortable feelings, therefore guided reflection may help the practitioner from becoming embroiled in negative responses. Boud *et al.* (1985) suggest that reflective techniques take time and practise to develop into an effective learning mechanism, and the nurse must find a model which suits them.

There are many models aiding practitioners to reflect in a structured way. Carper (1978) formulated a framework for nurses to become familiar with 'ways of knowing', that is to explore their practice using four categories of knowledge: empirical, aesthetic, ethical and personal knowledge. These categories are for nurses to become familiar with the full spectrum of their practice while working with their patients adopting humanistic values (Johns, 1995). Empirical knowledge prepares the nurse for the practical aspects of the job. Johns (1995) describes this knowledge as finding solutions according to the rules which govern practice. In her account of the 'advanced beginner', Benner talks of nurses learning about their role in terms of taking temperatures, recognising postoperative patient responses and prioritising workload. This would appear to be attending to practitioners' empirical knowledge needs. Nurses new to oncology are described as being task orientated and being acutely aware of making mistakes (Emery, 1993). Using Carper's framework for reflection, those nurses in oncology could not only attend to sorting and understanding empirical knowledge, but also find out more about why they respond to a particular situation in the way they did. This is aesthetic knowledge, much is being written about this often untapped source of knowledge which is sometimes referred to as intuition. Johns (1995) explains how difficult it is for nurses to describe practice involving intuition and for that reason it is often not taken seriously, however it is proving to be a rich source of learning and skilled care. Intuition may not come easily to some and therefore it may take experience to be able to practise using this knowledge. Frameworks like that of Carper help new and experienced staff to begin addressing this important aspect of care, and be able to describe it effectively through encounters during their careers.

According to Benner the next stage for staff after 'advanced beginner' is the 'competent practitioner'. Benner (1984) believes nurses at this phase have usually been in post for 2–3 years and are beginning to understand their actions in terms of long-range goals. Nurses with some experience plan care with some perspective, but still have difficulty in being able to recognise the overall picture in a situation (Benner, 1984). In the study by Hinds *et al.* (1994) comparing causes of stress and different grades of staff, it was found that nurses with at least 12 months of experience of paediatric oncology were concerned with why children had cancer and how they would cope with the treatment. They were also troubled by too many tasks and not enough time to complete them, and when stressed they were disappointed to discover that their coping strategies failed them. Benner (1984) suggests nurses at this stage require practice at coordinating complex patient demands to help them make the transition to becoming a proficient nurse. Nurses in the survey in Plymouth and Bristol at D grade level discussed having problems with caring for children who were dying in hospital (I accept that some D grade nurses have a great deal of experience and therefore do not fit with Benner's description of 'advanced beginner', however there were nurses who did fit the criteria). Hainsworth (1996) described how nurses caring for terminally ill patients in hospital expressed difficulty and feelings of stress, due in some way to hospital care being focused on curing patients. Bearing in mind what Benner suggests about nurses being unable to perceive all of the implications in a situation, it is understandable that nurses with limited experience may find it difficult to accept the end of active treatment and the beginning of terminal care. Hainsworth (1996) believes that little time is spent in nurse education preparing nurses for the care of dying patients, and when put into such situations nurses find it unbearable. Using Carper's reflective framework, nurses caring for terminally ill children can explore ethical implications as well as why they are reacting in a particular way to a situation. Experienced nurses are vital in these situations, as they will have experienced patient death and coming to terms with the end of active treatment.

Of course all nurses are affected by patient death, and in a study by Hainsworth (1996) it was established that the death of a loved one often determined how nurses perceived future deaths. It does however appear that although stressful, death and dying are found to be stressful in different ways. Hinds *et al.* (1994) found that nurses of considerable experience were stressed by lack of time to help children and their families face the realities of dying. They were also distressed by others' lack of care and support; however in examining how more junior nurses adapt to their roles, a perceived lack of care may in fact be an inability to cope with certain situations. Benner (1984) identifies that proficient and expert nurses are able to perceive situations as wholes rather than aspects. Their perception comes from experience and provides them with a holistic understanding of patient care. Differences between these two groups of nurses are the depth of experience and knowledge, Benner believes that proficient nurses learn from the use of reflection using critical incidents, comparing good experiences and bad. The same form of learning is advocated for expert nurses, however Benner feels that expert nurses need to take this further so that others can learn from their wealth of experience by the documentation of their practice. In using Carper's framework nurses are able to address all aspects of their knowledge, including personal knowledge. Reflection on positive and negative experiences throughout a nurse's career not only helps to find solutions to stress but also highlights the patient's lived experience of cancer. It can be argued that this creates a rich source of knowledge for nurses to carry forward to help other patients and nurses new to the speciality.

The rules which govern practice and give nurses a structure to their care can, if followed rigidly, hinder practice from developing (Benner, 1984). With the rich experiences nurses encounter their care is no longer solely dependent on rules and tasks. Nurses are able to use past experience to provide care that has proved effective, but to keep practice fresh and innovative a certain amount of rules are required in the form of theory and research (Benner, 1984). As previously mentioned the Scope of Professional Practice (UKCC, 1992b) offers nurses the chance to enhance their practice and take their skills forward in partnership with their patients and carers. It also gives nurses the opportunity to keep moving forward to make the necessary changes to help them through Benner's stages of experience. It would appear that nurses need support at all phases of practice from other nurses, benefiting from their expertise and personal interpretations of situations. Peplau (1988) describes some of the roles a nurse is expected to fulfil for patients, helping them to reach their own goals through teaching, counselling, previous experience and caring. All of these roles and many more can also be used to help nurses reach their potential, however it can be argued that to do this nurses need the time and resources to achieve all of this. It would seem that nurses are aware of their duty to care at whatever stage they are in their career, but are often stressed by the limitations imposed upon them as already identified.

Used effectively, reflection can help nurses make sense from their practice and can enhance practice. Literature reveals that nurses find value in discussing their stress. While it is acknowledged that this is important, at times it could be more structured in the form of reflection. This may be helpful to nurses who feel unsupported and contemplating leaving the speciality, especially if led by staff experienced in paediatric oncology.

Specific stressors and effects on nurses in paediatric oncology

Bond (1994) concluded in a study of work-related stresses that paediatric oncology nursing is a stressful speciality, and especially so when caring for dying children. This section does not intend to provide proof of evident stress in paediatric oncology, it is presumed through various studies to be a stressful occupation, but to establish what other authors and researchers have found and what effects of stress have been identified. Many studies illustrate causes of stress in cancer care, and although patient death evokes intense negative reactions with ongoing distress, it may also have a positive response (Saunders and Valente, 1994). Positive stress is growth producing and has been reported as getting nurses through difficult situations (Cohen et al., 1994). It is therefore important for nurses to be able to recognise stress and its negative effects, but also to realise the positive aspects and use them as a motivating force, with direction and guidance from ward managers. If stress is unrecognised there is the potential for nurses to enter the burnout stage, described as emotional exhaustion (Jenkins and Ostchega, 1986). This can be potentially serious for staff, their patients and the hospitals employing them. The consequences include deteriorating quality of care, increased absenteeism and, eventually, job exodus. Several nurses in the

Bristol survey experienced increased stress as a direct result of other nurses taking time off and the poor skill mix that resulted from staff shortages. It would be fair to suggest that nurses taking time off as a result of stress affects nurses remaining on the ward, especially if the gap is not filled in some way. Emery (1993) believes that management must be aware and responsive to stress experienced by paediatric nurses, in order to offer support and, hopefully, prevent situations which nurses perceive as stressful from progressing further.

Emery (1993) acknowledged anxiety resulting from the administration of drugs that cause numerous physical side effects such as hair loss, nausea and time spent in hospital as creating upset for the child and family. In addition to this the nurses were also aware of their own personal exposure to carcinogenic chemotherapy drugs. In regional centres like Bristol, nurses with the ENB 240 certificate were responsible for administering chemotherapy (Harding, 1994). A study by Tyler and Ellison (1994) identified nurses in oncology with a postregistration qualification experienced more stress through lack of support and a heavier workload. It could be reasonably suggested that some nurses have more exposure to chemotherapy, supporting Emery's findings (1993) that nurses have added emotional pressure and concerns for their own safety. This of course does not mean nurses without the paediatric oncology certificate experience less stress. Morse *et al.* (1992) believe that general nurses cannot physically escape from the patient's experience of suffering and some of that suffering is not under the direct control of the nursing profession. This can be further compounded by the perceived ineffectiveness of other members of the MDT who do not appear to be attending to the patient's needs. Jenkins and Ostchega (1986) argue that the number of deaths on a ward greatly influenced the amount of stress nurses experienced. This may be of significance for nurses in regional centres. Harding (1994) recognised that children came from all over the South West for treatment in Bristol, therefore the nurses there saw a higher proportion of children with cancer and also a higher number of deaths compared with nursing staff employed in DGHs. Yasko (1983) identified a link between the number of deaths on a ward and the lack of psychological support causing an increase in stress levels for staff. Saunders and Valente (1994) found that oncology nurses in the absence of support felt unable to verbalise grief, resulting in some nurses doubting their professional identity and self esteem. It may be that nurses doubting their role are not able to attend fully to the needs of children in their care. The survey of nursing staff in Bristol revealed that not attending fully to the needs of children and their families was a significant source of stress. The causes and effects of stress are closely linked and not always in the control of the nurse, this would endorse the opinion that support may be best suited to come from outside of the nurses' own networks (Yasko, 1983).

Closely linked with causes of stress are the effects and reactions experienced by nurses. Cohen *et al.* (1994) reported that symptoms of hypertension, infections due to altered immune responses and even cancer could be contributed to prolonged stress in oncology nursing. Psychoneuroimmunology is a relatively new field of study that investigates the interactions between neuro-endocrine and immune systems in response to such events as stress (Caudell, 1996). Studies show how stress affects the immune system in many ways, including suppression of antibody responses and cellular immune mechanisms (Caudell, 1996). Cognitive functions such as retention of information, calculations, etc. can also be affected (Benner and Wrubel, 1989). Nurses in the survey identified problems with their memories and lacked concentration, which creates even more of a problem if mistakes are made or more time is taken than required to carry out a task.

Unresolved stress may result in a condition known as 'burnout' (Allanach, 1988). Harris (1989) believes working closely and intensely with patients over long periods of time can lead to burnout. However research appears to show conflicting results when addressing levels of stress and burnout in cancer care. For example, Jenkins and Ostchega (1986) and Wilkinson (1994) concluded that oncology nurses do not experience high levels of stress and are not at great risk of burnout. These studies were not entirely taken from a paediatric nurse population and therefore not entirely appropriate to the paediatric oncology experience. Variables differ between the two disciplines, for example nurses encounter difficulties when trying to administer unpleasant chemotherapy, children require explanations and reassurance that the treatment is not a form of punishment and will make them better despite side effects (Waters, 1985). It would appear there are many causative factors in paediatric oncology which create stress for nurses even if they are experienced staff. However for those who remain in oncology it may be through accepting there will be sad and stressful times and being prepared to deal with these occasions effectively using well-rehearsed coping mechanisms.

Personality types and the relevance to coping mechanisms

Coping mechanisms vary according to the situations and individual personalities (Cohen *et al.*, 1994). It is suggested that adaptive coping is task orientated and deals with the problem or feelings associated with the problem. Maladaptive coping is thought to be a defence-orientated mechanism using techniques such as social isolation, drugs, alcohol and overuse of strategies that are normally adaptive (Cohen *et al.*, 1994). It is therefore recommended that a variety of adaptive coping mechanisms are identified and used. Jenkins and Ostchega (1986) implied in a study that lower burnout scores may partly depend on oncology nurses employing a range of coping strategies. Results from the survey carried out in Bristol revealed on average individual nurses identified between two and three coping mechanisms. Harding (1994) reported that despite nursing children with a terminal illness being considered stressful, some nursing staff felt they could cope because overall they enjoyed their work.

Mosely (1988) believes that sharing responses to issues such as patient death reduces feelings of isolation. Cohen *et al.* (1994) suggested that the process of talking about work leads nurses to take stock and recognise changes required to help them in their work. By doing so it may be seen that nurses are closer to developing what Benoliel (1988) described as an 'emotional muscle'. By understanding theory, using support and recognising their own mortality, nurses will be able to cope with caring for terminally ill patients (Benoliel, 1988). However it can be argued that without support and guidance to understand theory being provided by a ward, the nurse will not be given the chance to develop an effective coping mechanism such as an emotional muscle. The ward environment is one important factor in providing support and helping nurses to feel able to discuss their feelings when stressed (Lynn, 1992). Wilkinson (1994) who explored ward management issues, reported that staff valued a positive ward environment created by ward managers who were approachable and enthusiastic. This factor significantly helped to reduce perceived stress in oncology nursing (Wilkinson, 1994). Therefore it may be of value for staff to discuss research such as Wilkinson's at ward level to present differences in styles of management and environment to improve ward staff morale.

Nursing staff from the Bristol survey felt their families were a source of support to turn to in times of distress. Those nurses without a family are seen to exhibit more psychosomatic symptoms and resort to maladaptive or avoidance coping strategies (Tyler and Ellison, 1994). This may be of significance for nurses taking up posts away from family and friends. Browner (1987) suggests that social support set up at work reduces perceived job stress and its negative consequences. The promotion of support in the ward environment can be viewed as an important process to accept and assist new staff to settle in their posts, and also taking time to find out if new staff have family and friends in the area. The survey carried out in Bristol did not identify any formal support groups. Scully (1981) reported that outside experts such as psychologists involved in support groups can prove beneficial. However they may have difficulty identifying or understanding the feelings and perceptions expressed by nurses (Scully, 1981). Therefore individuals with a nursing background may be helpful to lead support groups. It should be remembered that nursing staff do not always have the facility to talk about problems when they arise. Workloads may prevent nurses from seeking help and therefore they may view formal support groups as impractical. Emery (1993) argues that if nurses are to deal with stress at ward level, they should be afforded the support of managers to nurture any positive advances.

Other methods of coping mentioned in the survey were issues of gaining access to information about children no longer on treatment or being treated on an outpatient basis. Harding (1994) reported staff were often not told of the progress of children treated in Bristol who then returned to their own areas. Link nurses may be a way of maintaining contact with the progress of children once back in their own areas. Results from research by Harding (1994) showed that nurses felt rotating to the outpatient department would give them the opportunity to see children off treatment or in better health than often seen on the wards. Rotating staff to other areas or keeping in contact with hospitals sharing care may encourage relations and sharing of knowledge. Hanson (1994) comments that the thread holding together the development of a paediatric oncology unit is the collaboration and close cooperation of all its members.

Literature supports the use of humour as an effective coping mechanism (White and House, 1991). One nurse in the survey identified humour as an aid to reducing stress on a ward. Theorists describe laughter as a necessary component of normal human psychological and physiological wellbeing (Smith, 1989). Simon (1989) states that laughter excretes secretions which contain bio-chemicals to deal with the accumulation of hormones and steroids produced as a result of stress. It is concluded that laughter is a catharsis which provides the body with a biological mechanism to release the tension (Simon, 1989). A study by White and House (1991) concluded that nurses might accept humour as a positive intervention to build group support which may buffer job strain. The study did not disclose information on the type of nursing sampled and therefore what relation to cancer care. The study concluded that humour may be judged as disparaging and there-fore how humour functions depends on how it is evaluated. It can be understood that while humour and laughter are effective when caring for children, parents may feel it inappropriate. It must be left to the nurse to judge the situation but be encouraged by the merits of laughter and humour.

It is interesting to note that when exploring the issue of stress and coping there appears to be less information on the role of personality and how it is illustrated through nurses' behaviour patterns when faced with consistently difficult situations. Earlier when dealing with the effects of stress it was mentioned that cancer may be attributed to prolonged stress. There is a considerable body of literature debating the existence of a cancer-prone personality (Benner and Wruble, 1989). That is to say cancer patients who have certain personality characteristics which can be perhaps linked to them having cancer. The link being made at this point is, interestingly, some of these traits can be seen in the way some nursing staff behave when dealing with stress that comes with caring for cancer patients.

Evidence and research into this subject matter extends some way back into history. Literature from the eighteenth and nineteenth centuries describe emotional distress as a cause of cancer (Greer, 1984). Personality types have been categorised into groups; coronary patients are placed into a 'Group B' detailing behaviour which may be responsible for their condition, cancer patients are classified as being in a 'Group C' (Guex, 1989). 'Type C' personality traits are described as repressing emotions, inhibition of aggression and relationships without conflict (Guex, 1989). Guex (1989) states that a significant number of studies have shown that individuals who repress their emotions can only deal with stress by exercising increased physiological control, therefore do the biological reactions have a pathogenic effect culminating in cancer? A stress response can be activated by anxiety and other emotions which have an effect on the sympathetic nervous system; increasing blood flow to skeletal muscle and acting upon endocrine function (Caudell, 1996). If the stress response continues, elevated hormone levels can lead to increased physiological and emotional reactivity and immunosuppression (Caudell, 1996). Physical and psychological effects from stress have been identified in the accounts given by nurses in research and literature dealing with stress. The problem appears to be when these effects occur and individuals try to distance themselves from the feelings or suppress them. Peplau (1988) believes nurses are unable to vent their true feelings as it would be considered unprofessional, therefore what do they do when feeling stressed or unhappy? Guex (1989) reports that those individuals able to speak about their feelings experience less stress at a physical level, for they regain a state of equilibrium. Benner and Wruble (1989) believe that part of stress management is to recognise feelings and not control them so rigidly that nothing can be learned from the experience. They go on to suggest that stress is alerting the individual that something important is at stake and needs to be attended to.

As Guex (1989) states, theories around a cancer-prone personality are divided, with evidence to suggest that cancer patients' behaviour may be a result of the disease and not the reverse. For example, the theory is difficult to apply to children with cancer who have not encountered life events which create stress in the way in which they are suggested to do in adults (Guex, 1989). From exploring research and literature it was difficult to find evidence to suggest that cultures where women have little power or choice in their own lives had a higher ratio of cancer, however, this may be due to the conditioning response of a particular culture nevertheless, it is interesting and valid to explore personality in relation to nurses and other members of the MDT caring for children and adults with cancer. The message from this section is not to suggest that by ignoring and suppressing feelings one will develop cancer (research is inconclusive), but the importance of attending to emotions and accepting them as part of a stressful occupation. However nurses will need guidance and support from experienced staff to be able to do this effectively and feel secure and safe. Purandare (1997) speculates on the absence of staff communication at an emotional level and the effect this has on honest and open communication with patients.

Conclusion

Perhaps the most striking feature of paediatric oncology is the stress involved in providing care for children and their families. The causes of stress appear to be varied, with individuals perceiving the causes and effects in different ways. It is accepted that caring for children with cancer and leukaemia is a stressful occupation and because of the nature of the work those causes of stress are likely to remain. Recent changes in the way in which nurses care are thought to bring additional stress from long and intense relationships. However, there are those who believe that relationships become stressful when nurses fail to care through remaining distant in an attempt to protect themselves from becoming too involved (Benner and Wruble, 1989). Relationships may also prove stressful because professional boundaries are blurred, with nurses becoming so close that they find it difficult to become objective about the role they serve in caring for a child with cancer. It would seem that it is a difficult balance for nurses to strike when so closely connected to a child's care, providing more than just physical nursing and dealing with not only personal emotions but also feelings and emotions displayed by family and other members of staff. However, families need effective nurses, someone who can be a friend in a professional sense, and paediatric oncology needs nurses to exercise self preservation to stay in the speciality to continue to care.

Other changes within health care are expanding nursing practice. Initiatives to reduce junior doctors' hours in the Calman Report (Department of Health, 1993) have given nurses more to do, helped by the Scope of Professional Practice (UKCC, 1992b) to ensure nurses are able to carry out new tasks. The Calman–Hine report (Department of Health, 1995) has also placed more responsibility on nursing staff to ensure patients receive a holistic approach to their care using the MDT. So it is understandable how, without the appropriate support, nurses have additional stress brought about by the multifaceted role they now have to adopt. Various research shows how many nurses are lost from paediatric oncology due to stress and subsequent lack of guidance. If the future of paediatric oncology nursing is to match the progress being made in the treatment of childhood malignancies, it is fair to assume nurses and nursing management must acknowledge the impact that caring makes on individual nurses. Advances in the treatment of cancer are becoming more intensive and complex with children surviving longer (Pinkerton *et al.*, 1994), therefore it is imperative that a growing speciality has a sufficient amount of skilled nurses to provide care and to pass on knowledge.

Experienced nurses in paediatric oncology have stated that, despite stressful situations, overall they enjoy their work and therefore feel able to cope effectively with stress (Harding, 1994). Although not directly suggested in the literature, these opinions may be linked with evidence to show nurses specialising in cancer care have taken time to consider issues of suffering, pain, dying and death before taking up posts in oncology. In recognising these factors, nurses are able to cope with the work they do and can move on from the initial responses of pity and sympathy to forming relationships with children and families which are productive, and the level of emotional involvement on the nurse's behalf is controlled to prevent burnout or excessive stress (Morse *et al.*, 1992). These are obviously important qualities which need to be utilised and taught to more junior nurses so that they may decide to specialise in paediatric oncology.

Boykin and Schenhofer (1990) assert that caring begins for nurses with knowing oneself and the care which has been received personally, at that point the nurse can move on to recognising others as worthy of care. It would be fair to assume from the evidence discussed in this chapter that caring can be stressful, especially when those being cared for die. Benner and Wruble

(1989) describe the stressful aspect of caring as being 'over-involved' and happens when the carer tries to control and dominate a situation to ensure they are protecting their interests. In cancer care, trying to control the inevitability of death is impossible and if left unresolved the carer may feel vulnerable and useless. Benner and Wruble (1989) suggest that practitioners instead help the patient to realise their own problems and anxieties and together try to go some way to solving them. Using reflection may be a way for nurses to re-evaluate their own caring abilities and enhance them further. However, as already established, nurses new to practising reflection may require help to make use of clinical incidents in oncology which appear to be negative or be encouraged to reflect upon good experiences exploring why the experiences were good (Hainsworth, 1996).

Wherever caring for children with cancer and leukaemia takes place there are difficulties to be dealt with. Nurses working in regional centres and district general hospitals all show their own types of stress which appear to be specific to their own particular situation. Regional centres have a higher proportion of deaths due to the specialised work they do and nurses recognise this as a factor contributing to their stress. Nurses working in district general hospitals also feel stressed by the comparatively fewer deaths they are exposed to. They felt less equipped to deal with death as they believe they have less experience. Although not mentioned by either groups of nurses, access to a counsellor may help as a coping mechanism to discuss feelings associated with caring for dying children. The counsellor may have the expertise to guide nurses with their feelings, to make use of them and not simply try to avoid sad or frustrating emotions. Some research found that nurses find it difficult to relate to a counsellor who does not have a nursing background and therefore would be unable to understand situations or experiences peculiar to nursing. There are of course other problems of not having someone to talk to when the need arises due to shift work or a heavy workload. Also there are still problems in getting nurses to talk to a counsellor as they do not want to appear to be unable to cope, yet as nurses we would assist families to find help in coming to terms with the loss of a loved one. It would appear that in choosing paediatric oncology nurses must accept a certain amount of stress is inevitable and therefore should seek the best way to deal with it. In doing so it could be argued that more junior staff will not follow the same patterns and bring to an end taboos surrounding stress and the inability to deal with it.

There are of course other sources of stress not discussed in this chapter, for example there is a large body of literature exploring the issue of shift work and its impact on nurses. Sources of stress

- What causes you most stress in your job? i.e., death of a child, demands on your time etc.
- What physiological and/or psychological effects do you experience when stressed? i.e., increased smoking, poor memory, etc.
- What coping mechanisms do you use to combat the effects of stress?

are often out of nurses' control, some due to changes within the health service or the advancement in treatments for cancer which impacts on nursing care. Coping methods are however within the realm of nursing practice, and need to be addressed at all levels of the nursing hierarchy from newly qualified staff to management in a bid to help nurses care more effectively and remain within this ever-growing speciality.

References

Allanach, E.J. (1988) Perceived supportive behaviours. *Advanced Nursing Science*, **10**, 73–82.

Bailey, R.D. (1985) *Coping with Stress in Caring*. Oxford: Blackwell Scientific.

Benner, P. (1984) *From Novice to Expert*. Reading: Addison Wesley.

Benner, P. & Wrubel, J. (1989) *The Primacy of Caring: stress and coping in health and illness*. Reading: Addison Wesley.

Benoliel, J. (1988) Health care delivery: not conducive to teaching palliative care. *Journal of Palliative Care*, **4**(1), 41–42.

Bond, D. (1994) The measured intensity of work-related stressors in paediatric oncology nursing. *Journal of Pediatric Oncology Nursing*, **11**(2), 44–152.

Boud, D., Keogh, R. & Walker, D. (1985) *Reflection: turning experience into learning*. London: Kogan Page.

Bowlby, J. (1973) *Attachment and Loss*, vol. II: *Separation, anxiety and anger*. London: Penguin.

Boykin, A. & Schoenhofer, S. (1990) Caring in nursing: analysis of extant theory. *Nursing Science Quarterly*, **3**(4), 149–153.

Browner, C.H. (1987) Job satisfaction and health: the role of social support at work. *Research in Nursing and Health*, **10**, 93–100.

Carper, B. (1978) Fundamental ways of knowing in nursing. *Advances in Nursing Science*, **1**(1), 13–23.

Casey, A. (1988) A partnership with child and family. *Senior Nurse*, **8**(4), 8–9.

Casey, A. (1995) Partnership nursing: influences on involvement of informal carers. *Journal of Advanced Nursing*, **22**, 1058–1062.

Caudell, K.A. (1996) Psychoneuroimmunology and innovative behavioural interactions in patients with leukaemia. *Oncology Nursing Forum*, **23**(3), 493–502.

Children Act (1989) London: HMSO.

Clarke, J. & Wheeler, S. (1992) A view of the phenomenon of caring in nursing practice. *Journal of Advanced Nursing*, **17**(11), 1283–1290.

Cleary, J. (1992) *Caring for Children in Hospital: parents and nurses in partnership*. London: Scutari Press.

Cohen, M.Z., Haberman, M., Steeves, R. & Deatrick, J.A. (1994) Rewards and difficulties of oncology nursing. *Oncology Nursing Forum*, **21**(8), 9–16.

Corner, J. (1988) Assessment of nurses' attitudes towards cancer: a critical review of research methods. *Journal of Advanced Nursing Care*, **13**(5), 640–648.

Coyne, I.T. (1995) Partnerships in care: parents' views of participation in their hospitalized child's care. *Journal of Clinical Nursing*, **4**, 71–79.

Darbyshire, P. (1994) *Living with a Sick Child in Hospital: the experiences of parents and nurses*. London: Chapman & Hall.

Davidson, L. & Lucas, J. (1995) Multiprofessional education in the undergraduate health professions curriculum: observations from Adelaide, Linköping and Salford. *Journal of Interprofessional Care*, **9**(2), 163–176.

Dear, S. (1995) Breaking bad news: caring for the family. *Nursing Standard*, **10**, 31–36.

Department of Health (1991) *The Patient's Charter Raising the Standard*. London: HMSO.

Department of Health (1993) *Hospital Doctors Training for the Future. The Report of the Working Group on Specialist Medical Training. (The Calman Report.)* London: HMSO.

Department of Health (1995) *A Policy for Commissioning Cancer Services. A Report by the Expert Advisor on Cancer to the Chief Medical Officers of England and Wales. (Calman–Hine Report).* London: HMSO.

Emery, J. (1993) Perceived sources of stress among paediatric oncology nurses. *Journal of Pediatric Oncology Nursing*, **10**(3), 87–92.

Evans, M. (1994) An investigation into the feasibility of parental participation in the nursing care of their children. *Journal of Advanced Nursing*, **20**, 477–482.

Fradd, E. (1994) Power to the people. *Paediatric Nursing*, **6**(3), 11–14.

Geen, L. (1986) A special friend. *Nursing Times*, **3**, 32–33.

Greer, S. (1984) The psychosocial dimension in cancer treatment. *Social Science and Medicine*, **18**, 345–349.

Guex, P. (1989) *An Introduction to Psycho-oncology*. London: Routledge.

Hainsworth, D. (1996) The effect of death education on attitudes of hospital nurses toward care of the dying. *Oncology Nursing Forum*, **23**(6), 963–967.

Hanson, E.J. (1994) An explanation of the taken for granted world of the cancer nurse in relation to stress and the person with cancer. *Journal of Advanced Nursing*, **19**, 12–20.

Harding, R. (1994) *Causes and Management of Stress for Trained Nurses Caring for Children with Cancer and Leukaemia*. Bristol: Avon and Gloucester College of Health.

Harris, R.B. (1989) Reviewing nursing stress. *Advanced Nursing Science*, **11**, 12–28.

Hinds, P.S., Fairclough, D.C., Green, R.H., Maynall, J. & Day, L.A. (1990) Development and testing of the stressor scale for paediatric oncology nurses. *Cancer Nursing*, **13**(6), 354–360.

Hinds, P.S., Quargnent, A.G. & Hickey, S.S. (1994) A comparison of the stress response sequence in new and experienced paediatric oncology nursing. *Cancer Nursing*, **17**(1), 61–71.

Hooton, M. (1994) Clinical supervision. *Paediatric Nursing*, **6**(7), 8–10.

Jenkins, J.F. & Ostchega, Y. (1986) Evaluation of burnout in oncology nurses. *Cancer Nursing*, **9**(3), 108–116.

Johns, C. (1995) Framing learning through reflection within Carper's fundamental ways of knowing in nursing. *Journal of Advanced Nursing*, **22**, 226–234.

Kennedy, P. & Grey, N. (1997) High pressure areas. *Nursing Times*, **93**(29), 26–28.

Kerstetter, N. (1990) A stepwise approach to developing and maintaining an oncology multidisciplinary conference. *Cancer Nursing*, **13**(4), 216–220.

Kunkler, J. & Whittick, J. (1991) Stress management groups for nurses: practical problems and possible solutions. *Journal of Advanced Nursing*, **16**, 172–176.

Langstaff, D. & Gray, B. (1997) Flexible roles: a new model in nursing practice. *British Journal of Nursing*, **6**(11), 635–638.

Lansdown, R., Pike, S. & Smith, M. (1990) Reducing stress in the cancer ward. *Nursing Times*, **86**(38), 34–38.

Lynn, C. (1992) Where can I go? *Nursing Times*, **88**(20), 52.

Mast, D., Meyers, J. & Urbanski, A. (1987) Relaxation techniques: a self-learning module for nurses. *Cancer Nursing*, **10**(3): 141–147.

Morse, J.M., Botorff, J., Anderson, G., O'Brien, B. & Solberg, S. (1992) Beyond empathy: expanding expressions of caring. *Journal of Advanced Nursing*, **17**, 809–821.

Mosely, J.R. (1988) Developing a bereavement program in a university hospital setting.

Oncology Nursing Forum, **15**, 151–155.

Norris, E. (1995) Achieving professional autonomy for nursing. *Professional Nurse*, **11**(1)

Peplau, H. (1988) *Interpersonal Relations in Nursing*. London: MacMillan Education.

Pinkerton, G., Cushing, P. & Sepion, B. (1994) *Childhood Cancer Management: a practical handbook*. London: Chapman & Hall Medical.

Platt, H. (1959) *The Welfare of Children in Hospital. Report Committee on Child Health Services*. London: HMSO.

Purandare, L. (1997) Attitudes to cancer may create a barrier to communication between patient and caregiver. *European Journal of Cancer Care*, **6**, 92–99.

Robertson, J. (1958) *Young Children in Hospital*. London: Tavistock.

Robinson, C. (1985) Parents of hospitalised chronically ill children: competency in question. *Nursing Papers*, **17**(2), 59–68.

Saunders, J.M. & Valente, S.M. (1994) Nurses' grief. *Cancer Nursing*, **17**(4), 318–325.

Scully, R. (1981) Staff support groups: helping nurses to help themselves. *Journal of Nursing Administration*, **11**(3), 48–51.

Selye, H. (1980) *The Stress of Life*. New York: McGraw-Hill.

Sepion, B. (1990) Teamwork. Caring for the child, the family and staff *in* Thompson, J. ed. *The Child with Cancer*. London: Scutari Press.

Simon, J.M. (1989) Humour techniques in oncology nurses. *Oncology Nurses Forum*, **16**(5), 667–670.

Smith, P. (1989) Nurses' emotional labour. *Nursing Times*, **85**(47), 49–51.

Stutzer, C. (1989) Work related stresses of bone marrow transplant nurses. *Journal of Pediatric Oncology Nursing*, **6**, 70–78.

Tyler, P.A. & Ellison, R. (1994) Sources of stress and psychological well-being in high dependancy nursing. *Journal of Advanced Nursing*, **19**, 469–476.

UKCC (1992a) *The Code of Professional Conduct*. London: UKCC.

UKCC (1992b) *The Scope of Professional Practice*. London: UKCC.

Waters, A.L. (1985) Support for staff in a paediatric oncology unit. *Nursing*, **43**, 1275–1276.

Wheeler, H.H. (1997) Nurse occupational stress research 2: definition and conceptualization. *British Journal of Nursing*, June.

White, C. & House, E. (1991) Managing humour: when it is funny and when it is not. *Nursing Management*, **24**(4), 80–96.

WHO (1988) *Learning Together to Work Together for Health*. Technical Report Series 769. Geneva: WHO.

Wilkinson, S.M. (1994) Stress in cancer nursing: does it really exist? *Journal of Advanced Nursing*, **20**, 1079–1084.

Wilson, J. (1996) A look up the scope. *Nursing Management*, **2**(8), 16–17.

Yasko, J. (1983) Variables which predict burnout experienced by oncology clinical nurse specialists. *Cancer Nursing*, April, 109–116.

Coping mechanisms 7

MERVYN TOWNLEY AND STUART WELTON

Key points
- Use of defence mechanisms
- Common coping strategy in response to stress
- Benefit to child and family
- Simple model of stress
- Illustrates facets involved in stress
- Helps in understanding of stress from cancer
- Play
- Crucial to normal development process
- Helps to reduce anxiety in children
- Support groups
- For children with cancer
- For families of children with cancer
- Assistance in long-term emotional stability
- Family roles and responsibilities
- Alternation of roles when child has cancer
- Consideration of principles from family therapy
- Complementary therapies
- Principles
- Potential uses
- Psychosocial support
- As benefit for child and family

Introduction

The purpose of this chapter is to examine the various coping strategies that may be utilised by children who have cancer and their families during what may be long and sustained periods of illness. A range of methods may be employed, including those that may be of a unique nature to each child or the family and those that may be offered from a range of different professionals. The methods examined in this chapter form only a small number of those that may be available and serves to give the reader some insight into their use. Following some thoughts on coping strategies in general there will be some discussion on the use of play, support groups, family therapy, complementary therapies and some forms of psychosocial support

Firstly, it is important to understand what may be meant by 'coping'. Every one of us is faced with difficulties and problems on an almost daily basis. Coping is how we respond to these and may take the form of a range of thoughts, feelings and actions. For many situations we are able to deal with them with ease and without undue stress. However, there are also situations that provoke varying degrees of stress which cause unpleasant feelings of anxiety. There are a number of ways in which this may then manifest itself. Atkinson (1993) gave details of two main forms in which we cope in these situations.

The first form is known as problem-focused coping and involves either tackling the problem in an attempt to resolve it or developing strategies to avoid it altogether. For example a girl who is in her GCSE exam year may fail her mock exams unexpectedly. If she seeks extra help from her teachers and devises a study plan with her parents at home she is responding to the stressful situation by focusing on the problem itself.

The other way in which we might respond is known as emotion-focused coping and entails dealing with the emotions that may be experienced as a result of the stressor. The aims of these strategies are to reduce the unpleasant feelings that may be associated with being stressed (Beresford, 1993). For example the girl above may choose to avoid her feelings of anxiety resulting from her failure by convincing herself that it is unimportant to pass her exams and that they will serve her no useful purpose, as the job she wants to do does not require them. Alternatively, she may socialise at every opportunity in order that she can avoid having to think of her predicament.

It may be that both these strategies are used for coping either at the same time or at different times, and from the example given it is not difficult to imagine a combination of responses from the girl.

Sloper and While (1996) suggest that although the research is not as prolific with children as it is with adults, there would seem to be some significance, in terms of outcome, of the coping strategy that is used. However, it is only too easy to judge outcome from the perspective of the professional, and what may be seen as good coping strategies by them may not necessarily be good for the child or for other members of the family. In any discussion involving issues such as these the uniqueness of each individual's stress should always be remembered.

The higher the level of stress or anxiety that we are experiencing the more likely it is that the emotion-focused strategies will be used and, likewise, episodes of moderate levels of stress are

- We all experience situations that we find traumatic. Think back to a recent example of when you have been stressed by events in your life.
- How did this make you feel?
- What were the methods you employed to deal with this?
- Now read on and see if your method of coping is similar to any that follow

more likely to be dealt with by using problem-focused methods. As health professionals there are a number of other strategies that we may be in a position to offer the child or their family, of which several are dealt with later in the chapter.

Freud wrote about emotion-focused coping strategies that he called defence mechanisms. These are attempts to defend ourselves against potential threat from stressors by distorting how we might perceive things. He saw this as an unconscious process, and from Table 7.1 below it is easy to identify with the examples given and at some stage it is likely that we use some of these mechanisms as strategies to deal with our stress.

It is important to acknowledge that these mechanisms and indeed others not listed are used by all of us to varying degrees. They are important in helping us through difficult phases of life when the level of stress is high and allows us to then deal with the stress at a later time. However, if these mechanisms are used in such a way that the stress in not being dealt with, i.e. the distortion or deception of reality is a long-term coping mechanism, then this is viewed as both unhealthy and undesirable (Gross,

Table 7.1   Some classic psychological defence mechanisms (adapted from Gross (1992) and Atkinson (1993))

Mechanism	Explanation	Example
Denial	When reality is too difficult to face up to we might deny it exists at all	Parents of a child with a malignant tumour refuse to admit anything is wrong despite being fully informed
Repression	This involves being able to forget and exclude from conscious awareness thoughts and feelings that are too painful or frightening to deal with at the time	A 14 year old who has been told that a bone marrow transplant is the best course of treatment for him Is able to carry on without thinking about it at all
Rationalisation	This involves carefully analysing problems so that a logical and socially acceptable explanation can be found in order that we can show that we have acted rationally. This often entails searching for a sound reason rather than the real reason for one's behaviour	A colleague may fail to attend a series of ward meetings. The 'rational' reason being that there is always too much to do on the ward. The actual reason may be the fear that if she attends she will get into conflict with her colleagues. However, the reason given may be seen as quite acceptable

Table 7.1   (cont'd)

Mechanism	Explanation	Example
Displacement	Freud suggests that we all have a number of basic drives which are experienced in response to various situations. Where it would cause too much anxiety to direct these drives to the person or people who provoke the feelings in the first place, they are 'displaced' or directed elsewhere	Parents of a child who feel that they have been neglected or mistreated by the medical staff may vent their anger on the nursing staff when minor incidents of frustration or conflict arise
Reaction formation	This involves being able to substitute thoughts or feelings about what we really think or feel, often with those that give strong expression of the opposite	The mother who thinks that her child should die rather than be put through vigorous treatment regimens may deal with this by being overprotective, overindulgent and appear enthusiastic with the progress in treatment
Projection	Feelings that are difficult to handle and not wanted are attributed to someone else	A nurse who finds the nature of a child's illness distressing may suggest to the parents that it must be very distressing for them
Intellectualisation	Dealing with stressful situations by being very matter of fact and discussing it in intellectual ways	Dealing with a child undergoing chemotherapy who is suffering enormously by way of side effects by seeking information on drug half-lives or discussing with colleagues the various attributes of different drug regimens.

1992). Most adults have developed mental mechanisms in some form or other and to some extent may have support networks involving competent adult peers. Additionally, adults may have formed spiritual beliefs, have personal decision-making power and perhaps alternative physical activities that may help them cope with stress and crisis and avoid serious problems.

Children, on the other hand, often experience changes or crises in life which they are not able to fully understand and for which they cannot foresee beyond the short-term consequences of the situation. The younger the child the less likely they will have developed the coping mechanisms available to adults, have less support from emotionally stable peers and less autonomy in decision making. A relatively small change in adult perception, such as changing schools, may be extremely traumatic if the child has no support and limited life experience. Dealing with cancer and the many traumatic issues and experiences associated with it is therefore likely to have an even higher impact on younger and not well supported children. This may lead to a severe adjustment disorder, which includes exaggeration of normal childhood stress reactions such as crying, depression, anxiety, hyperactivity, sleeplessness and lethargy that may persist for months or that are extreme in their presentation. Indeed, it is known that children with life-threatening illnesses are more prone to mental health problems and disorders (Rutter, Taylor and Hersov, 1994; Department of Health, 1995) (Table 7.2).

Having talked about stress it is important to recognise those situations that may trigger such behaviours and emotions that have been described. From the above activity you are likely to have developed a list which shows a number of key life events that are known to cause stress reactions in many people. Monat and Lazurus (1985) discussed the work of Holmes and Rahe, who developed what they termed 'The Social Readjustment Scale', which identified those life events that were deemed to be associated with future illness. The interesting thing to note from this work is that those events normally seen as positive such as marriage or changing jobs (promotion for example) are also

Earlier you were asked to consider one event that you found stressful. Now spend a few minutes thinking about the most stressful times that have occurred in your life to date and write them down beginning with the most severe.

Table 7.2 Mental health problems and disorders (reproduced with permission from Department of Health 1999 Crown copyright material is reproduced with the permission of the Controller of Her Majesty's Stationery Office)

Mental health problems	Mental health disorders
Nocturnal enuresis	Emotional disorders with onset in childhood
Sleep difficulties	Major depression
Feeding difficulties in children	Conduct disorder
Abdominal pain without organic cause	Tic disorder
	Obsessive–compulsive disorder
Severe tantrums	Hyperkinetic disorder
Simple phobias	Encopresis
Educational difficulty	Anorexia nervosa
	Bulimia nervosa
	Attempted suicide/deliberate self harm
	Suicide
	Substance misuse

Case study 7.1

Becky was diagnosed as having ALL aged 7 years. She was treated for some time and was described as a happy and cheeky girl. Her condition relapsed and a bone marrow transplant failed. Her family spent a lot of time and money in travelling abroad in search of the treatment that would cure their daughter. Becky eventually ended up in hospital at a crisis point in her illness. It was being questioned whether a second transplant would be the appropriate course of action. It was at this point that Becky became uncommunicative and closed herself off from the staff and her parents. The culmination of several years of treatment and periods of isolation had been an emotional battering for Becky. She remained in this almost catatonic state for several weeks. One particular nurse had an exceptional relationship with her and this was utilised to help Becky and regain her confidence, motivation and regain her self esteem. Unfortunately, Becky died before a second transplant was possible but some compensation for relatives and other carers was her progression from what was a severe emotional reaction to her illness.

sources of stress as a result of the degree of readjustment that may be required. For the significance to families who have a child with cancer the importance of this should not be underestimated. From the list in Box 7.1, personal injury or illness and major health changes in a family member feature as having high mean values in potential effects on future health. It is not unusual to experience major financial implications as a result of childhood illness of this nature, and this too appears in the top 16 events. It is thought that the higher your score within the previous 2 years the more susceptible to illness you are likely to become in the following years. This should highlight to all health professionals that we have a responsibility to develop an awareness when families are subjected to highly scored life events and to consider offering some of the coping strategies outlined in this chapter, and reinforces the importance of the philosophy of family-centred care.

The research in Box 7.1 was completed using data from adults. While many of the life events may be equally applicable to children, there are also a range of stressors that are likely to have a particular impact on them (and these will vary depending on the developmental stage of the child) or will be perceived very differently in terms of severity. For example, the death of a pet is likely to feature as a particularly stressful life event for some children.

Whether stressors are enough to produce behavioural-focused

Box 7.1   The Social Readjustment Rating Scale: 16 of 43 items listed (adapted from Monat & Lazurus, 1985)

Life event	Mean value
1. Death of spouse	100
2. Divorce	73
3. Marital separation	65
4. Detention in jail or other institution	63
5. Death of a close family member	63
6. Major personal injury or illness	53
7. Marriage	50
8. Being made redundant/loss of job	47
9. Marital reconciliation	45
10. Retirement from work	45
11. Major change in health or behaviour of family member	44
12. Pregnancy	40
13. Sexual difficulties	39
14. Gaining a new family member (birth, adoption, relative, etc.)	39
15. Major business readjustment	39
16. Major change in financial state (for better or worse)	38

responses or emotional-focused responses, or indeed if they should lead to mental health problems or disorders, will depend on how each individual perceives the particular event. Similar events experienced by two different individuals may produce very different responses.

Having acknowledged that children with cancer and their families are likely to be under more stress than usual, it is important to examine the various mechanisms or strategies that may be employed to reduce the impact of this. The psychological mechanisms that may be used have already been outlined (and the long-term use of these recognised as usually unhealthy) and the potential range of mental health problems and disorders identified. However, there are a number of strategies that may be used to help minimise the potential negative responses to the illness.

There are a number of models which could be utilised in relation to stress and coping. The model for stress and coping by Lazurus (in Ellerton *et al.*, 1994) and that in Aitken and Hathaway (1993) are two such models, and they have been adapted to produce the model shown in Figure 7.1, which we believe to have particular relevance to the coping strategies of children with cancer. There are key features to this model that are of particular note. It is important to recognise that the most important place

Figure 7.1 Stress model for children with cancer (adapted from Lazarus (1984) in Ellerton, Ritchie and Caty (1994) Factors influencing young children's coping behaviours during stressful healthcare encounters. *Maternal-Child Nursing*, **22**(3), 74–82. and Aitken & Hathaway (1993) Long distance related stressors and coping behaviours in parents of children with cancer. *Journal of Pediatric Oncology Nursing*, **10**(1), 3–12.)

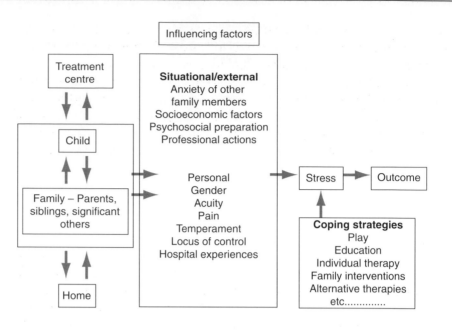

for the child is at home with the family members or significant others. The significant others could even include pets, which may have a special emotional attachment for the child. As a result of diagnosis the treatment centre becomes of particular significance to the child and family as well. Close relationships with some personnel may develop and it is likely that several different geographical services will be involved. Unless the family happen to live within close proximity to the specialist centre, the local hospital, the GP and perhaps community nurses are likely to all form part of the 'treatment centre'.

The effect and ultimately initial responses to illness will be determined to a large degree by a range of factors, some of which are identified in Figure 7.1. There are clear implications for the professionals involved at the diagnostic stage, as this model demonstrates. These issues are dealt with elsewhere in this book, but much can be done at this stage to minimise the longer-term emotional turmoil that can potentially occur.

There will be a level of stress that results from the illness. To what degree this develops will be different for all children and families. Consequently the strategies that may be employed to help alleviate some of the stress will also be different for them. Some of the options available are listed, but this of course is only a small list of possibilities.

The level of stress, together with the degree of use of coping strategies, will determine the outcome. What is meant by outcome is essentially the level at which the child and family are functioning at a personal and social level. How they perceive the illness, the emotional response, morale and how well they are functioning socially may all be markers used to determine outcome.

As professionals we have a responsibility to determine what may be available to these children and their families and to have some understanding of how such coping strategies may be of some help. This chapter will now explore a range of these strategies in an attempt to illustrate the potential benefits of them.

Play

Play is a term that encompasses a wide range of activities and for some time has been acknowledged as having a vital role in social, cognitive and emotional development. Just because a child becomes sick in some way does not take away the need to develop in these areas. The sick child may, however, be disadvantaged, as a number of circumstances may lead to the reduction of opportunities for play. The child in isolation, for example, is going to be limited in the range of play activities available. For some children with cancer there are a number of situations where the use of play can be of particular significance in sustaining development.

Examples of these will be illustrated, but in order to understand these better it is important to remember that there is an important link between the developmental stage of the child and the types of play that may be appropriate. It is also important to recognise that the developmental stage of an individual child may not correlate to their chronological age and this may result from differences prior to an illness but can also be a result of the illness. Frankenfield (1996) discussed the importance of using humour with children with cancer and identified various activities that made children laugh and that might be seen as fun. By expanding her list to include a range of other play activities, those listed in Table 7.3 may be seen as a rough guide.

The importance of play cannot be underestimated and in many hospitals there are play leaders specifically employed to help coordinate and promote various play activities. It should be remembered, however, that with more care needs being met within the home setting, those professionals involved at this level should also develop skills in recognising the play needs of children in order that they may be able to offer appropriate advice or guidance. It has been recognised in a number of key reports (Department of Health, 1992; Hogg, 1996) that specialists in play should be available to children in hospital.

The following examples of how play may benefit children in

Table 7.3 Activities that may be used to encourage humour in children with cancer (adapted, from Frankenfield, 1996)

Piaget's stage of development	Developmental activities: humourous and others
Sensorimotor Birth to 18 months	Familiar voices and people, motion of body parts, tickling, toys that make a noise, peek-a-boo (4–8 months), bubbles, humorous routines
Preoperational thought (preconceptual phase) 2–4 years	Pretend, make-believe play, fantasy, imaginary friends, playing dressing up, funny stories and pictures, intense activity in group games (running, jumping, etc.)
Preoperational thought (intuitive phase) 4–7 years	Silly songs/cartoons, playing with word rhymes, made-up words, tongue twisters, 4 year olds laugh in reaction to behaviours that deliberately violate social norms (father putting on child's hat), practical jokes, drawing funny pictures, laughing at mishaps and playing pranks, school age children imitate teachers
Concrete operations 6–12 years	Interested in ready-made jokes and riddles, capable of understanding more abstract and implied incongruities and not just those that can be immediately perceived, understands the double meaning of words, 'oh gross', stage-slime, whoopie cushions, fake poop, etc., Nintendo computer games
Formal operations 13 years to adult	Peer-related laughter, sexual overtones, funny films, writing funny stories, irony, sarcasm

hospital are taken from the experiences of the play specialists at the Bristol Children's Hospital.

Reducing the effects of isolation

The effects of isolation are well documented (Wong, 1997) and, combined with the effects of intensive care, the restrictions imposed on children are immense. In a bone marrow transplant Unit both these situations combine to produce a highly stressful environment for a child to endure for a long period of time. It therefore requires some innovative and creative thinking to help reduce this stress. In Figure 7.2 the results of a particularly creative project with children can be seen. This arose from ideas developed by the children themselves and was developed on a daily basis with the play specialist and the unit staff. The project became a focal point for the children, their families and for staff.

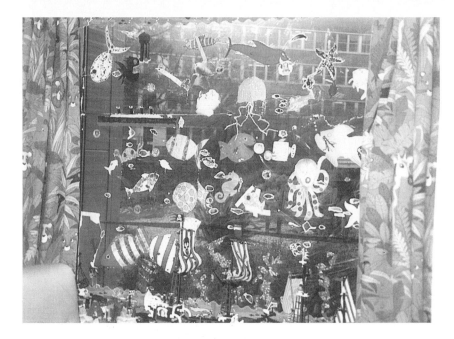

Figure 7.2   A mural which was developed in a play project for children in hospital (reproduced with permission of the Play Department, Bristol Children's Hospital)

The role of the play therapist in cooperation with other staff is crucial to the process of reducing the harmful effects of the isolation and intensity of treatment. Her continued presence in helping the children create these window pictures was essential. Experience in developing play in a sterile, restricted environment where no peers are available meant that the three children involved were allowed to retain some normal developmental experiences. However, it is important to remember that there are going to be times in the day when children undergoing treatment are too tired to engage in or concentrate on play (Wilson, Kendrick and Ryan, 1992).

Preparing children for surgical and other procedures

The benefits of preparing children for various procedures or for surgery by reducing their anxiety is well documented (Thornes, 1991; McMahon, 1992; Hogg, 1994). This can be achieved in a variety of ways and depends on the age of the child. For example, the use of a doll to explain the care required for a longline was used in Case study 7.2.

Story telling is one of the play activities that many children enjoy, and when this is combined with a visual set of cues children can build up a better understanding of what is being explained. It is no surprise then that this method of preparation for children can be very effective (Dwivedi, 1997).

Figure 7.3 is an example of pages from a book that has been

Case study 7.2

Jo was 9 years old and had returned home following a lengthy spell of treatment. She adamantly refused to allow anyone to touch her longline (wiggly) and consequently there was a serious risk of infection. The play leader visited Jo and left a doll to one side while spending some time with her. On getting up to leave the play leader mentioned that she had this doll that needed caring for but had no one to do it. Jo immediately jumped at the opportunity to care for the doll. The play leader explained that the doll had a wiggly and that it was important to look after this as well. She went on to demonstrate what was needed for the doll and why this was important for the doll's well being. Subsequent visits from nurses presented no problems provided the doll had the same care as Jo.

developed and utilised in the past by staff at the Bristol Children's Hospital. The book can be coloured in and provides a basis from which children may be able to ask questions. Parents sometimes also benefit from a simple explanation of such procedures and help make sense of the technical jargon that may have been used with them. There are many examples of such books, produced both nationally and locally, which are often developed by staff from play specialist departments.

There are occasions when models can be used as part of a package to prepare children for procedures. A superb example of this is written up by Pressdee *et al.* (1997), who describe how a model of a scanner with playpeople can be used to demonstrate the processes involved. To further the understanding of such procedures photographs can be used to show what various equipment actually looks like and even the use of tape recorders to demonstrate what various pieces of machinery sounds like (such as the sounds of a scanner) is very effective. All these fall within the range of activities that most children consider play, and therefore the effect is to reduce the level of anxiety surrounding them by presenting them in a familiar medium.

The needs of adolescents

It is sometimes difficult to meet the needs of adolescents who have cancer. It is clear from the evidence available that the adolescent population fare badly generally within the health care system (Action for Sick Children, 1990; Department of Health, 1991) and provision for adolescents with cancer is no different. Many trusts who fail to provide appropriate resources (Audit Commission, 1993) and it is often left to the goodwill of play leaders and

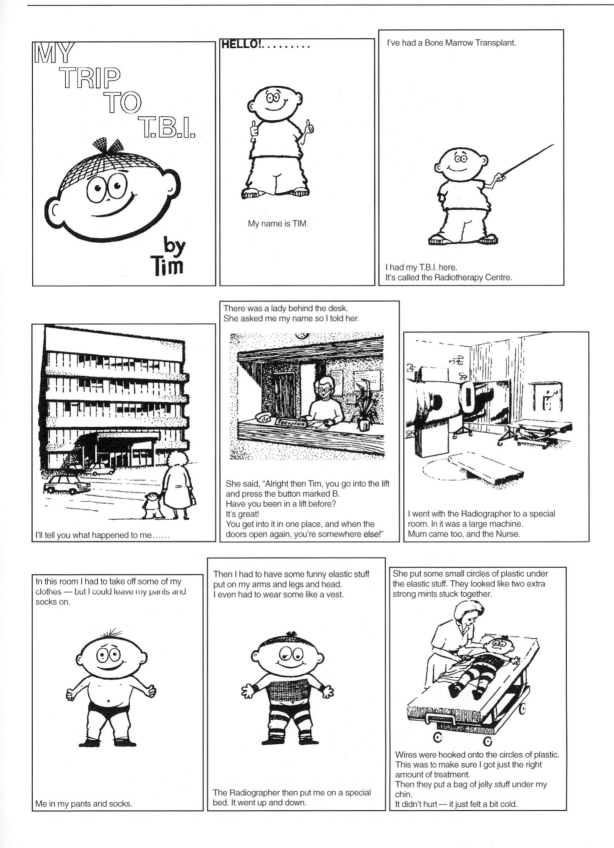

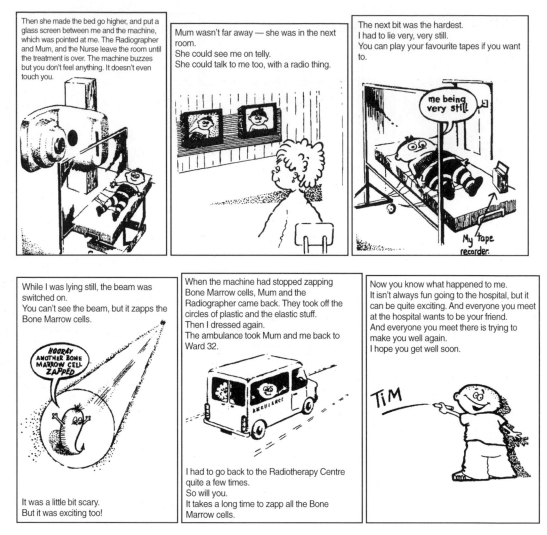

Figure 7.3   My trip to TBI (total body irradiation) by Tim (reproduced with permission of the Play Department, Bristol Children's Hospital)

nursing staff to help bridge the gap. There are a number of ways of achieving this, but one effective method is to utilise the known benefits of setting up opportunities for peer support (support group reference).

Although adolescents may not use the term 'play' as such, there is still an important need for them to be able to have leisure time and appropriate activities. Computer games, televisions, snooker tables and a selection of appropriate board games should be viewed as essential items in the same way that teddies and dolls and Lego are for younger children.

Support groups

Support can be divided into four broad categories (Murray, 1995):

- Emotional support – this involves giving love, being empathetic, encouraging, caring and showing understanding, as well as being trustworthy.
- Instrumental support – this involves providing financial support or giving direct help which enables someone to function better.
- Informational support – by providing information or guidance, a better understanding of the illness and various related issues can be achieved which may assist changes or adjustments to be made to someone's life.
- Appraisal support – there is often a need to have one's own beliefs and interpretation of situations confirmed as being appropriate.

Methods for children and their families to obtain the support they require will vary enormously, but it is important to acknowledge that all members of a family are likely to need support and may respond to support in different ways.

> Although the diagnosis of cancer in any family member can be a devastating experience for the entire family, when the family member is a child the experience seems even more traumatic. (Murray, 1995)

The use of groups to provide support in all the categories identified above is not a new concept. There are a large number of support groups that could be accessible to children who have cancer and their families. Many of these will be local to the hospital from where the child is being treated as a network develops between other children similarly affected.

Support from the type of groups described in Case study 7.3 can be very effective and exist in various forms for children with cancer, siblings of these children and for parents. It should be recognised that some individuals do not want this type of support and clearly when this is the case this should be respected.

The needs of siblings of children with cancer is now well documented (Harding, 1996) and there is clear evidence that demonstrates the impact on them (Walker, 1988; Murray, 1995). It is therefore appropriate that these needs are met in a number of ways. Support groups for siblings is one such method. Oakhill (1988) described how a group set up for siblings who were presenting with regressive or angry interpersonal behaviour at home or with problems at school was particularly successful in that the behaviours described had diminished to minimal level. This was after a 5-week period of regular groups which allowed the siblings

- Consider what you would want in the way of support if you were either diagnosed or a member of your family was diagnosed as having cancer.
- It is likely that if you then compared your thoughts with someone else there would be many similarities but your emphasis may be slightly different.

Case study 7.3

John, aged 15 years, had just completed a course of chemotherapy for the first time. He was experiencing the whole range of emotions that are not uncommon with adolescents having treatment – anger, confusion, fear and sadness. Also in hospital at the same time was Laura who was about to embark on her third course of treatment. Laura was particularly empathic and spent a lot of time talking to John. In the course of the conversation she suggested that he join her at the 'club' that was organised within the hospital for teenagers with cancer. This was run on a monthly basis for both hospitalised and non-hospitalised teenagers. A set of videos is collected from the nearby rental shop, a bar with soft drinks set up, the lights dimmed and adults kept at bay. The degree of support in all four areas identified above is high and for this group is highly valued. John returned to the ward that evening knowing that there were others who had and were still going through similar emotions and this provided the basis on which he developed the coping strategies to deal with these.

to explore three key areas (resentment of the special care the sick child obtained, embarrassment when talking about the illness and when using words like cancer, and education relating to the illness).

The use of groups with children must be managed in a way that is age appropriate. Support groups can conjure up an image of sitting around in a circle with a facilitator in a formal therapeutic manner. Clearly this approach would not be appropriate with someone like Paul in Case study 7.4, and an informal atmosphere can be generated with little structure apart from perhaps the time parameters.

Case study 7.4

Paul was 6 years old when his brother died 4 months after being given a diagnosis of ALL aged 8 years. Paul was at home when his brother died and attended the funeral with his family. For a variety of reasons Paul was not able to discuss his brother for some time. Two years following the death Paul had become difficult to manage at school, was not sleeping well and his parents had split up. He began to attend a support group for siblings of children who had died, and this helped him discuss and say some of the things about his brother that he was unable to express previously. However, it was not until a picture of his brother disappeared that his behaviour and sleep improved dramatically. It turned out a new younger sibling had taken it and it had become lost. At a subsequent support group he was able to talk of the impact the photograph had on him and the emotional pain that this caused him.

Groups set up specifically for parents either informally by providing them with a network of other parents or formally by professionals with specific aims are also available to varying degrees. The needs of parents and the value of support from other parents is apparent from various studies (Lynam, 1987; Wells et al., 1990; Williams, 1992).

Several national charities provide support in a variety of ways, including running local support groups. Sargent Cancer Care for Children and Cancer and Leukaemia in Childhood (CLIC) are two of the more well known examples that provide a range of support services. In addition, modern technology has opened up a huge number of resources on the Internet. While one should exercise some caution with material gained via this route, there is nevertheless information that may be of value and help support children and families. Examples of these, together with the two mentioned above, can be found at http://www.ncl.ac.uk/~nchwww/guides/clinksl.htm#menu.

Family therapy

Family therapy can be of use to both families and professionals in a variety of ways. The first step, as with any considered intervention, is to assess. Here there are a number of factors to consider, not least the developmental stage of the child: 'This assessment should include not only general developmental issues but also the child's comprehension of time, the human body and death …' (Adams-Greenly, 1991). We might also assess under several broad headings, which are discussed further below.

Family history
The family that sit with the therapist bring with them all of their joint experiences of coping as a family group but also their past experiences as individuals. How an individual has coped with a major crisis in the past will have a direct effect on how they cope in the present.

In parents past or current marital conflict will have a negative effect on their ability to cope with the diagnosis of cancer (Weiner, 1970; Weisman, 1976). In the child it is said that past problems with peers and also a history of poor academic attainment will have an effect when the child returns to school.

Communication
Koocher and O'Malley (1981) found that more open family communications lead to better psychological recovery. Assessing this not only means listening to the facts but also hearing the

Before we proceed, think of a time when your family faced a crisis. How did you all cope? Did you need professional help? What help do you think you might expect from a family therapist?

meaning behind the words. Does the family have a climate that allows for the expression of emotion?

Cohesion

Cohesion is an important factor. How close to each other do individual family members feel? How similar are the coping mechanisms employed by family members. Sometimes children find it difficult to verbalise these kind of sophisticated feelings and here it is the therapist's role to help facilitate this. Take the case of Emily, a 7-year-old cancer sufferer who was having difficulty saying how close she felt to Mum and siblings but how distant Father felt to her. The therapist asked if she would find it easier to draw how this was for her, and Figure 7.4 shows how Emily was able to graphically illustrate the situation. This enabled her whole family to talk about this and Emily's father was able to change his work patterns to allow him to spend more time with his family.

How can family therapy help?

'All family members suffer when a child is diagnosed with cancer' (Spinetta, 1984). The way in which the family may suffer has been discussed earlier in this chapter as well as elsewhere (Carr-Gregg and White, 1985; Greer, 1985; Van Dongen-Melman and Sanders-Woustra, 1986; Lansdown and Goldman, 1988; Pinkerton *et al.*, 1994).

Not every family of a childhood cancer sufferer will have contact with a family therapist but they will perhaps encounter professionals using some family therapy techniques:

Health care professionals caring for children with cancer have recognised the complexity of providing care for the child and the family. No one health professional can completely meet

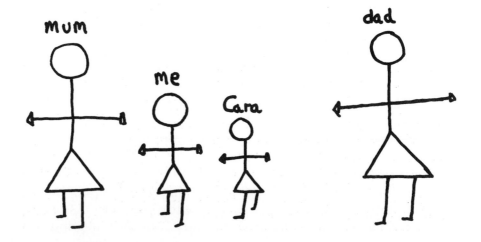

Figure 7.4 Cara diagram

a family's needs and a multidisciplinary approach is more likely to be able to provide comprehensive care that supports the family through the disease and its treatment (Herch and Wiener, 1989).

Perhaps the most important work to be done with families is to normalise the feelings that they are experiencing. This acknowledgement and validation of emotions are invaluable, '… these feelings are not abnormal and may require permission or the provision of appropriate facilities to express them, e.g. privacy to cry or open spaces to scream and shout' (Pinkerton *et al.*, 1994). Black (1989) talks of the problem of non-compliance with treatment and illustrates how family therapy can help. The patient in Case study 7.5 has chronic renal failure, but we suggest that

---

☞ Case study 7.5

Tony, 9 years old and the middle of three children, has had years of teasing for short stature, overactive behaviour and learning difficulties, and was diagnosed recently as having chronic renal failure. He was referred as an emergency case to the child psychiatrist because of difficulty in getting him to take his medication. His mother related with some pride how it would take her one and a half hours to get his tablets into him. His father, who was as taciturn as his mother was garrulous, said it took him only half an hour. Hannah (11 years old) was clearly a parental child and completely bustled about keeping the 6 year old in check. None of them when invited to explain why Tony was having to take medication could do so. They had a hazy notion it was to do with his kidneys not working but did not know why they were not, what kidneys did or even where they were. This boy had a congenital disease which had been missed by his previous physicians although the evidence was there. However Tony had always been very energetic and so nobody had suspected he was ill. Because straightforward techniques (rewards and punishments) had not improved Tony's compliance it was necessary to look at the systemic factors maintaining this dangerous behaviour. A strategic intervention produced a dramatic response.

Tony was congratulated on his courage in maintaining his energy level all these years in spite of often feeling rotten. The therapist appeared impressed at the way he had 'fought' his illness. Now everyone knew he was ill they were trying to protect him but he felt it was important to go on with the behaviour that had helped him deal so effectively with his problems before, i.e. fighting. Of course his parents were fighting too – for his life – so there was bound to be a battle, he fighting against the tablets they fighting to give them. It was important they all went on fighting because not to fight was like giving up … Tony caught by a prescription of the problem (Haley, 1978) responded in his negative way by spitting a liquid medicine at a nurse and demanding it in tablet form which he swallowed readily.

Can you remember an instance of non-compliance? List all the ways in which you might have helped the client and their family.

the principles underlying the intervention could be applied in childhood cancer.

All of this work must go on in the light of a child's chronological and developmental status: 'individuals perception of cancer will be dependent upon their age education development culture economic status and race. All these variables thus create a unique situation for each child and family.' (Pinkerton *et al.*, 1994).

Complementary therapy

Perhaps the first question we need to ask is, why do people turn to complementary therapy? Before we go further make a list of as many possible reasons why you think people do this.

The literature in this area gives three main reasons:

- 'Resorting to complementary medicine is perhaps an attempt to revert to traditional remedies, those of the origins and roots of humanity.' (Guex, 1994)
- 'Some use complementary therapy when orthodox medicine has failed.' (Thomson, 1989)
- Some are said to come to complementary therapy to fight against the side effects of orthodox treatments, or to improve their prognosis as well as enhancing general health; this is supported by Arkko *et al.* (1980).

Homoeopathy

Based on the principle that like is cured by like, homoeopathy was discussed and practised in ancient times as far back as Hippocrates. This was developed further by Dr Samuel Hahnemann in 1842 (Kunzli, Nande and Pendleton, 1983).

There are a number of underpinning concepts in homoeopathy:

Make a note of all the complementary therapies you have heard of. Briefly note how you think they are used.

Your list may look something like this:

- homoeopathy
- healing
- aromatherapy
- herbalism
- acupuncture
- reflexology
- visualisation/ imagery.

- The organism is in a constant state of self repair, and all organs and parts are constantly renewing themselves. This means that there is a considerable capacity for overcoming the cause of disease, if that capacity can be stimulated into activity.
- The cure can only be achieved by the organism through its own devices. This means that the homoeopathic definition of cure may be different to more common uses of the word.
- The organism becomes sensitive to that which will stimulate cure: i.e. that which is homoeopathic to the patient. The extreme degree of sensitivity of the organism to the unique (homoeopathic) stimulant is appreciated by those who are familiar with the amount of dilution involved with most homoeopathic remedies.

Healing

Perhaps where a cure is not possible prayer may help receive pain, distress and discomfort. It has been used for centuries in the pursuit of cure and it has played a large part in the religious rituals and customs of all cultures throughout the world.

Aromatherapy

This is the therapeutic use of concentrated essential oils. These oils are usually taken from medicinal or aromatic plants and are generally applied externally by massaging them into the skin. Oils used include neroli, juniper, eucalyptus and lavender.

It is generally said to be one of the fastest growing therapeutic techniques in Europe. This growth has resulted in an increase in research in the area. In the treatment of cancer aromatherapy has been used and found to help relaxation, calmness and general comfort.

Herbalism

Some western doctors are trained in medical herbalism and lay herbalists may work alongside doctors. People sometimes mistakenly believe that they may use herbal remedies without recourse to a trained practitioner, but care must be taken as they are not without adverse effects. The administration of herbal remedies in children should be used with caution and the use of herbal teas in children is thought to be unwise. (Newell, Anderson and Phillipson, 1997).

Acupuncture

Some orthodox doctors are now trained in the use of this technique. Acupuncture sets out to treat the whole being and not just the disease. Research shows its use for both pain control and as an antiemetic to be significant (Richarson and Vincent, 1986; Dundee, 1988).

Reflexology

This form of foot massage has been used for thousands of years in China and Egypt. Tension and stress are helped by this technique. As with other therapies it should be administered by a trained practitioner. In practice this technique's advocates count the fact that it can be applied easily in most clinical settings as a real advantage.

Reflexes are found mainly on the soles of the feet but also on the top and sides. The right foot represents the right side of the body and the left foot represents the left. When the therapist massages a part of the foot it can have an effect on a part of the body quite removed from the foot. Patients feel no side effects and are often left feeling revitalised and refreshed.

Visualisation/imagery

The following is drawn directly from *Life Choices and Life Changes Through Image Work* by Glouberman (1989) and we feel is the best illustration of this technique:

> …One little boy with a brain tumour thought to be incurable was, following the advice of a doctor who believed in the value of imagery, practising visualising shooting the brain tumour with little rockets. One day he announced that he had just taken a trip through his head in a rocket ship and could not find the cancer anywhere. To everyone's disbelief he was absolutely right: the cancer was gone.

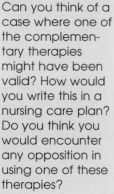

Can you think of a case where one of the complementary therapies might have been valid? How would you write this in a nursing care plan? Do you think you would encounter any opposition in using one of these therapies?

Psychosocial support

Any support offered whether on an individual or group basis must take into account the child's developmental stage. Perhaps the most important part of this process is an assessment of the child's understanding of the concept of cancer and death, which is outlined in Table 7.4.

Having looked at the developmental issues described above and established the level of understanding of the child, we can now examine psychosocial support. Elsewhere in this chapter we discussed play therapy, here we concentrate on:

- psychotherapeutic support
- cognitive-behavioural methods
- physical techniques.

Psychotherapeutic support

This can take several forms and may be immediate and in response to a critical moment in time such as at the moment of diagnosis or at the point of a relapse (crisis intervention) or as a part of longer-term planning of care. This commonly takes one of the following settings:

- Individual psychotherapy – this may be supportive only or involve a more intense approach.
- Group therapy – groups might be based on problem-solving theory or might be a patient support group.

What models of individual psychotherapy have you come across? List them and briefly note whether each one would be appropriate to use in childhood cancer?

Your list may look something like this:

- counselling
- psychoanalysis
- play therapy
- art therapy
- Gestalt therapy.

Individual psychotherapy

Here we will consider only counselling. The use of play has been explored elsewhere in this chapter and the use of art is a familiar method of working with children in health care settings. The specific use of art therapy in working with children with cancer

Table 7.4   An assessment of children's understanding of the concept of death and cancer (adapted from Foley (1986) and Pinkertan et al. (1994))

Age	Understanding of time	Understanding of the body	Understanding of death
Baby	No concept of time	No concept of cancer	No concept of death
Preschool	Understands morning and night-time. Does not understand the future but has started to understand yesterday and tomorrow	Can name external parts of body but has no knowledge of internal body parts	Attributes life processes and consciousness to the dead (e.g. dead people eat and get wet when it rains)
6–8 years	Learning to tell the time; understands yesterday and tomorrow. Future is a long time away. May know birthday but not how long away it is	Knows location of some of the large organs. Has some knowledge of body processes, e.g. digestion and climination	Perceives death as an external malevolent event, e.g. man with a knife. Personifies death, e.g. the bogey man
9–13 years	Time and events are mastered. Starting to identify self as part of future but may not be realistic, e.g. football star or prime minister	Understands circulation and respiration and enjoys learning. Becomes anxious about body changes as puberty approaches	Knows that death is irreversible. Is concerned about culture and rituals as social vehicles for sharing feelings. May use religion for this purpose
14–18 years	Sense of identity is established. This leads to academic and career choices	Becomes increasingly easy with own body; groups disease and ageing as concepts	Realises that everyone dies at some point in time

is something that does not appear to have been explored much in the literature although, of course, many play therapists will use art in a therapeutic manner. Gestalt therapy is an interesting area of work when dealing with children and we would commend Violet Oaklander's work as being of specific worth (Oaklander, 1978). Psychoanalysis is another area of special note, but in the context of this chapter it is best left to others to explain and expand on that particular theme.

Briefly note your
definition of
counselling.

Counselling

Here are some definitions of counselling quoted in the literature:

- Tschudin (1991) quotes from a BBC Radio 4 programme: 'Counselling is … a way of relating and responding to another person, so that that person is helped to explore his thoughts, feelings and behaviour; to reach clearer self-understanding; and then is helped to find and use his strengths so that he copes more effectively with his life by making appropriate decisions, or by taking relevant action. Essentially then, counselling is a purposeful relationship in which one person helps another to help himself.'
- 'It (counselling) fills the gap between psychotherapy and friendship, it has become a recognised extension of the work of almost everyone whose business touches upon the personal, social, occupational, medical, educational and spiritual aspects of people.' (Anon)
- Crompton (1992) notes her definition of counselling children as: 'The purposeful interaction between adults and children/young people within the context of an agency or organisation, statutory or voluntary, concerned with social, educational, occupational, spiritual and/or health care and welfare.'

Two models of counselling are considered and are briefly described (Box 7.1).

Let us take a closer look at Egan's model;

- Egan gives *problem definition* as the first stage here, and the client's opportunities as well as problems are explored. This is called the 'present scenario'.
- *Goal development* is the next stage and Egan states that the goals should be action oriented. Egan calls this the 'preferred or future scenario'.
- The third and final stage given by Egan is *action*. Here strategies aimed at achieving goals are devised and implemented. This is 'getting the new scenario on line'.

Box 7.1   Models of counselling

Egan	**Nelson-Jones**
Problem definition	Describe and identify the problem
Goal development	Operationalise the problem
Action	Set goals
	Intervene
	Exit and consolidate self-help skills

The Nelson-Jones model is made up of five stages:

- *Describe* – Here the task is to build a relationship to the point where a therapeutic alliance is formed. One must also assist the client in firstly revealing, identifying and describing their problem.
- *Operationalise the problem* – This stage is concerned with gathering relevant information for defining and stating the problem.
- *Set goals* – Working goals can now be set and client and therapist must negotiate interventions to attain them.
- *Intervene* – The task here is to decrease skills deficits and also to build skills resources in any identified problem areas.
- *Exit* – Here the whole process is reviewed. The therapeutic relationship is terminated when the client has enough self-help skills.

One might say that there are problems relating this model to children with cancer. One of the basic premises is that the client must own the problem and it may be questioned as to how a child may be responsible for having cancer. This is clearly absurd and we suggest that professionals use this model with a view that the child's illness has resulted in some poor adaptation to their situation. This model we suggest may be best used with older children. If we think of the child's developmental status it would not be appropriate for everyone we meet.

Take for instance the hypothetical case of George, a 5-year-old boy diagnosed with a terminal illness. During the stage of describing we might expect him to be preoccupied with his own mortality. In fact it would be unusual if he were not. However, as the relationship progresses we may find that this is only part of the picture of how he may be feeling. He may be experiencing feelings about his lost potential and perhaps about leaving his parents or siblings. It may be that at the heart of his difficulties is that he is unable to talk to his family about his impending death. A worthwhile goal in this instance may be to be able to describe how he feels to his parents. The therapist's task once this goal is set is to negotiate interventions with George. This could include writing them down or practising on the therapist. Using this approach to increase his skills he may eventually be able to go on and be able to talk to his parents with support. The exit phase would then be when both George and the therapist review the whole process.

Cognitive-behavioural methods
Here treatment focuses on new learning and on producing changes in therapy which can be generalised outside the clinical

environment. The work is dependent on an alliance between the child and the therapist. All aspects of the treatment are made explicit to the patient and together they endeavour to discover more about the problem, thus enabling them to develop strategies to deal with the now clearly detailed problem.

This magnification which Luke in case study 7.6 experienced is known in cognitive-behavioural terms as a cognitive distortion.

The following list will provide a definition of cognitive distortions and illustrate this with examples.

- *Selective abstraction* – Basing a conclusion on isolated details while ignoring contradictory and more salient evidence. For example: 'I just can't control myself. Last night when I had dinner in a restaurant, I ate everything I was served, although I had decided ahead of time that I was going to be very careful. I am so weak.' and 'The only way I can be in control is through eating', or 'I am special if I am thin'.
- *Overgeneralisation* – Extracting a rule on the basis of one event and applying it to other dissimilar situations. For example: 'When I used to eat carbohydrates, I was fat: therefore, I must avoid them now so I won't become obese', or 'I used to be of normal weight and I wasn't happy. So I know gaining weight isn't going to make me feel better.'

Case study 7.6

Luke aged 15 is suffering from common ALL. As a result of treatment Luke started to lose his hair. He became withdrawn and started to refuse treatment and eventually refused to leave his bedroom. Eventually Luke was referred to a clinical psychologist and during the course of several sessions they managed to define the thoughts surrounding his 'problem'. It transpired that Luke had been involved with his first girlfriend. This important relationship had been severed by the girl just at the same time as Luke had started to lose his hair. Perhaps this was coincidental, but this was magnified in his thoughts. Based on this one experience Luke was certain that no one would find him attractive ever again. Gradually the therapist was able to get Luke to challenge this distortion. He asked Luke to consider how logical it was to take one instance and let that instance govern his thinking for the rest of his life. Luke also opted to test the reality of his thoughts and started asking some of the significant people in his life whether they found him attractive. All this started to change Luke's view of himself and this was further helped by discussion with his therapist about beauty and attractiveness as an issue. Luke concluded that people would find him attractive. If they did not and they let that affect their relationship with him then they were not worth bothering with anyhow.

- *Magnification* – Overestimation of the significance of undesirable subsequent events. Stimuli are embellished with surplus meaning not supported by an objective analysis. For example: 'Gaining five pounds would push me over the brink' and 'If others comment on my weight again, I won't be able to stand it', or 'I've gained two pounds, so I can't wear shorts any more'.
- *Dichotomous or all-or-nothing reasoning* – Thinking in extreme and absolute terms. Events can only be black or white, good or bad, right or wrong. For example: 'If I'm not in complete control, I lose all control. If I can't master this area of my life, I'll lose everything' and 'If I gain one pound, I'll go on to gain a hundred pounds', or 'If I don't establish a daily routine, everything will be chaotic and I won't accomplish anything'.
- *Personalisation and self-reference* – Egocentric interpretations of impersonal events or overinterpretation of events relating to the self. An example might be: 'Two people laughed and whispered something to each other when I walked by. They were probably saying that I was unattractive. I have gained three pounds ...', or 'I am embarrassed when other people see me eat', and perhaps 'When I see someone who is overweight, I worry that I will be like her'.
- *Superstitious thinking* – Believing in the cause–effect relationship of non-contingent events. For example: 'I can't enjoy anything because it will be taken away', or 'If I eat a sweet, it will be converted instantly into body fat'.

In all the initial stages of cognitive therapy the first task is establishment of the therapeutic alliance. This rapport building is vital to the efficacy of the therapy and without success here progress is unlikely to be made. Another aspect of these early stages is that cognitive distortions are only noted they are not challenged, this comes later. It is common to ask the client to keep a record of their eating behaviour and their feelings around food in the form of a diary. This should be viewed at each session.

As the therapeutic relationship builds the therapist may start to challenge the distortions presented in sessions alongside the belief systems of the client that these distortions support. The use of therapeutic tasks or homework is also common. This may be employing a strategy to cope with the need to vomit after a meal. For instance a client living with their family might be encouraged to play a board game with a sibling or parents as a way of distracting themselves at a time when one can predict that they will be vulnerable. As the therapy progresses further the task of cognitive restructuring becomes important. By now the therapist and client have a trusting relationship which will enable them to challenge the cognitive distortions.

Physical techniques

Listed here are relaxation techniques. These are said to help counter the side effects of treatment and to relieve stress. These techniques can be used by and taught to children. Sharman (1997 p. 81) gives an excellent example of guided imagery and a muscle tension-relaxation session. We have found this type of technique to be of value and Case study 7.7 presented here involves Keith, who had recovered from major surgery to remove a brain tumour.

Conclusion

This chapter has explored some of the ways in which children and families might respond to stressful situations that are only

Case study 7.7

After major surgery to remove a brain tumour, Keth, a 16-year-old was left with some behavioural problems which were worse when he was stressed. Part of the nursing care plan stated that Keith would have regular relaxation sessions from his nurse. This consisted of two half-hourly sessions per week. In early sessions Keith was encouraged to lay comfortably on a mat and close his eyes. He was taken using guided imagery to places that were peaceful, where Keith could feel safe and secure, where he knew that things moved calmly along at a gentle pace. These places included sunny fields, beaches and woodland. All places that Keith had told us he liked. All along Keith was encouraged to be aware of different muscle groups and, as in Sharman's example, he was directed to tense and then relax these groups. After several sessions Keith asked to select a special place of his own that he could go to in the guided imagery. We encouraged this and Keith started to tell us of his special place. We were surprised to find that it was not a remote quiet spot but a park in an inner city. When we asked about this choice Keith explained that he needed a spot that he could get to in his mind very quickly and he felt that since parks were in reality nearer to him then in fantasy they would be too. Keith continued to tell us of his special park and in later sessions we used his detail. Keith was now starting to generalise the work we had been doing to his real world and this was having a profound effect on his behavioural problems. Staff began to note that Keith would ask to leave a room where he was having difficulty and would stay away for a while before reappearing in a calmer frame of mind. When we quizzed Keith about this he told us he was sitting quietly going to his special place.

too common when serious illness such as cancer is present. By exploring possible mechanisms that are used psychologically by children and families it is hoped the reader will increase their ability to understand and consequently be more empathic with them. A simple model of stress and coping is offered, and it is hoped this will provide a basis for the consideration of many factors that may have a part to play in determining the outcome or effect of the stress resulting from serious illness. As part of this model, coping strategies have been identified that professionals may have a big part to contribute towards in helping to reduce the negative effects of the stress. Those examined briefly in this chapter include play, support groups, family therapy, complementary therapies and some forms of psychosocial support. It is not the view of the authors that any particular approach is any better than another, and it should be stressed that those described here are but a few in comparison to the range of methods that can be available.

The aim of this chapter has been to provoke some thought and increase the insight of readers into the options open to help prevent and manage stress that may develop as a result of a serious illness such as cancer. It is well known that if we take care of the mental health of our children this will help equip them to cope with the stressors that will confront them in later life. Similarly we know that the way in which parents and other family members deal with the stress of a child with cancer will have a direct impact on the way the child is able to cope. There is no question that examining ways in which we can provide healthy coping mechanisms for children and their families is a worthwhile exercise.

References

Action For Sick Children (1990) *Setting Standards for Adolescents in Hospital*. London: Action for Sick Children.

Adams-Greenly, M. (1986) Psychological staging of paediatric cancer patients and their families. *Cancer*, **58**, 449–453.

Adams-Greenly, M. (1991) Psychosocial assessment and intervention at initial diagnosis. *Paediatrica*, **18**, 3–10.

Aitken, T.J. & Hathaway, G. (1993) Long distance related stressors and coping behaviours in parents of children with cancer. *Journal of Pediatric Oncology Nursing*, **10**(1), 3–12.

Arkko, P.J., Arkko, B.L., Kari-Koskinen, O. *et al.* (1980) A survey of unproven cancer remedies and their uses in an outpatient clinic for cancer therapy in Finland. *Social Science and Medicine*, **14a**, 511–514.

Atkinson, R. (1993) *Introduction to Psychology*, 11th edn. Fort Worth: Harcourt Brace Jovanovich.

Audit Commission (1993) *Children First: a study of hospital services*. London: HMSO

Beresford, B.A. (1993) Resources and strategies: how parents cope with the care of a disabled child. *Journal of Child Psychology and Psychiatry*, **35**(1), 171–209.

Black, D. (1989) Life threatening illness, children and family therapy. *Journal of Family Therapy*, **11**, 81–101.

Carr-Gregg, M.R.C. & White, L. (1985) The child with cancer: a psychological overview. *Medical Journal of Australia*, **143**, 503–508.

Crompton, M. (1992) *Children and Counselling*. London: Edward Arnold.

Department of Health (1991) *The Welfare of Children and Young People in Hospital.* London: HMSO.

Department of Health (1992) Hospital Play Staff. Executive Letter EL (92) 42.

Department of Health (1995) *A Handbook on Child and Adolescent Mental Health: mental illness key area.* London: HMSO.

Dundee, J. (1988) Acupuncture/acupressure as an antiemetic: studies of its use in postoperative vomiting, cancer, chemotherapy and sickness of early pregnancy. *Complementary Medical Research,* **3**(1), 2–14.

Dwivedi, K. (ed.) (1997) *The Therapeutic use of Stories.* London: Routledge.

Ellerton, M., Ritchie, J.A. & Caty, S. (1994) Factors influencing young children's coping behaviours during stressful healthcare encounters. *Maternal-Child Nursing,* **22**(3), 74–82.

Fairburn, G.C. & Cooper, P.J. (1989) *in* Hawton, K., Salvaskis, P.M., Kirk, J. & Clark, D.M. eds. *Cognitive Behaviour Therapy for Psychiatric Problems: a Practical guide.* Oxford: Oxford University Press.

Foley, G. (1986) Facilitating death discussions with children. *Paediatric Nurse, Update,* **1**, 2–8.

Frankenfield, P.K. (1996) The power of humor and play as nursing interventions for a child with cancer: a case report. *Journal of Pediatric Oncology Nursing,* **13**(1), 15–20.

Glouberman, D. (1989) *Life Choices and Life Changes Through Image Work. The art of developing personal vision.* London: Unwin

Greer, S. (1985) Cancer: psychiatric aspects *in* Granville-Grossman, K. ed. *Recent Advances in Clinical Psychiatry.* London: Churchill Livingstone.

Gross, R. (1992) *Psychology. The science of mind and behaviour,* 3rd edn. London: Hodder & Stoughton.

Guex, P. (1994) *An Introduction to Psycho-oncology.* London: Routledge.

Haley, J. (1978) *Problem Solving Therapy.* San Fransisco: Jossey-Bass.

Harding, R. (1996) Children with cancer: the needs of siblings. *Professional Nurse,* **11**(9), 588–590.

Herch, S.P. & Weiner, L.S. (1989) Psychosocial support for the family of the child with cancer. *Principles and Practice of Paediatric Oncology,* **42**, 897–913.

Hockenberry-Eaton, M., Dilorio, C. & Kemp, V. (1995) The relationship of illness longevity and relapse with self-perception, cancer stressors, anxiety, and coping strategies in children with cancer. *Journal of Pediatric Oncology Nursing,* **12**(2), 71–79.

Hogg, C. (1994) *Setting Standards for Children Undergoing Surgery.* London: Action for Sick Children.

Hogg, C. (1996) *Health Services for Children and Young People.* London: Action for Sick Children.

Koocher, G. & O'Malley, J. (1981) *The Damocles Syndrome: psychological consequences of surviving childhood cancer.* New York: McGraw Hill.

Kunzli, J., Nande, A. & Pendleton, P.J. (1983) *The Organon of Medicine,* 6th edn. London: Gollancz.

Lansdown, R. & Goldman, A. (1988) Annotation: the psychological care of children with malignant disease. *Journal of Child Psychology and Psychiatry,* **29**, 555–567.

Lynam, M.J. (1987) The parent network in pediatric oncology. Supportive or not? *Cancer Nursing,* **10**(4), 207–216.

McMahon, L. (1992) *The Handbook of Play Therapy.* London: Routledge.

Monat, A. & Lazurus, R.S. (1985) *Stress and Coping: an anthology.* New York: Columbia University Press.

Murray, J.S. (1995) Social support for siblings of children with cancer. *Journal of Pediatric Oncology Nursing,* **12**(2), 62–70.

Newell, C.A., Anderson, L.A. & Phillipson, J.D. (1997) *Herbal Medicines: a guide for healthcare professionals* London: The Pharmaceutical Press.

Oakhill, A. (1988) *The Supportive Care of the Child with Cancer.* London: Wright

Oaklander, V. (1978) *Windows to our Children.* Moab: Real People Press.

Pinkerton, C.R., Cushing, P. & Sepin, B. (1994) *Childhood Cancer Management: a practical handbook.* London: Chapman & Hall.

Pressdee, D., May, L., Eastman, E. & Grier, D. (1997) Use of play therapy in the preparation of children undergoing MR imaging. *Clinical Radiology,* **52**, 945–947.

Richardson, P.H. & Vincent, C.A. (1986) Acupuncture for the treatment of pain: a review of evaluative research. *Pain,* **24**, 15–40.

Rutter, M., Taylor, E. & Hersov, L. (1994) *Child and Adolescent Psychiatry – modern approaches.* Oxford: Blackwell Scientific.

Sharman, W. (1997) *Children and Adolescents with Mental Health Problems*. London: Baillière Tindall.

Sloper, P. & While, D. (1996) Risk factors in the adjustment of siblings of children with cancer. *Journal of Child Psychology and Psychiatry*, **37**(5), 597–607.

Spinetta, J.C. (1984) Measurement of family function, communication and cultural effects. *Cancer*, **10**, 2330–2338.

Thomson, R. (1989) *Loving Medicine: patients experiences of the Bristol Cancer Health Centre*. Bath:Gateway

Thornes, R. (1991) *Just for the Day. Caring for children in the health services*. London: HMSO.

Tschudin, V. (1991) *Counselling Skills for Nurses*. London: Baillière Tindall.

Van Dongen-Melman, J.E.W.M. & Sanders-Woustra, J.A.R. (1986) Psychosocial aspects of childhood cancer: a review of the literature. *Journal of Child Psychology and Psychiatry*, **27**, 145–180.

Walker, C. (1988) Stress and coping in siblings of childhood cancer patients. *Nursing Research*, **37**, 208–212.

Weiner, J. (1970) Reactions of the family to the fatal illness of a child *in* Schoenberg, Carr, Peretz & Kutscher (eds). *Loss and Grief; psychological management in clinical practice*. Columbia: Columbia University Press.

Weisman, A. (1976) *Coping with Cancer*. New York: McGraw-Hill.

Wells, L.M., Heiney, S.P., Swygert, E., Troficanto, G., Stokes, C. & Ettinger, R.S. (1990) Psychosocial stressors, coping resources and informational needs of parents of adolescent cancer patients. *Journal of Pediatric Oncology Nursing*, **7**(4), 145–148.

Williams, H.A. (1992) Comparing the perception of support by parents of children with cancer and by health professionals. *Journal of Pediatric Oncology Nursing*, **9**(4), 180–186.

Wilson, K., Kendrick, P. & Ryan, V. (1992) *Play Therapy*. London: Ballière Tindall.

Wong, D.L. (1997) *Whaley & Wong's Essentials of Pediatric Nursing*, 5th edn. St Louis: Mosby.

Bone marrow transplantation

TRACY LAWRANCE AND SARAH KIRK

Introduction

Bone marrow transplantation (BMT) has evolved from an experimental to conventional form of therapy, which frequently offers the best chance for prolonged survival and cure for many children with malignant disease. While published research issues related to the advancement of such treatments tend to focus on biomedical technology and outcomes, emphasis on the sequence of the families' coping strategies related to such intense therapy needs to be addressed. Twenty years ago Pfefferbaum, Lindamood and Wiley (1977) recommended a model of working with families undergoing BMT and encouraged nurses to meet with other disciplines to discuss family care. Despite many adaptations to these early recommendations, we feel that the perspective of those directly involved in the experience of BMT has not always been explored; partnership in care actually offers this insight as the multifaceted skills of today's BMT nurse takes a family-centred approach to care.

This chapter will discuss the main issues highlighted in the key points, and related to partnership in care, for the family undergoing BMT.

Overview of bone marrow transplantation

It is not the objective of this chapter to detail the specifics of the BMT process, side effects and outcomes, as there are many fine texts worthy of referral (Whedon, 1991; Forman, Blume and Oski, 1994; Buchsel and Whedon 1995). However a brief review of the principles of BMT will enable you to reflect and assess your current level of knowledge.

Abramovitz and Senner (1995) describe the goal of bone marrow transplantation (BMT) as the replacement of defective or non-functioning bone marrow with normal stem cells. There are several different types of transplant:

Key points
- Brief overview of BMT
- Evolution and current status of BMT technology
- Costs and benefits of BMT
- Recommendation and referral for BMT
- Experiences of life as a potential cause of uncertainty about BMT
- Pre-BMT information giving
- Legal and ethical issues affecting families consenting to BMT
- Bone marrow donation
- The child in hospital undergoing BMT
- Pre-transplant
- Early recovery
- Mid- recovery and discharge home
- Late recovery
- Interface between curative and palliative care during BMT
- Staffing issues

- Autograft, which involves having one's own bone marrow removed and returned post cytoreductive treatment.
- Allogenic transplant, which involves receiving bone marrow usually from a family member with an identical tissue type.
- Syngenic transplant, which is receipt of bone marrow from an identical twin.
- Matched Unrelated Transplant (MUD), the donation of bone marrow from a volunteer donor.

There are several variations on these themes dependent on the method of acquiring the stem cell and the degree of tissue type match or mismatch. For the child with cancer BMT is a means of restoring or rescuing normal haematopoeisis and immunological function after any residual cancer cells have been destroyed with high doses of chemotherapy and/or irradiation. The specific preparative protocol for conditioning treatment depends on the underlying disease and should be capable of eradicating malignancy, have tolerable morbidity without mortality and have sufficient immunosuppressive effects in allogenic BMT to avoid graft rejection (Figure 8.1). No ideal preparatory regimen exists and recurrence of the original disease still accounts for a significant number of treatment failures. Wiley and House (1988) state that infants, children and adolescents receive approximately half of all BMTs and from the literature reviewed BMT is identified as a treatment modality for children not only with malignancy but also with other previously considered chronic illnesses, hence this chapter may be of relevance to other groups (Brochstein, 1992; McDonagh and Nienhuis, 1993; Beutler and Sullivan, 1994; Forman, Blume and Oski, 1994).

The evolution and current status of bone marrow transplant technology

Modern technology continues to explore ways and means of acquiring the pluripotent stem cell and in recent years there has been a shift from conventional bone marrow harvesting techniques to the use of peripheral blood stem cell (PBSC) harvesting (Deméocq et al., 1994; Walker et al., 1994; Takaue et al., 1995). In addition Kurtzberg (1995), Wagner et al., (1995) and Gluckman (1996) suggest that umbilical cord harvesting/transplantation is now a recognised if not common procedure. Furthermore another fascinating advancement is gene therapy, whereby the stem cell is used as the vehicle for inserting normal genes and can also involve the use of in utero BMT during the first trimester (De

The timetable below indicates the conditioning treatment for a child following a relapse in both bone marrow and central nervous system ten months into a two year treatment for common acute lymphoblastic leukaemia.

Figure 8.1 Bone marrow transplant timetable

Day

-12   Admit to BMTU, consent for BMT, Comence Campath

-11   Campath

-10   Campath

-9   Campath, commence 1st cranial boost of radiotherapy

-8   Campath, 2nd cranial boost and testicular boost, 3rd cranial boost

-7   Commence total body irradiation (TBI) 08.00hrs, 16.00hrs

-6   Total body irradiation 08.00hrs, 16.00hrs

-5   Total body irradiation 08.00hrs, 16.00hrs

-4   Total body irradiation 08.00hrs, 16.00hrs

-3   Commence intravenous cyclophosphamide 60mg/kg/day

-2   Cyclophosphamide 60mg/kg/day

-1   Commence intravenous cyclosporin twice daily

0   Commence intravenous acyclovir, bone marrow infusion, commence intravenous immunoglobulin weekly

+1   Commence methotrexate 7.5mg/m^2/day

+3   Methotrexate

+6   Methotrexate

+8   Methotrexate, commence GCSF

Santas and Cowan, 1992; Moore, 1993). All new technologies will however bring with them ethical and moral dilemmas which need addressing if we are to fulfil our professional responsibility of ensuring the families' perceptions are considered and respected throughout the BMT procedure.

As BMT advances so does the progression of complications of toxicity of cytoreductive preparatory regimens, acute and chronic graft versus host disease (GVHD) (Ford and Ballard, 1988; Parr et al., 1991; Heiney et al., 1994). For these reasons BMT must be performed at centres where technology and multidisciplinary expertise and skills are available to manage both the physical and psychosocial consequences (Whittaker, 1995; International Society for Haematotherapy and Grafting Engineering (ISHAGE) and the European Bone Marrow Transplant Group (EBMT), 1997).

Costs and benefits of bone marrow transplantation

The reason we are addressing costs and benefits at this early stage in this chapter is a representation of the current impact that health care expenditures have within the National Health Service (NHS). With the increased utilisation of BMT there is also the pressure on NHS trusts to contain and reduce costs, as even though BMT is not as costly as other organ transplants, it is still an expensive use of funds (Whedon, 1991). At present most NHS trusts work within the constraints of regional or subregional contracts within the geographical regional location. Often these contracts are influenced by the availability of funds. We would argue that the current implications to practice mean that health care professionals cannot act without consideration to the financial implications of their decisions, a good enough reason we feel for us to be aware of the costs and benefits of such a procedure. Moreover this knowledge could in the near future be a key factor in leading to a more equitable and reasonable distribution of whatever resources are available.

Methods of costing health care and relating costs to benefits have however proved very controversial (Rees, 1985; Peterson, 1996). Beard (1991) argues that the cost of any disease and its treatment is almost impossible to assess, as is the social cost, consequent loss of life, mental and physical disability and disruption to family life. Moreover, all these factors are likely to be greater when an intensive therapy like BMT is applied to a young person. The case that aroused outrage when brought to the public's attention by the mass media, *Child B v. Cambridge Health Authority* (Dyer, 1995), highlighted the plight of a child who had previously been treated with BMT for acute leukaemia and then relapsed. The health authority refused to fund a second BMT on the grounds of costs outweighing the possible long-term benefits to the child. Subsequently Child B was treated in a private hospital with the costs being met by an anonymous donation. It could be argued that the depth of suffering would have been greater following the death of the child, and for that reason it seems appropriate to focus on intense treatment like BMT and to relate the monetary cost of the procedure to the life-years gained, and to their quality. Beard (1991) attempted to define the costs involved in carrying out BMT, determined by the quality of life gained, and to document subsequent annual costs using Quality Adjusted Life Years (QALYS).

You may find it of interest to look at you trust's business plan and contract for BMT and see if any costs and benefits or quality of life assessment has been determined?

Recommendations and referral for bone marrow transplantation

Lesko (1994) comments that BMT is being addressed as a treatment option at a much earlier stage in the child's disease. However only three empirical studies were found that addressed the initial link in the decision-making chain that progresses to the BMT process (Chauvenent and Smith, 1988; Singer and Donnely, 1990; Andrykowski, 1994). The literature suggests that the beginning of the BMT process is the point at which the physician introduces the option as a possibility or makes the relevant referral to the BMT consultant. It is our experience, however, that the family's personal acquisition of information has already begun and often the decision to go ahead with BMT has already been made.

Experience of life as a potential cause of uncertainty about bone marrow transplantation

Various sources of information relating to BMT are available at both specialist and shared care centres, in keeping with the philosophy of educating and empowering families to become informed (described in more detail in Chapter 3). Patient information booklets, videos, picture books, cassette tapes and text books all have a role to play as portrayal of treatment outcomes is presented (Anthony Nolan Bone Marrow Trust, 1995; United Kingdom Childhood Cancer Study Group (UKCCSG), 1996; Leukaemia Research Fund, 1997).

At our regional bone marrow transplant unit (BMTU) we have also observed the effects of the experience on individuals involved with other families proceeding through BMT. In the majority of cases this observation of others' experiences seems to bear a great weight in influencing unfavourable attitudes and fears towards BMT as a treatment option compared to those families that have no previous experience. This particular issue has been recognised at our centre, since families undergoing BMT are now treated within an oncology/haematology ward rather than, historically, a separate bone marrow transplant unit. Case study 8.1 encapsulates the intensity and implications of the experience of one family who lived through and shared the experiences of others and then faced the decision of BMT.

Case study 8.1

Sadie an 18-month-old girl diagnosed as acute myeloid leukaemia began treatment (Medical Research Council, 1997). Because of the distance from home, the failure of her disease to remit and gross toxicities from induction treatment, it was impossible for her to get home even for short reprisals and the family spent almost 6 months resident at the hospital. During that period of hospitalisation Sadie and her family had direct contact with 14 families involved in BMT: five of those children died and two suffered severe graft versus host disease (GVHD). As time progressed BMT was suggested as the most appropriate form of treatment for Sadie. Her parents were thrown into turmoil, and felt that, 'if we took the option of BMT it was an instant death sentence, whereas Sadie had proved she could get through the chemotherapy, so why not carry on as we are?' Despite all the literature, professional counselling and support Sadie's family had received they still followed their instinct, influenced by their perception of the lived experience.

We certainly believe that those exposed to such disturbing experiences quite often have a distorted understanding of the facts and from this point need the support of the transplant team to be able to put the irrational impressions in to some sort of factual sequence. The only study found acknowledging this scenario encourages staff to always be aware of the overpowering influence that other children dying on the ward may have on families in transplant, it may be the last factor to tip them over the edge emotionally (Heiney *et al.*, 1994).

Another dilemma apparent to professionals working with families referred to a new hospital or centre for BMT is the need to clarify information, determine facts and make plans. For families who may have received their treatment under a different consultant or at another regional oncology/haematology centre, shared care or mainly in the community, and have already established trusting professional relationships with a multidisciplinary team, they now face the challenge of getting to know the transplant team. Singer and Donnely (1990) found in a study of relevant information giving for BMT by referring physicians, that 80% of doctors believed that families had adequate knowledge and information to be able to consent to BMT, however divergent opinion about what information should be presented was apparent. This data was consistent with the practice of many BMT consultants who were found to select information primarily for therapeutic benefit and not for relevance for decision making. Thus information presented by the referring consultant is most likely to influence families' choice to undergo BMT and information presented by the trans-

plant team is most likely to enhance compliance with the treatment regimen (Tomlinson, 1986; Singer and Donnely, 1990.) The
results of these empirical studies then necessitate a strategy for
educating and training nurses and allied professionals working in
the community and shared care centres, to enable them to feel
confident in answering the inevitable questions from families
following consultation with the referring consultants.

Another entity worthy of consideration is the influence of information gathered from the mass media, support groups, libraries,
internet, or even families making direct contact with world-
renowned specialists. Despite what information has been acquired
there still needs to be a process of unravelling the 'known' from
the 'unknown', a difficult task by any means when there are many
uncertain and unpredictable outcomes of the BMT process.
Furthermore, Lee *et al.* (1994) recommend the need for the BMT
team to address the possibility of other life stressors, not just the
transplant. Therefore to enable some form of order, control and
empowerment for the family, the communication and information-
giving process starts as soon as the potential need for BMT is
known. We do however believe that the providers of this information need to be equipped with a deep professionally experiential,
empathic understanding and a great awareness of the legal, ethical,
advocacy, nursing care and dependency issues involved in the
information-giving process to enable families to make informed
decisions about BMT.

Information giving pre- bone marrow transplantation

Most paediatric BMT units in the UK use different tools for preparing the child and family for transplantation. The formation of
the Royal College of Nursing Paediatric Bone Marrow Transplant
Group in 1996, the United Kingdom group of nurse and allied
professional members of the European Bone Marrow Transplant
Nurses Group founded in 1997 and the collaboration of The International Society for Hematotherapy and Graft Engineering in
collaboration with The European Bone Marrow Transplant Group
in 1997 all recognise the need for standards and guidelines in this
fast-evolving speciality. We agree that guidelines need to be set,
if the child, family and carers needs are not to be lost among the
search for improving survival outcomes. At our regional centre
we feel that communication between professionals and the family
must be of the highest quality if the best care is to be achieved
(Department of Health, 1995). In our experience one of the most
important ways of communicating is through information giving
and preparation. This eases the child and family through a

Box 8.1

Information on Bone Marrow Transplantation is given under the following headings by the BMT Team. Both written and pictorial educational resources are used to back-up discussion and rationales for all prescribed treatments

- PROGNOSIS/POSSIBLE OUTCOMES OF BMT
- MAJOR RISKS OF BMT
- CHEMOTHERAPY USED FOR CONDITIONING
- RADIOTHERAPY USED FOR CONDITIONING
- PRE-BMT INVESTIGATION APPOINTMENTS AND CONDITIONING TIMETABLE GIVEN TO THE FAMILY
- SHORT TERM SIDE EFFECTS:
    - vomiting
    - mucositis
    - diarrhoea
    - risk of infection
    - risk of bleeding
    - anaemia
    - veno-occlusive disease
    - hypertension
    - convulsions
    - alopecia
    - eating/appetite problems
    - acute graft versus host disease
    - somnolence
    - regression
    - behavioural problems
- LONG-TERM SIDE EFFECTS:
    - chronic graft versus host disease
    - infertility
    - endocrine function impairment
    - growth and development delay
    - eating problems
    - skin hyperpigmentation
    - cataracts
    - secondary malignancies
    - current long term follow up strategies
- CYCLOSPORIN AND ASSOCIATED SIDE EFFECTS
- ANTI-LYMPHOCYTIC GLOBULIN/MONOCLONAL ANTIBODY USAGE
- GRANULOCYTE COLONY STIMULATING FACTOR (GCSF)
- ENTERAL/PARENTERAL FEEDING
- INFORMATION ON ANY SPECIFIC CLINICAL TRIAL OR RELEVANT RESEARCH STUDY
- THE USE OF PAIN SCALES, OPIATE BASED MEDICATION AND PATIENT CONTROLLED ANALGESIA TECHNIQUES
- PROTECTIVE ISOLATION MEASURES
- DIETARY RESTRICTIONS
- FAMILY ACCOMMODATION
- SIBLING NEEDS
- NAMED NURSE SYSTEM/INTRODUCTION TO BMT TEAM

distressing time if begun well in advance of the commencement of treatment. A large part of the preparation is done by the nurse transplant co-ordinator, whose main role is to ensure that all relevant family members are fully informed of all aspects of the transplant and its consequences (Box 8.1). Bass *et al.* (1996) retrospectively surveyed families about the role of the nurse BMT co-ordinator; all subjects responded by valuing and benefiting from the input. The UK members of the European Bone Marrow Transplant Nurses Group (Outhwaite, 1998) are also in the process of collaborating over facets of the nurse co-ordinator's diverse roles, with the general feel reflecting the development and advancement of the scope of professional practice (United Kingdom Central Council for Nursing, Midwifery and Health Visiting (UKCC), 1996a).

Preparation for the family is treated as a priority and all members of the multidisciplinary team will contribute. Timetabled appointments to pass on the individual's field of expertise, input and support throughout transplant are organised within the BMT timetable. Social workers, play specialists and the transplant co-ordination sister also become involved in home visits in order to acquire a full picture of the social and family network and support systems enabling the child and family to feel more relaxed, with a view to absorbing important information (Figure 8.2).

Grandparents

The role of the grandparents is crucial throughout the BMT process and they need to be included at appropriate stages as

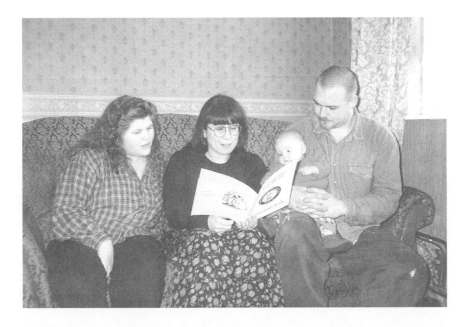

Figure 8.2 Bone marrow coordinator on home visit (reproduced with permission)

they are desperately trying to help their grandchildren but at the same time their need to support and protect their own children is overwhelming. They often express feeling left out, not only about the decision making but especially throughout the inpatient stay. Grandparents are often involved with caring for the grandchildren at home including the donor, therefore they often have the responsibility of being first in line for a variety of complicated questions. However they will prove to be of little use to their grandchildren when reassuring and answering their never-ending questions if they have not been involved in the decision-making process and kept up to date with the course of events in hospital.

Specific preparatory regimens are utilised: preparation for hospital admissions, isolation, central venous line insertion, naso-gastric tubes and feeding, bone marrow harvesting under general anaesthetic or peripheral blood stem cell harvesting methods, bone marrow donation, total body irradiation and cranial and testicular boosts of radiotherapy. All are planned, timetabled and pre-arranged with the family and health care professional to ensure the optimum understanding of all treatments related to the BMT process (Figure 8.3).

Legal and ethical issues affecting families consenting to bone marrow transplantation and nurses involved in the families' preparation

It is well established in English law that a person of sound mind and over the age of 18 years has the right to determine what

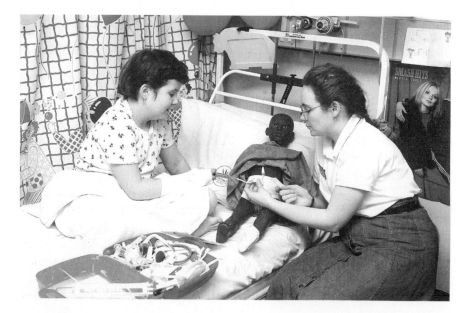

Figure 8.3 Play specialist prepares child for insertion of central line (reproduced with permission)

Case study 8.2

A 16-year-old girl describes for us her decision-making process. 'Having a bone marrow transplant was one of the biggest decisions I have ever made in my 16 years of living. I had been ill constantly, having blood transfusions, high fevers, taking tablets and several other problems – my life could not continue this way. I was asked about having a bone marrow transplant. I was dead against the idea, I did not want to think about it, let alone discuss the matter. I was forced by my parents to find out what it entailed. Still not convinced I blocked it all out of my mind completely. There was no way I was losing my hair, throwing up and making my little brother have an operation to try to make me better when no one on earth could tell me it would really work and that I would be cured for life. That was a year and a half ago now and since then things have only got better. My health has improved greatly, it's a strange but fantastic feeling of becoming "normal". Being able to plan for the future when before you took one day at a time.

should be done to his/her body (Dimond, 1995.) On this point Korgaonkar and Tribe (1993) suggest that a difficulty arises in the cases of the mentally impaired and children under the age of 16 years. Therefore as children are considered to be vulnerable members of our society changes in child law have evolved in an effort to protect and empower them to give or withhold consent to medical treatments. From this legal perspective The Children Act (Department of Health, 1989) states the authority that parents have over their child and in the eyes of the law children under 16 years are not considered competent to consent, although their cognitive maturity and understanding will be of the upmost importance. However for the purpose of preparation and consent for BMT we will refer to informed consent as a process of shared decision making between the family and the BMT team, based on mutual respect and participation (Lasagna, 1983).

It is our experience that the ambiguities of the many possible outcomes of BMT make it difficult to weigh up where this treatment lies within the ethical principles associated with informed consent. The difficulty in adhering to these principles has certainly been cause for concern, for health care professionals, therefore we feel that good information giving enables families to make the decision of what is in the child's best interest and promotes the principle of beneficence. Non-maleficence refers to the prevention of harm, which in the case of BMT is unpredictable as a paradox of BMT is to endure suffering in order to save life (Esbensen, 1996). Furthermore the pace of disclosure of information given in respect of the families' coping strategies requires individual assessment to avoid possible harm related to the emotive content of information discussed. Finally the principle of justice or non-exploitive treatment encompasses the availability of BMT as a treatment modality and the non-coercive approach to presenting this complex treatment. We therefore recommend that consent for BMT be addressed on an individual basis, taking into account the parents' unique experience of their own children, particularly when dealing with emotive issues with the sick child or siblings. The communication links already established with other health care professionals, named nurses, primary health care teams and shared care units offer an invaluable contribution here, at a time when the BMT team are in the early stages of establishing new partnerships with the family. Nevertheless if the law states that minors cannot give consent the decision will lie with those who have parental responsibility. Furthermore, the validity of surrogate or proxy decision making rests on the assumptions that the decision maker can gauge the individual's needs, views or interests with some accuracy (Delany, 1996; Kent, 1996; Mahaffey, 1996). Moreover it could be argued that when such choices need to be made in the context of a child with cancer requiring BMT, that the parents may not be in a rational position to make such a proxy decision (Peck, 1992; Turner, 1993; McCarthy, 1996).

It is also debated by Thomas (1983) and Carney (1987) that it is expecting too much of perspective families undergoing BMT to fully comprehend the potential hazards associated. Given the gruelling nature of the BMT procedure and the associated morbidity and mortality, the decision and consent for the family, particularly parents on behalf of their child, is bound to be difficult and one of significant distress. Furthermore, Andrykowski (1994) states that distress compromises the consent process by: inhibiting communication with the informer, limiting rational consideration of the cost and benefits of BMT and inhibiting comprehension or memory of information communicated during the consent process. It is therefore our philosophy to begin informing as soon as possible to allow time to work through the emotional angst associated. The investment in recruiting, training, retaining and supporting a core group of multidisciplinary experts, pulled together by the co-ordination of the transplant timetable, can therefore not be undervalued as a key facet of sustaining the families' coping strategies when dealing with the massive amount of information required. Home visits and nurse-led clinics can also help families to feel more receptive to discussion and the use of models to introduce the possible care pathways and outcomes may help to clarify some of the ambiguities and uncertainties that go hand in hand with BMT (Figure 8.4).

Many also debate that the decision for BMT is made solely on

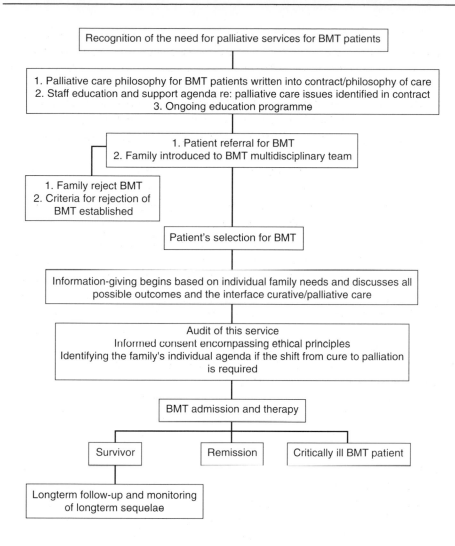

Figure 8.4 Possible care pathways for children undergoing bone marrow transplantation

Figure 8.4   (*Cont'd*)

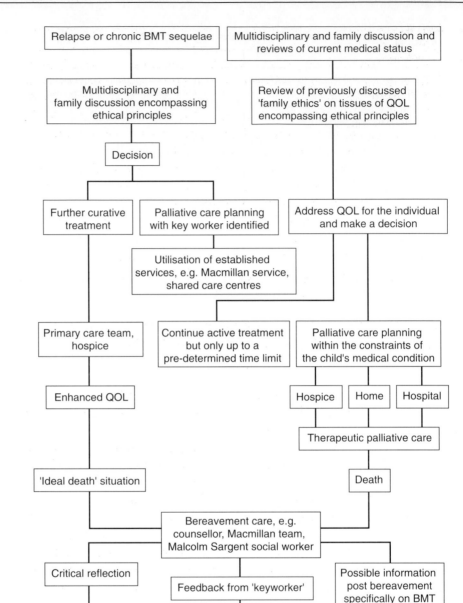

the option of life and death and, if so, is this informed consent? It is our perspective that despite information being discussed on all facets of BMT during the pre-BMT preparation period, fundamentally families are consenting to a curative treatment, with the possibility of palliative care for the future being a difficult concept to comprehend. Moreover no literature could be found regarding an appropriate timescale for addressing the information needs for informed consent in BMT, hence we would argue that there could never be too much time allocated to creating good relationships with families, assessing individual's needs and empowering families to make decisions that are informed.

In recent years empirical qualitative research is evolving in a bid to enable BMT professionals an insight into the view of the family and the impact and usefulness of information pre-BMT (Crook and Hopkins, 1996; Hostrup, 1996; Lawrance, 1997).

Family and health care provider relationships and information giving in preparation for bone marrow transplantation

Many studies have highlighted how parental and family involvement with the sick child has changed in recent years (Department of Health, 1989, 1995, 1996; Association for Children with Life-threatening or Terminal Conditions (ACT) and their Families and The Royal College of Paediatrics and Child Health (RCPCH), 1997). One of the major features of these reports and recommendations is the sharing of care by parents and professionals, which it is suggested should commence prior to admission. Striving efforts have also been made to promote normality for the child and family within the limitations of the hospital environment, a concept known as 'family-centred care', discussed in detail in Chapters 1 and 2. More recently the terms 'parental empowerment', 'shared care' or 'partnerships in care' have been used and reviewed by those attempting to conceptualise the notions of family involvement in the care of the child. The model we feel is more appropriate for utilisation when empowering families undergoing BMT is that described by Gibson (1995), who states that even the most challenging situation for a family can be adapted to, and defines empowerment as a process of recognising, promoting and enhancing a person's abilities to meet their own needs, solve their own problems and mobilise the necessary resources in order to feel they are in control. Generally however the drawback to these suggested models is the lack of guidelines for adaptation to different health care scenarios, and little material to guide nurses on the practicalities (Rennick, 1986; Pass and Pass, 1987).

Success of parental involvement depends on the willingness of the professionals and the enthusiasm of parents (Cleary, 1986; Fradd, 1987; Brown and Ritchie, 1990). However Brown and Ritchie (1990) suggest that most nurses seem unaware that parents might have a very different view of their role, needs and what was best for their child. Garbett (1996) implies the uneven balance of power between consumer and provider as a possible facet of this phenomenon. Melvers (1991), Shelley (1992) and Rudman (1996) all highlight the importance of using people's experience of health care to improve nursing and client education. Furthermore, Wiles (1996), Mallet (1996) and Lawrance (1997) promote methodology to uncover the families' own experience of BMT. Gibson (1989) asserts that the main emphasis on pre-admission preparation for BMT is the development of a relationship with the BMT co-ordinator. Hence the role of supporter and assessor of parents' attitudes to involvement in care can be established, in an aim to empower parents to gain confidence and form a link from home to hospital.

Hostrup (1996) carried out a thorough retrospective investigation of the experiences of parents whose child had survived autologous BMT and their experience of nursing care. The study began with a qualitative approach, by inviting parents to a workshop and using focus group interviews to extract statements and themes from respondents. The next, quantitative part of the study, utilised a questionnaire to measure the weight of various problems previously highlighted in the focus group evaluation and received a 66% return rate. The third stage involved a deep analysis of the data from the focus group from a phenomenological view, and the fourth and final stage was making changes in nursing care practices. Indeed, Hostrup (1996) concludes 'that parents can find a bearable way of existing with their anxieties if they have support and specific information and guidelines'.

The conclusions drawn here are an emphasis on mutually acceptable relationships between families and health care provider if families are to be empowered to participate in decisions and care throughout BMT. Nevertheless the next major issue to enable the BMT process to proceed is the selection and availability of a compatible donor.

Bone marrow donation

Once BMT is voiced as an option for further treatment the avid search begins for a compatible human leucocyte antigen match (HLA). As mentioned earlier, an allogeneic transplant may come from a variety of sources – sibling, parent, extended family member or a matched unrelated donor (MUD). There is a one in four chance of each sibling being a possible match, hence the immediate family will initially be tissue typed, the results shaping the course of the subsequent treatment. The initial waiting period and uncertainty for the family as they 'hope and pray' for a match is often the time when the family's fears are voiced about the potential donor and the effects of donation. If none of the close family members are found to be a match a search of the volunteer donor registers begins, triggering further anxiety related to this uncertainty. If a MUD donor is found the potential donor can withdraw their consent to donate at any time, and in unfortunate circumstances be deemed unfit for donation following the strict medical examinations required. Case study 8.3 presents the devastating position one family found themselves in after a MUD transplant was proposed.

Sibling donation

There are some important points to consider in sibling donation:

- If there is *more than one sibling* in the family, there may be the added pressure of only one being a match and the other feeling rejected, often with the manifestation of behaviour changes.
- There is a possibility that the *siblings may hope to be a match* so they can 'save' their brother or sister's life. On the other hand, they may secretly hope not to be a match but may not admit this to the rest of the family for fear of seeming selfish.

Case study 8.3

John, a 10-year-old boy who had relapsed in both his bone marrow and his central nervous system 2 weeks following completion of 2 years of treatment for acute lymphoblastic leukaemia (ALL), was a prime candidate for a BMT. None of the family members were found to be a match so a search of the voluntary registers was initiated. No UK donors were identified and as this case was considered to be one of urgency an international search was begun and a donor found in the USA. Plans for treatment to commence were progressing to coincide with the availability of this US donor, only for the BMTU to be informed 2 weeks before the transplantation that the donor had been found to be unfit to donate now or in the future. Consequently the recipient's family were devastated, all their hopes for a future for their child were wiped out. Added to their concerns were the fact that their child had not had any treatment for a number of weeks and the genuine fear that the disease could reoccur unless further treatment was given. Try and imagine how this family must have felt?

Using your past experiences within the speciality think of a family you have nursed and discuss with colleagues how you would deal with this situation and what specific skills would be required to plan the supportive care of the family facing such a crisis.

Sometimes *siblings may feel resentment* towards the BMT recipient, as once again they are the one who requires the attention.

There can be problems associated with *parents secretly wishing for one child to be a match as opposed to the other*, however this is a rare occurrence as most parents are so relieved at the discovery of a match at all after the endless uncertainty and waiting (see Case study 8.5)

Case study 8.4 illustrates these points.

Eleanor was a 3-year-old little girl who was to have a transplant for relapsed ALL. She had two sisters, one slightly older and the other about 8 months old. The baby turned out to be a match and the older sister found this extremely difficult to cope with, exhibiting disruptive behaviour at school and regression at home. With the involvement of the play specialists and ward nursing team, the affected sibling was present at all of Eleanor's preparation for BMT. This enabled her to feel informed, involved and valued as an individual family member who too was dealing with the trauma of a member of the family facing a potentially life-threatening procedure.

Case study 8.5

Three-year-old Emma was scheduled to have a transplant for high-risk ALL and had two potential sibling donors. Her parents were secretly wishing that her elder sister would be the match as she had coped much better in the past with her own illnesses, and with Emma's disease and treatment. Tissue typing results revealed it was the younger sister who was the match. She coped very well with the process and if anything enjoyed playing the 'sick role', showing attention-seeking behaviour towards her family and peers by insisting that she should have two nights in hospital as she had arranged for many of her school friends to visit.

- There is also the fear, particularly if there are just two siblings, of *one of them not being the donor* and therefore feeling left with no role to play in the proceedings.

Once a sibling donor has been identified, the interests of all the children involved must be protected in the same way. This is vital at a time when the donor, whatever their age, is very vulnerable to family and outside pressure and is invariably and unintentionally coerced into donating. It is imperative that donors have a sound, full and honest preparation and explanation of the procedure that they will have to endure, especially their understanding of the re-generation process of their marrow. Pinkerton, Cushing and Sepion (1994) said that the sibling's ordeal should not be 'belittled' in terms of comparing it to the sick child. They must feel that they have an important role to play and be encouraged to express their fears and worries. This will rely on sound professional preparation prior to the donor being admitted to the hospital to ensure an

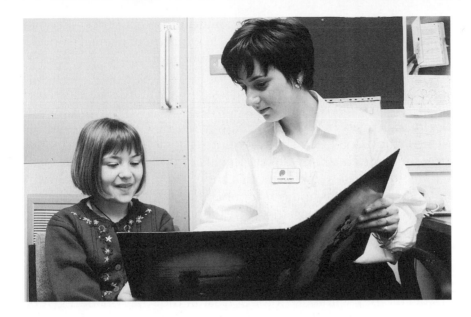

Figure 8.5 Sibling donor preparation by play specialist (reproduced with permission)

adequate understanding of the whole situation, procedures and their implications (Figure 8.5). The peaks and troughs often seen in the sibling's psychological health can be influenced by their sick sibling's physical status as well as fears for their own welfare.

The siblings inevitably have to cope with the outcome of the transplant whatever it may be, however being told of the risk of relapse, graft failure and GVHD is very different to the scenario of watching one's brother or sister going through the painful, unsightly complications associated with BMT. Downs (1994) emphasises that the physical risks are minimal to the donor but the psychological risks could be devastating, this must not be forgotten or taken on lightly.

Downs (1994) states that during hospitalisation of the sibling donor the nursing staff may feel very torn between which individual, the donor or the recipient, needs greatest support; we feel that considerations of both individuals are equally important. We try to ensure the nurse caring for the child receiving the transplant also cares for the donor on the day of transplantation. This relies on sound staffing organisation but hopefully assists in communication and partnership between family members, allowing them to stay in regular contact with both children. In particular at this stressful time the parents feel very torn as to which child to be with. In practice the parents tend to stay with one child each and then swap so that the donor feels less abandoned.

Often the family are physically split during this process, sometimes a long distance from home, leaving their normal support systems behind. In many cases this means that following donation the donor returns to the family home the day after, and is often cared for by grandparents or extended family. Some can feel neglected and feel resentment towards the sick child. One 6-year-old little girl was heard to say 'Now what do I do? I've done my bit now they don't need me anymore'. Doyle (1987) felt siblings were the last to hear any developments of the sick child's progress leading to fantasies and fears that they had caused the problems and then been left at home as a punishment. Children can imagine all sorts of things unless they are kept informed regularly, and they must be encouraged to visit as often as time allows, despite the fact that they may not be allowed to go into the cubicle. It is also vital for the siblings to maintain physical contact with their parents. If changes in the sick child's condition are not relayed frequently they will loose a lot of trust in their information givers, which may well be detrimental to their future relationships with both their siblings, their parents and the BMT team.

The extended search

As the extent of conditions that are treated with BMT expands so does the use of HLA mismatch transplants. At the time that the siblings are tissue typed the parents are tested too. Should one parent prove to be a potential donor the stress on the family's relationship, which is often already being pushed to its limits in having to cope with caring for a child with cancer, may reach breaking point. The enormous guilt that parents have to cope with should the transplant fail inevitably tests their relationship to the limit; fears of relapse or failure of the BMT procedure and the fact the recipient may not survive is a huge burden to carry while also trying to care for the affected child and the family.

Often paediatric transplant centres are within children's hospitals, meaning the parent will often have to donate in an alternative adult hospital, dividing their loyalties at a time when they feel their child needs them most. This calls upon their maternal/paternal feelings to be put in the background, while someone else cares for their child during their own hospitalisation for donation. This can be extremely upsetting, and in some cases means that the parent discharge themselves earlier than would be advised in a bid to get back to caring for their child. This relies on the BMT nurse's supervisory observation of the donor parent in a discreet supportive manner to ensure that the parent takes adequate rest, a vital facet if they are to be of continued benefit to their child throughout the transplant process. At our centre allogeneic PBSC

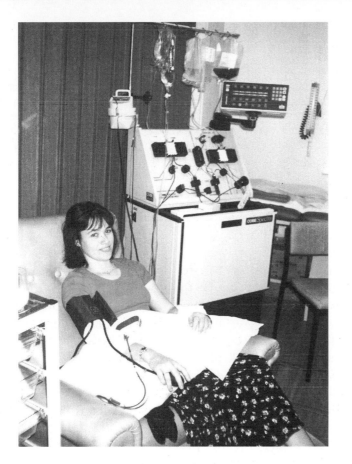

Figure 8.6 Mother donates her peripheral stem cells (reproduced with permission)

harvests of adults including parent donors is carried out by skilled nurses who are part of the BMT team, and therefore are already familiar to the family (Figure 8.6). This cuts down the anxieties mentioned above, has the benefit of an outpatient procedure and it is done at the children's hospital in a private area. (This technique will be discussed in more detail later.)

Matched unrelated donors

The clinical definition of the donor in BMT is rapidly expanding to encompass those beyond the nuclear family (Ruggiero, 1988). There are two volunteer donor panels available, The Anthony Nolan and the Bristol Blood Transfusion Service; they both work closely searching firstly the UK and if requested, the international panels. For some families however the time taken to search is unbearable and it is not unknown for families and their local communities to become very preoccupied in a desperate bid to help to find a match.

Case study 8.6

Adam, a 4-year-old little boy with ALL, was found not to have any family matches. His dad, a policeman, chose to try to establish some community involvement by recruiting colleagues in an attempt to discover a match for his son. This proved to be a very emotive issue placing a lot of strain and pressure on the family, particularly when local press became involved and were intrusive of the family's privacy. However the positive effect on the register, as far as new recruits were concerned, helped the family psychologically as they felt they were putting something back into society.

The endless wait

When the only hope of a match is through the register, it poses the additional burden of time that the child may not have. Should an extended delay occur in the searching for a match the probability of disease relapse and health deterioration increases. With the identification of a compatible donor, however, the transplant team then have the task of juggling the emotions of the family's elation with the need to explain all the risks of transplantation.

With the advent of technology and the easier access to international registers, there has obviously been an increase in the use of international donors. The team and the family however are still acutely aware of the precise timing of the conditioning programme in relation to the arrival of the donor marrow. A recent case at our centre was of a little boy waiting for the marrow to arrive from Australia. The family found it extremely difficult to focus on the day-to-day issues, instead focusing on what could happen to the marrow during transportation, such as spillage, transport problems or contamination, especially as the conditioning regimen was almost complete. Hostrup (1996) describes how parents have fears and fantasies surrounding marrow donation and delivery of the product to the donor.

Bone marrow transplant techniques

Both autologous and more recently allogenic BMT techniques are gradually being replaced by peripheral blood stem cell transplants (PBSCT), this requires the administration of donor conditioning pre-harvest in order to ensure there are an adequate number of stem cells in the peripheral blood for collection, referred to as the 'mobilisation' period. Granulocyte colony stimulating factor (GCSF) is at present the drug of choice, and there has been much debate about the ethics of administering GCSF to healthy donors (Anderlini *et al.*, 1996; Russell, 1996.) Due to the short time that GCSF has been used it is unclear what long-term implications it may have on a healthy individual. We must therefore rely on stringent honesty and the non-coercive approach during the informed consent procedures. The alternative, however, is for the donor to undergo a general anaesthetic for the bone marrow harvest as was traditionally used. At present the administration of GCSF to healthy sibling child donors is not authorised.

The future of bone marrow transplantation

As described earlier the future for BMT is very exciting and is involving some revolutionary treatments. Umbilical cord blood which is rich in stem cells, can now be stored and used to transplant should the cord blood prove to be an HLA match. As parents are becoming more aware of the possibilities of these technologies, inevitably the 'consumer demand' is increasing and the question of whether to conceive to bring about a means to an end is a potential issue. Some families deliberately conceive to potentially find a donor, placing incredible tension on a family already under stress. Sometimes, however, couples have a difference of opinion about the feasibility of this option and outside support or counselling may be warranted.

T-cell re-infusion

The use of T cells from a previous donor has recently become an option for children who have relapsed following transplantation and relies on a second donation. The risk of coercion becomes

Case study 8.7

Elizabeth, a 5-year-old little girl, was diagnosed with ALL but unfortunately relapsed during treatment, and was subsequently HLA tissue typed. There were no family or MUD compatible donors identified, Elizabeth's mum was however expecting a baby at the time, and an umbilical cord harvest was set up for the delivery, with a view to immediate transplantaion if the cord blood was compatible. The results proved to be negative and once again all hopes were dashed as there was little alternative treatment for Elizabeth now that her disease was progressing rapidly; palliative care was therefore introduced. The feelings towards the new baby were difficult, particularly for mum who experienced anger towards her for not being a match. Numerous offers of independent counselling about these negative feelings were offered, however by this time Elizabeth had died and the parents were grieving, desperately stuck in the 'blame stage', directing this negative emotion at the new baby.

The implications for where the baby in Case study 8.7 fits into the family and the reasons for conceiving are massive. Do they tell the child in the future? Is the child really wanted for the individual they are? Retrospectively would a positive tissue type match have lessened the ethical dilemma? Further professional discussion and reflection at this stage may prove beneficial for you.

Is the mother in Case study 8.8 capable of making a rational decision?

Case study 8.8

Timothy, a 2 year old, required a transplant and his mother Susan was the closest HLA match. During the initial discussions about BMT it was established that Susan was fearful about going into hospital and having a general anesthetic but proceeded to donate. Timothy relapsed 6 months post BMT and after all options of further treatment were discussed Susan was called upon to donate her T cells using PBSC harvesting techniques. Susan was already in a desperate situation and facing the fact that her child would probably die, she thinks only about Timothy and not how this second procedure will affect her.

an issue, particularly in relation to the ability of parents being able to make rational decisions at this time of immense stress and if the donor is a child who is under the age of consent. However the donor may see it as a second chance to do good, but equally so it may be a second chance for BMT to fail and if so has the donor then failed twice?

The hospitalised period

Pre transplant

This is a timed and planned admission when all facets come together, such as donor availability and planned conditioning regimens. Admission occurs 7–14 days prior to transplantation in order for the child to begin their conditioning regimen (Figure 8.1). This is a stressful time for the whole family, particularly as they feel it is now the point of no return and often suggests feelings of 'no control'. These feelings can be exacerbated if the family are transferred to another unit or hospital. The uncertainties encountered during this period can become overpowering, even for those families with good understanding and support networks, as despite the extensive preparation period it is not until the admission to hospital that BMT becomes reality.

The post-transplant period is divided into three separate phases:

- Early recovery – the neutropenic phase pre engraftment.
- Mid recovery – the post engraftment phase, usually 2–3 months post BMT.
- Late recovery – the period beyond 3 months as cellular and humoral immunity recover (United Kingdom Childhood Cancer Study Group, Bone Marrow Transplantation Sub Group (UKCCSG), 1996).

Early recovery

All children experience in varying degrees the side effects from the conditioning treatments, many of which are predictable. The whole family require a great deal of support and help through what can be a very daunting process, parents experience feelings of helplessness and loss of control (Whedon, 1991), as the severity of symptoms peak at approximately 7 days post BMT. No two children present in the same way, and many families express devastation at the impact of seeing others going through the same process, but at a different stage. As discussed earlier, the BMT nurse must be astute to the impact of another child's experience on the family throughout the BMT process. Lesko (1994) advises that parents need an identity within the BMT team to help promote better communication and stability when it appears that only uncertainty looms. This relies upon the continuation of open, honest and frequent communication, as there has never been a more important time for the family and the ward team to work together. The expected parental participation in care at a time when the child is highly dependent must not be exploited and the BMT nurse must reflect on their personal expectations of the parents to ensure an equal partnership that is acceptable to both parents and nurse. There may be times when the parents will be unable to act as their child's advocate and communicate for them, thus relying on the BMT nurse to take on the role as child and family advocate until they feel confident to re-establish self care.

Isolation and the psychological implications

As the child's full blood count begins to fall and the child becomes pancytopenic, one of the major risks post transplantation is the complication of life-threatening infection due to neutropenia and prolonged immunouppression (Foley, Fochtman and Mooney, 1993). The child is therefore nursed in protected isolation which aims to eliminate normal microbial flora and prevent colonisation of the patient by new micro-organisms from the hospital; however

Figure 8.7 Parents learn the isolation techniques (reproduced with permission)

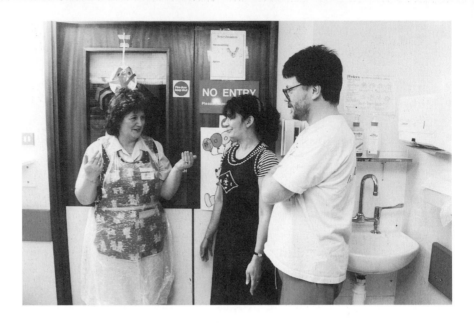

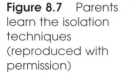

Spend some time reflecting upon your experience of nursing children in isolation.

Discuss with your team the advantages and disadvantages and future possible changes in isolation principles and practices and how they might affect the management of your nursing resources.

endogenous flora plays a large role as a source of infection in the neutropenic child. The isolation procedure itself poses a great deal of anxiety and apprehension for the child and the whole family. The overall goal should be to minimise the impact of isolation on an already stressed family (Foley *et al*. 1993), thus maintaining good psychological health. Not only is the transplantation approaching rapidly but the family are now empowered to take on the responsibility of maintaining protective isolation. Both the parents and the child will have had specific formal preparation for isolation, however the day that the child goes into isolation can be particularly stressful for the family (Figure 8.7). They are required to prepare all the clothes, belongings and food, plus try to physically get the child bathed and into clean clothes before they can go in – an exhausting schedule!

Minimal empirical research exists on the argument of isolation versus non-isolation, however within the UK alone many different techniques are adopted. You may argue, is isolation really necessary? Ask yourself the following: what difference would it make to the long-term outcome if children were nursed in a cubicle with the use of stringent hand-washing techniques as opposed to filtered air or laminar flow cubicles? Are we fostering dependence by exaggerating the importance of isolation? Are we therefore increasing the stress put on the family by enforcing the isolation issue?

Once in isolation, there never seems to be enough space. Lack of natural light, fresh air and seeing the same faces contribute to a dreary, long and uncertain road ahead. The child's activities are very restricted, which can prove to be difficult especially for the initial days if the child is reasonably physically well and needs

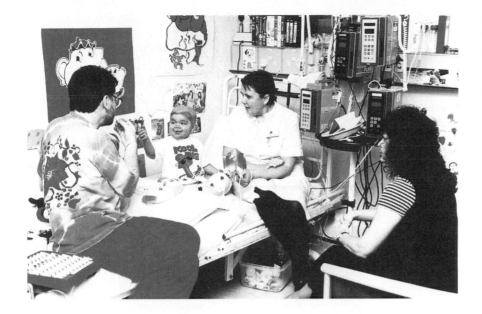

Figure 8.8   A child can still have fun despite the restrictions of isolation (reproduced with permission)

lots of occupying. Isolation is not however all bad and most of the children do have fun (Figure 8.8). Nevertheless discipline and initial boundary setting needs to be established to enable the nursing staff to give appropriate care. Therefore negotiation and organisation must occur with the children at an early stage, preferably when they are still feeling well enough to make their own decisions. Keeping the momentum of an agreed partnership however becomes difficult for staff when there is low compliance.

The infants

Much literature concentrates on the effect on child development while the child is in isolation. Lesko *et al.* (1984) advise careful consideration for the developing infants who need to smell, handle and touch. At our BMT unit we have the facilities to enable parents to sleep with their children while in isolation (Figure 8.9).

The younger child

The younger age group may display signs of overdependence and behavioural regression, which may be brought about by sensory deprivation. This calls on the multidisciplinary team to be routinely involved, for example the play specialist, the physiotherapist and the school teachers, on a daily basis.

An 8-year-old little girl described isolation as 'I feel like a caged animal because I can't talk to anyone properly and play with the other children. I wish there was a door so I could look out like in Alice in Wonderland'.

Remarkably the majority of the children and their families cope

Figure 8.9 *Parental contact is vital throughout isolation (reproduced with permission)*

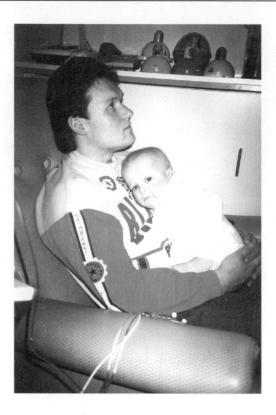

extremely well with isolation if they feel supported and informed. In our experience we have only had one child who physically tried to get out of the isolation room – a reflection of the impact of appropriate preparation and occupation for the isolated child.

The adolescent

Teenagers in isolation, particularly the adolescents, often complain that it is like an intrusion into their privacy when suddenly they have to return to being dependent on others. Suddenly their control and autonomy are taken away from them, which invariably leads to differing opinions, often with long-suffering parents. For BMT nurses it is a common intervention and large part of the routine psychological support of teenagers to reinforce the routines and rationale of isolation, enabling them to make informed decisions regarding their care. Abramovitz and Senner (1995) advise allowing active participation for the adolescents and choice where possible within a structure of daily care. Moreover many teenagers comment positively on the peace and quiet in a cubicle, which they appreciate when they are feeling unwell.

During the protective isolation period we put a restriction on visitors to a maximum of three main carers, which we recognise can put additional stress on the sibling relationships. Both the sick child and young siblings can become encapsulated in their own worlds if they are not kept up to date with what is happening to each other. Until empirical guidelines are available we will continue this practice with the rationale that school age children are at risk of being in contact with infectious disease, hence the physical risks to the sick child outweigh the possible psychological manifestations.

The importance of normalising the child's routine while in isolation cannot be overemphasised, as the expectations are that the child will recover from transplantation. In order to display some individuality the children are encouraged to help decorate their room and bring in photographs or any other momentos from home to help them feel more settled. Isolation is surprisingly rarely seen as a negative issue and some families even described positive feelings of being attentively cared for while in isolation (Lesko, 1994).

The day of the bone marrow infusion is often described as an anticlimax; however, from then on the pathway to the individual's final outcome of BMT is unpredictable. The child relies on structured, routine and thorough daily care during the period of profound immunosuppression until engraftment. Much of the routine care encompasses personal hygiene, which can be quite upsetting for the child, and non-compliance can become a major issue unless dealt with in a way which is acceptable to the child and family. The play specialists are an invaluable member of the BMT team and are a great help at this time by encouraging and motivating through age-appropriate play, for example by designing star or sticker charts for help with procedures, in particular mouth care.

Non-compliance

During this acute pancytopenic period many of the principals used to care for the critically ill child do apply. The parents are put into an extremely difficult position once their children start to refuse to comply with treatment that on the surface seems to be non life threatening, but all the same very necessary. Whedon (1991) encourages a family-centred approach with open and honest communication, involvement of the patient and family in the care and ongoing education. Daily negotiation of care is imperative, so that the parents have a choice regarding what care they wish to be involved with for that day. The degree to which the parents wish to be involved will vary considerably within a family and tends to be linked to how well their child is at the time.

Tesno (1995) found that if the nurse assumed responsibility for difficult treatment it proved less frustrating and emotionally less draining on the family members; however, difficulties may become apparent if the parents or carers begin to see the BMT nurse as pushing their child to the limits in attempting to nego-tiate compliance. The use of the 'named-nurse system' is useful at this time as it encourages continuity of care and helps to restore the balance of partnership as the parent then continues to be the person to give the comfort and reward and is not seen to be the perpetrator of inflicting pain and upset. The issue of adherence to treatment or strategies for non-compliance in the paediatric BMT setting has been addressed thoroughly (Phipps and De Cuir-Whalley, 1990).

Atkins and Patenaude (1987) comment particularly on the difficulties parent donors have in setting limits on their child's behaviour, as there is the fear that the recipient would not survive. This situation relies on an independent person to help lay down ground rules if the family are to maintain appropriate family roles and daily routine care is to be achieved. This relies upon excel-lent pre-BMT planning, preparation and organisation to include contingency plans for parents, such as taking it in turns to be the main carer and the use of family accommodation away from the BMT unit and the encouragement of regular breaks.

As the child's full blood count begins to recover the rehabilita-tion process from the dependent state of isolation needs consi-deration. This creates additional worries that the parents usually dwell upon themselves well before the time arrives. The feelings most commonly expressed are not being able to wait to get out of the cubicle, where as others would rather stay in isolation until they are discharged. Each individual will have differing views and the situation relies upon much support and encouragement for all.

Although the transplant process is unpredictable there are a number of side effects that one can guarantee the majority of the children will experience. Many of these side effects are caused by the complex conditioning regimens. If you have limited expe-rience of BMT nursing, it is essential that you do some further reading around the issues identified in Box 8.1 and the related nursing care issues. When reading about these side effects always consider how these acute symptoms can impact on the psycho-logical health, for example mucositis leads to severe pain which often requires opiate pain relief which may cause sleepiness. The side effect of sleepiness however can impinge on the child's ability to carry out self care, therefore compliance is hindered.

Always in the parents' minds is the possibility that the marrow will not engraft or be rejected. Parents become particularly tuned into the results of the daily full blood counts, continually looking for the first neutrophil. They become extremely concerned if they spot any changes, particularly drops in the neutrophil count once the marrow has started regenerating. White (1994) reported on the physical and emotional stress associated with the full blood count results, one parent said 'there is nothing more anxious than waiting for the count, you sit there and literally shake waiting'. Once the consultant decides to perform a bone marrow aspirate they hope that the wait is over to discover whether the marrow is that of the donor, and then in some cases still the wait goes on as the confirmation through chromosome studies can take weeks to complete. There is also the possibility that the disease will recur before the marrow has had a chance to engraft which in itself has major implications, not least that the disease is resistant to the high-dose treatment and therefore what is the future for their child?

GVHD is the donor T lymphocyte cells mounting an immune reaction against the patient (host), resulting in clinical disease (Foley *et al.*, 1993). Clinical GVHD seen most frequently is that of the skin, gut and liver, and it has a distressing impact for the child's family as the child's condition appears to be deteriorating, despite the fact that the BMT has worked, yet again exacerbating the uncertainty of the final outcome. Such acute complications can become chronic long-term problems and involve numerous unpleasant treatments to halt the donor cells' immune reaction of the host.

In turn this treatment will cause more adverse side effects, so the original focus of treatment fades into the distant past. At this time the BMT nurse's insight is extremely important, the skills to predict and anticipate the potential problems the children may encounter enables prompt intervention which we believe is an art acquired through experience and practice.

There is a possibility that children undergoing BMT require intensive care (ITU) treatment, which will once again shift the focus of outcome of the BMT. Some paediatric ITUs have filtered air or laminar flow cubicles, but in most cases the child will be nursed in a single cubicle or on the main unit. The family are suddenly plummeted into an alien environment with people they do not know and their child is extremely unwell usually requiring ventilation. Families experience feelings of insecurity and abandonment at an emotionally and clinically challenging time (Buchsel and Whedon, 1995). Their worst fear is now that the child will not survive and in the short term what will the future hold? It is vital to keep up the relationships with the ward/unit to provide support for the parents and for the ITU staff who may well be unfamiliar with the care of transplant patients. Collaborative partnerships which provide mutual support for both sets of staff are encouraged (Buchsel and Whedon, 1995) and can only prove beneficial for all concerned, not least the child and family.

McConville *et al.* (1990) found that many of the older children who had experienced the ITU expressed concerns when further complications arose and often requested not to be left alone. A recent experience at our unit reciprocated this; Mohammed, a 15-year-old boy, required ITU treatment with full ventilation and sedation. He later returned to the BMT unit but became so anxious he could not settle down, relax or sleep, and became prone to panic attacks, eventually returning to the ITU. When coming back to the unit for a second time he was so frightened at being left alone that he needed one-to-one care plus lots of support and reassurance for a number of days to regain his confidence. Long-term impressions of ITU treatment must not be underestimated for the lasting effects it may have on the child and the family. On return from the ITU the family's priorities may be very different from when they left the BMT unit, so the importance of a thorough handover from the ITU staff is essential for continuity of care.

As the length of stay for transplantation continues the parents' abilities to cope can deteriorate with lack of sleep and the ongoing worry of the condition of their child. Once again the BMT nurse must be aware and encourage the parents to take regular rests, especially when the children are sleeping, and let others help out with the care if necessary. Lee *et al.* (1994) found that the parents' ability to cope or not tended to serve as a model for the child's coping strategies. Financial insecurities can also develop as an additional worry, despite many employers responding compassionately to the family's dilemma.

Late recovery

Leading on from the acute transplant phase where the child experiences rapid and uncertain fluctuations in their condition, they proceed to a late recovery phase, up to day +100 post BMT. By this stage engraftment has often been documented and from that respect there is a huge sense of relief. After weeks of being totally focused on blood count recovery the family now see stability, and a general improvement in their child's condition. From this stage two common pathways emerge: one of recovery, rehabilitation, planned discharge advice and home with close follow-up; the other the onset of GVHD and associated complications. If the latter pathway is followed obviously emotions go on a downward spiral and nursing interventions increase accordingly.

The first line of treatment for GVHD is often immunosuppressive therapy, resulting in an increased risk of infection, more prophylactic antimicrobials and active treatment if the child becomes febrile. This relies on the excellent communication skills of the BMT nurse to clarify the parents understanding of GVHD, its treatment and the side effects, but most importantly the uncertainty of the effectiveness of these treatments.

Phipps and De Cuir-Whalley (1990) comment on the extended hospital stay requiring greater efforts at maintaining adherence, which invariably deteriorates over time. Frequent negotiation in care is essential as the child's condition peaks and troughs, and the family's coping mechanisms are challenged. McConville *et al.* (1990) found that parents of children who had unexpectedly high complications showed more psychological distress patterns than for those who had survived up to 1 year after BMT. It is essential that the team do not assume that the parents' coping abilities are static the longer that they are inpatients.

All these contribute to a very frightening and uncertain future as the child's dependence on supportive care increases rather than decreases, despite the length of time since the transplantation. Inevitably the families will also see other children recovering far quicker with minimal complications, which can only burden them further and increase their fears as they struggle to cope with the extended stay and the seriousness of their child's condition. White (1994) found parents' relationships with other transplant families proved to be especially significant in the support they provided. It is helpful to acknowledge these benefits, but we must not forget the potential reverse effects that these relationships may have.

The length of time between engraftment and discharge is very variable. Because of the uncertainty of GVHD there is no set date for discharge post BMT. These families are placed in a phase where their child is not visibly recovering neither are they rehabilitating. In addition the child may well be experiencing the somnolence caused by the radiotherapy, an expected side effect which invariably coincides with the symptoms of GVHD.

Many of the younger children display symptoms of withdrawal, not wanting to play, not sleeping properly and at times refusing to verbalise. At this stage non-compliance can present itself again as the need to carry on daily care extends and the child and the family are unable to visualise any end to the problems. Inevitably they also pick up on their parental worries which can only add to their distress. Continued involvement of the whole team, especially the teachers and the play specialists, is vital at this stage.

The discharge

The decision when to discharge must be made in partnership with the family. The medical staff must be content that the child is stable and the nursing staff must feel confident that the parents/carers are capable of coping with their child's care at home, but most importantly the family must feel confident. Buchsel and Whedon (1995) said that the goal of discharge planning should be that the patients and carers need to feel knowledgeable, comfortable with daily routines, medications and symptom reporting.

As there is so much to cover, discharge planning begins as soon as possible to enable the families to learn at their own pace. Buchsel and Whedon (1995) found parents overwhelmed with the number of medications required; however it is imperative that both the child and parents are made aware of non-compliance and the consequent grave complications.

Cultural, religious and language barriers are becoming more of an issue in multicultural communities. This puts immense pressure on all concerned and adds additional stress to the family and relies on thorough preparation and discussions throughout the transplantation. In some cases this factor has extended the stay of the child due to the time needed to prepare the family for discharge through an interpreter.

The families must be assessed on an individual basis. Brown and Kelly (1976) talked about the parents' ambivalence prior to discharge, they were happy but insecure about leaving the hospital and how their lives had been altered by the transplant. Many families at this stage are eager to leave hospital, usually due to the extended stay and lack of normalcy in their lives, however they also experience feelings of fear, panic and isolation as they leave the one place where they have felt secure, protected, understood and 'loved'. This relies on re-establishing partnerships of care with health professionals in the community to provide the continued support that is so vital after such a stressful experience. Before they leave, however, it must be clarified and communicated exactly who is to continue the overall management of their care. The families are always reassured that they can contact the unit at any time however minor the problem. Many families say that they did not use this service but that it was comforting to known that it was available should they run into difficulties.

Try and list all the interventions and skills that parents will need to be confident with prior to the child being discharged. Which skills would you consider to be nursing skills and which are parenting skills?

The post-discharge period

Post-transplant care

Children post BMT receive close follow-up care at least on a weekly basis. If the families live a long way away from the hospital, as is often the case with regional centres, then the links with the shared care hospitals and community professionals must be negotiated pre discharge. Atkins and Patenaude (1987) discussed the shared care staff's relief and joy of survival of the child which may overshadow the reality of how precarious the medical condition is.

Many parents however are quite happy to have continued support from the transplant centre and feel reassured by the concerns for their child, however individualised patient care must be considered and the potential for fostering continued dependence on the transplant centre is a consideration that professionals need to address. Moreover the regional BMTU continues the responsibility for long-term follow up according to UKCCSG long term follow-up guidelines.

Settling back into a routine

Despite the initial anxieties pre discharge, once the family arrive home there is a sense of euphoria as they are a 'survivor of BMT'. However often the family soon discover the child is experiencing restricted ability compared to their previous 'well' status and they often begin to realise they have unrealistic expectations of the length of time it will take to return to normalcy. The family need support and reassurance post discharge regarding the pace of activity and the rehabilitation process, often home visits from a member of the BMT team can be worthwhile.

Altered body image

The child's altered body image continues to be a worrying issue for a long time post transplant. Jennifer, a 16-year-old girl said, 'I hated the sight of myself, my skin was darker, drier and flaky, I would cover myself up totally'. This illustrates the intensity of feelings they experience, which we as a team often accept as a part of BMT without empathy related to the reactions of others. The team must be sensitive to the child's reaction to their altered body image and sensitively address them, particularly with adolescents who have survived transplantation and are then expected to slot back easily into their peer groups, a very daunting prospect. The same girl talked about buying girls magazines: 'all they would feature was pretty, thin girls with a head of long silky hair, beauty advice and places to go with your mates'. All this adds to their stress as they try to rediscover their place back to the 'body beautiful society' that we live in.

Many children are discharged on steroid treatment leaving them cushingoid, carrying extra weight and they could potentially be hairy due to the cyclosporin. They may still require nasogastric feeding and many children develop dark pigmentations of their skin caused by some conditioning therapies and GVHD. At last they are free to go out only for people to stare and comment, friends and close family may even comment on not being able to recognise them. The family continues to require support and reassurance, especially if the children begin to refuse to go out because of their physical appearance.

Buchsel and Whedon (1995) found many families fatigued and confused as to what to expect of the patients post discharge. This varies greatly from one child to the next and the difficulty some children experience in returning to 'normal' must not be under-emphasised, some distress levels will remain very high whereas others will slot back in quickly and easily.

The return to school

If BMT has gone smoothly the child will return to school after about 6 months, which is a major stepping stone to recovery. Close communications with the school are vital so the teachers are aware of any necessary restrictions, and often a visit from the BMT co-ordinator may alleviate concerns and worries. The uncertainty of how the children will be received back at school is a huge worry for all concerned. Invariably the child's form or year and close friends are a great support, it is the children in other years who are unaware of the circumstances who poke fun and tease adding to the child's list of experiences that they have to find their own way of coping with. Jennifer, the 16-year-old who described her feelings about body image above, also commented on going back to school:

> Going back to school was hard work, I had actually returned to school in the November to take my mock GCSEs but the work was so hard I felt under pressure and it was a relief when my head of year said I didn't have to take them. I hated having no hair and having to wear a hat, everyone in my year knew why I was wearing a hat and was really caring, whilst those in the year below just thought it would be funny to make comments about me.

White (1994) describes the vulnerability of returning to normal which was accompanied by a need to know what the future holds as identified by parents concerns post-BMT discharge. Many complications may occur months to years after transplantation, such as cataracts, interstitial pneumonitis, relapse, secondary malignancies and infertility; all these warrant further reading to give an overall idea of what long-term psychological stresses the children and their families are asked to cope with. The majority of families have not allowed themselves to think any further than the BMT. The long-term effects on parents coping with a child undergoing BMT has also been likened to a post-traumatic stress disorder (Heiney *et al.*, 1994):

- degree of life threat
- duration of the trauma
- degree of bereavement or loss of significant others
- displacement from the home community
- potential for re-occurrence of disease
- role of parent in the trauma
- exposure to death.

With the passage of time families become less dependent on hospital- and community-based staff, whether fully recovered or suffering the long-term sequelae of BMT. White (1994) provides the groundwork for future research into the post-BMT experience by giving caregivers an insight into the impact of various situational factors on a family passage through the transitional period from dependency to independence. However for some children the outcome of BMT is not successful.

The interface between curative and palliative care for children undergoing bone marrow transplantation

Earlier we mentioned how strategies for improving cure rates continue and outcomes of BMT are reported in number or type of response, or length of disease-free survival. However in an effort to bring together and balance all outcomes of treatment, ACT and RCPCH (1997) suggest that information be gathered identifying the missing qualitative data on issues of morbidity as well as mortality. Moreover for those children whose outcome of BMT is not cure, palliative interventions are essential. It is not however the purpose of this section to discuss the therapeutic care needs of BMT families, but to address the ambiguity of BMT as the main hindrance to the transition from curative to palliative treatment goals.

Palliative care for children and young people with terminal illness encompasses an active and total approach to care, embracing physical, emotional, social and spiritual elements. It focuses on the enhancement of quality of life for the child and support for the family, and includes the management of distressing symptoms and the provision of respite care through death and bereavement (discussed further in Chapter 12). The latest UK document on palliative care services for children delineate four broad groups of children with life-threatening conditions: Group 1 includes those with conditions for which curative treatment may be feasible but may fail, true of the group of children undergoing BMT for malignant disease (ACT and RCPCH, 1997). It is our experience that a variation in palliative care provision exists for some BMT patients.

If a child becomes terminally ill following the relapse of a malignant condition or following long-term sequelae post BMT, planned palliative care enables a dignified comfortable end to their life; 'the ideal death situation' (Parkes, 1977). Proven and established plans of care are in use at most regional oncology and haematology centres, originating from earlier 'oncology models' and discussed later in Chapter 12. However it is our observation that a group of children exist, who suffer acute adverse effects

Case study 8.9

Regimen for Jason, a critically ill child following BMT:

Day −14: admission to hospital for insertion of triple lumen central line and back-up bone marrow harvest.

Days −12 to −1: all pre- BMT conditioning completed, prophylactic anti microbial and anti rejection therapy commenced.

Day 0: allogenic BMT administered, filtered air isolation cubicle and dietary restrictions started.

Day +2: onset of pyrexia with neutropenia requiring 1st line antibiotic therapy.

Day +4: persistent pyrexia and rigors with negative microbial cultures, hence antibiotics changed. Thrombocytopenia with little platelet increment following transfusion. Intravenous morphine started for severe mucositis.

Day +5: commenced on total parental nutrition.

Day +8: persistent pyrexia, commenced on IV antifungal therapy. Hypertension and tremor diagnosed as cyclosporin toxicity.

Day +9: acute renal failure requiring haemodialysis.

Days +10 to +15: continuation as above.

Day +16: macular, papular rash confirmed as acute GVHD.

Day +9: neutrophil count persistently up, isolation relaxed.

Days +21 to 26: raised serum bilirubin, skin GVHD worse, started on high-dose IV steroids.

Day +27: liver biopsy confirms severe GVHD liver, antilymphocytic globulin started. Bone marrow aspiration shows engraftment. Requiring increased doses of IV morphine for control of abdominal pain.

Day +30: liver failure diagnosed, requiring massive doses of coagulation therapy tor gastrointestinal and urinary tract bleeding. GVHD skin deteriorating.

Day +32: rapid deterioration of respiratory function, chest X-ray shows pneumonia, all active treatment continues.

Day +33: discussion with parents of the inappropriateness of cardiopulmonary resuscitation or artificial ventilation if required. All active treatment continues, clergy informed and visited family.

Day +34: Jason dies with all active treatment continuing.

following BMT, whether due to failure or complications of the procedure consequently becoming acutely ill and often terminal. Esbensen (1996) describe the side effects of BMT as often worse than the underlying disease being treated. Buchsel and Whedon

(1995) acknowledge the fact by recognising the related morbidity of BMT as an ethical dilemma caused by the application of such an advanced technology as BMT. This scenario is demonstrated by Case study 8.9 Jason, a 14 year old, who received BMT as treatment for ALL.

As with all facets of BMT there are no guidelines or criteria for acknowledging the need to move from curative to palliative care for the children who become critically ill. Emphasis for cure therefore may continue until a few days or even hours before death, resulting in an undignified end to the life of the child and a lifetime of trauma for the family in remembering the events that preceded their child's, brother's/sister's death. Often initially the parents express guilt as they equate the suffering with the conditioning therapy and complications of transplantation, and feel a great responsibility for committing their child to 'a death sentence' by signing a consent document on their behalf.

We find ourselves asking why there is a variation in the approach to palliative care intervention for some children when there exists considerable empirical evaluation and research on the general needs of families dealing with the dilemma of moving from curative to palliative care (Soutter *et al.*, 1994; Beresford, 1995; While *et al.*, 1996). However no guidelines exist to guide families or health care professionals facing this outcome of BMT, which relates to the relative infancy of BMT as a treatment compared to other specialities, and leaves a massive gap between the theories of therapeutic palliative care interventions and practice in the paediatric BMT setting. The dilemma is exacerbated by the perceptions of the family in relation to the ambiguity of outcomes of BMT, as despite balanced information being discussed pre-consent, fundamentally the family are consenting to a curative treatment. Furthermore, there is a lack of educational or support resource for health care professionals on this very specific issue (Shedd, 1991; ACT and RCPCH, 1997). Shedd (1991) also comments on the noticeable avoidance of communication/discussion on issues related to quality of life among health care professionals dealing with this situation, and suggests personal attitudes or coping strategies could be responsible for evoking this response. However whatever the reasons for the lack of research or guidelines, we feel that the accumulation of informal data from the clinical field through retrospective reflection rationalises a need for further exploration of this ethical and professional dilemma. It is therefore the BMT nurse's professional responsibility as part of the BMT team to acknowledge possible reasons that hinder effective palliative care 'act always in such a manner as to promote and safeguard the interests and well-being of patients and clients' (UKCC, 1996a).

Take a few minutes to reflect on your own experiences of caring for a child in the terminal stages following BMT. Jot down the palliative care interventions the child had. Did you feel this was satisfactory? If not reflect on what you learnt and clarify what could have been done more effectively.

Some of the ambiguities that may stand in the way of palliative interventions are clarified below.

Ambiguity of outcomes of bone marrow transplantation identified during the informed consent process

The ambiguity and uncertainty faced by families undergoing BMT originates from the time of referral for BMT selection and may continue until cure or death, placing an immense strain on the coping capacity for families who can be given few concrete answers during this time of immense crisis. At this stage during the BMT process the nurse as advocate has a demanding role to play in reiterating and explaining the ever-changing clinical condition of the critically ill child. The family will also certainly need a listening ear, as they attempt to justify their past and future decisions. However no matter what decision is made, whether it be to continue in the curative mode or to explore palliation, the family need to continue their partnership with the professionals with whom they have a secure trusting relationship, as both choices have uncertain outcomes.

Ambiguity of diverse opinion and attitudes of health care professionals at the time of moving from curative to palliative treatment goals

For nurses caring for a child undergoing BMT one of the greatest disappointments is the realisation of a failed curative attempt. Familiar common side effects can be dealt with as they are an expectation of BMT (Box 8.1); however the unexpected, severe uncontrollable adverse effects often blur the way forward. During this period we acknowledge the expression of concerns by BMT nurses over the continuation of 'the curative mode' and the inevitability of death. This is the time when most will challenge their own agreed personal ethics for working in such a speciality (Ellis, 1992). The two key emotional dynamics present in nurses working in the BMT environment that require clarity essential to their emotional functioning are: guilt as the person administering the agent that may cause the side effects, for example the infusion of the bone marrow product that subsequently engrafts but then causes graft versus host disease, resulting in a loss of perspective of the original disease, and the reason for BMT. (Issues surrounding staff emotional coping and involvement is discussed in detail in Chapter 6.)

Ambiguity of professional opinion and attitudes having effect on relationships and partnerships within the family

Another possible hindrance can be the issues of professional conflict about the interface between curative and palliative care.

This problem can only be addressed openly if good team foundations exist. Forman *et al.* (1994) describes the relationships between the staff and family throughout the BMT process as a psychological system, however others state that this system can fray, resulting in a detrimental effect on patient and family care. Futterman and Wellisch (1990) state that the breakdown of this psychological team system is seen more commonly surrounding conflicts in sight of the dying patient. Often nurses see that patients have been selected inappropriately on the grounds of research goals or outcomes and doctors often feel that nurses lack vision or proper scientific perspective necessary to advance the speciality. We would argue that effective education and the comfort of sharing professional perspectives in a comfortable informal setting would enable a shared vision to be presented to the family.

Ambiguity of resistance to changing treatment goals

There are many views on the inability of health care professionals to resist a move from curative to palliative measures. A shared opinion is that many experienced health care professionals feel uncomfortable at identifying the point at which medical intervention is no longer useful (Vianello and Lucamante, 1988; Emery, 1990). Some doctors also see death as a failure (Olin, 1982). Others feel justified that they are doing the family a favour by withholding information, on the assumption that they will not cope (Dickenson and Johnson, 1993; Fallowfield, 1993). Frank dishonesty or evasion however may add to the family's distress and prolong the adjustment process from curative to palliative care. Lichter (1984) states:

> silence may be eloquent ... But if we do not tell it is not just the prognosis we withhold, we have not told the family that we understand the illness, understand how they feel and that we shall support them and keep them comfortable, the essence of palliative care.

Ambiguity and misconceptions by health care professionals of the family's perception of events

A recurrent dilemma originates from the misconception that parents understand things in the same way as health care professionals, and are aware of the shift from the curative mode before receiving explanations. Pinkerton *et al.* (1994) established that this is untrue. In the case of Jason's family in Case study 8.9 intuition and experience alerted many BMT nurses to the near-death situation; from day + 27 onwards, however others felt that the family were also intuitive of the situation. We feel that if BMT nurses are to carry on working as advocates as discussed earlier, then they must be involved with other members of the BMT team in information giving to empower the family to make informed choices. The information required at this turning point has to be honest and realistic if partnerships already established are to be of continued benefit. At this point the care pathways already familiar to the family can prove invaluable in clarifying and communicating that cure is no longer attainable, but supportive palliative intervention is (see Figure 8.4). The tool can also be an asset in encouraging ethical debate and appreciation of others as well as one's own personal perception/beliefs, hence strengthening team support and improving patient care.

Staffing issues

Kiss (1996) recognises that little attention has been given to the psychosocial side of staff working in the area of BMT and therefore makes recommendations. We will utilise the identified model to address issues within our BMT team that are specific to paediatric transplantation and will highlight the stresses, possible criteria for preventing problems and future challenges.

Specific stressors

Specific stressors can be identified:

- The BMT nurse is continuously coping with treatments that cause high morbidity and mortality.
- The continuous advancement of BMT technology and the associated ethical dilemmas.
- Misconceptions about BMT nursing: by answering the question of what BMT nursing entails, an opportunity is given to alleviate misconceptions often expressed by those not directly involved in nursing care, and consequently this raises the profile of BMT nurses.
- The potential for the loss of perspective of the original disease.
- Financial and human resource restraints affecting patient care and job satisfaction.
- Physically and psychologically demanding nursing care issues.
- Attachment to long-term patients.
- Dealing with loss and bereavement.
- The risk of overinvolvement.
- The continuous need for education and updates.
- The extended scope of practice increasing the degree of professional responsibility and accountability. DiSalvo (1996) describes BMT nursing as a profession with maximum accountability and responsibility, but with varying degrees of authority.

- Professional conflict from within the ward team, BMT team and others outside of the direct care environment. Bacon (1993) describes 'on the job conflict' as a clash with personal beliefs.

Burnout

High stress levels, emotional exhaustion, low personal accomplishment, development of negative self concept, negative job attitudes and loss of ability to be concerned for clients are all identified as factors related to burnout in BMT nursing (Maslach, 1979).

Molasiotis *et al.* (1994) carried out a study of 15 BMTUs in the UK to evaluate the psychological effects, burnout syndrome and job satisfaction in nursing and medical staff. As a result of the increased work-related stress, 73% of nurses and 53.8% of doctors mentioned that they had experienced difficulties in their daily personal life and social life. The BMT working environment proved to be very stressful for both doctors and nurses; many respondents suggested that intervention techniques should be introduced. In conclusion it was felt that working stress and psychological problems, combined with low job satisfaction in BMT health care professionals, decreased patients' quality of care and increased the number of nurses giving up their jobs, or being unable to cope with their stresses.

Preventing burnout

Staff coping mechanisms will be discussed as personal and establishment or professionally organised initiatives:

- *Personal initiatives* tend to focus on self reflection of coping strategies and the responsibility for recognising stress and the appropriate management, whatever is suitable for the individual.
- *Establishment initiatives* must begin with the assessment and recruitment of the 'appropriate personality' type (described in detail in Chapter 6) and the recognition of the existence of stresses in the BMTU, as well as the importance of stress management.

The following mechanisms can be adopted to prevent burnout:

- For nurses new to the speciality preceptorship programmes (UKCC, 1996b) linking a newly qualified or appointed nurse (the preceptees) to a nurse with extensive BMT experience is recommended, as is the use of clinical nurse specialists or clinical educators to ensure nurses are acquiring the relevant educational input from the onset of their experience.
- Setting agreed standards of care and policies related to

specific procedures can also enable nurses to feel they are working within defined objectives.

● Establishing a shared vision for the future also promotes a proactive approach to the future challenges within the speciality.

● Performance management strategies offer an opportunity for all staff to recognise and discuss difficulties, as well as planning and setting objectives for the future.

● An ongoing educational update helps to empower nurses.

● Partnership in care with families undergoing BMT can offer many rewards for nursing staff, who with experience and confidence can develop a professional but humoured relationship with the family. Particularly when the family are in isolation the BMT nurse is often relied upon to be the link with the outside world and the person that will ease the loneliness. Even though we have acknowledged the potential here for overinvolvement, we also recognise that there is a place for humour, sharing jokes and experiences, that to a degree helps to bridge the gap between the professionals and the patient and brings some normalcy to a very unnatural existence.

● The use of 'in-house' humour serves a purpose in alleviating stress from very stressful situations. For those looking in from outside of the immediate care arena there may be the assumption that there is nothing to laugh at working in such an area when considering all the specific stresses identified above. However for those experienced in working in emotive high-stress situations, you will agree that often the most emotive of situations can sometimes become funny, humour being a coping mechanism in itself.

● Structured professional support and counselling sessions are available for team members as a group or 'one-to-one' sessions. We have found it useful to use an 'outsider' such as one of the hospital counsellors or psychologists who are only indirectly involved with the BMT team. A chairperson for group meetings takes a neutral approach and enables the discussions to stay focused, which avoids the meetings turning in to moaning sessions. ACT and RCPCH (1997) in the guidelines for paediatric palliative care services recommend that staff support should be a hospital-led initiative and included in service contracts.

● At our unit, debriefing sessions encouraging reflection, particularly following a crisis or a particularly distressing death, have proved useful. However as mentioned earlier the BMT team has to rely on strong team foundations if honesty in opinion is sought, and the appropriate support offered.

- Seeing families post BMT and particularly at long-term follow-up clinics has also proved to be an invaluable experience for unit-based nurses.

The forgotten team members

The BMT team consists of more than the permanent 'hands-on' people such as nurses and doctors. Often team members such as cleaning staff, laboratory staff or voluntary workers are left out of support networks, with the assumption that all groups have a recognised departmental support strategy, when often this is not the case.

Future developments that may influence coping strategies for nurses

For nurses working in the BMT environment, the following may influence their coping strategies:

- The changing socioeconomic climate of health care and the possibility of BMT becoming 'consumer demanded'.
- The expansion of BMT contracts without increased resource or enlarging the BMT team, which will add pressure to carry out more transplants. This may possibly mean the lowering of nursing care standards, resulting in frustration and demoralisation for the BMT nurse.
- As technology advances so do the ethical dilemmas associated.
- The difficulties of nursing science keeping up with advanced technology.

Conclusion

We have established that BMT is no longer considered to be an experimental therapy, but a treatment of choice for many children with malignant disease. However the endeavour to accelerate and finely tune specific procedures and protocols within the BMT arena continues. For families and the BMT team involved this treatment is therefore advancing medical technology in practice.

The application of BMT and the outcomes do however bring new medical dilemmas. Furthermore professionals involved need to feel 'comfortable' with the way these legal, ethical and advocacy dilemmas are dealt with, as the nurse plays a major role through partnership in ensuring the family understands the choices involved throughout the procedure.

The phenomenon of partnership in care within the paediatric BMT setting offers a rich natural insight into both the physical and psychosocial effects of BMT on the child, family and staff. Moreover, the profile of BMT nursing will be raised if nurses apply relevant research methodologies in an exploration of these experiences and draw scientific conclusions, subsequently being able to influence policy and procedures and advance nursing practice.

References

Abramamovitz, I. & Senner, A. (1995) Pediatric bone marrow transplantation. *Oncology Nurses Forum*, **22**, 107–115.

ACT & RCPCH (1997) *A Guide To The Development of Children's Palliative Care Services – Report of a joint working party*. London: ACT and RCPCH.

Anderlini, P. *et al.* (1996) Biological and clinical effects of granulocyte colony-stimulating factor in normal individuals. *Blood*, **88**, 2819–2825.

Andrykowski, M.A. (1994) Psychosocial factors in bone marrow transplantation: a review and recommendations for research. *Bone Marrow Transplantation*, **13**, 357–375.

Anthony Nolan Bone Marrow Trust (1995) *You Too Could Save a Life Become a Bone Marrow Donor*: public information leaflet. London: The Anthony Nolan Trust.

Atkins, D.M. & Patenaude, A.F. (1987) Psychosocial preparation and follow up for pediatric bone marrow transplant patients. *American Journal of Orthopsychiatry*, **57**, 246–252.

Bacon, C.A. (1993) On the job conflict, how to survive. *AAOHN*, **41**, 529–532.

Bass, G., Pratt, J., Mahendra, P. & Marcus, R. (1996) Is the role of BMT co-ordinator nurse beneficial to the patient? Abstract of presentation from The European Bone Marrow Transplantation

International Conference, Vienna, Austria. *Bone Marrow Transplantation*, **17**, 160.

Beard, M.E.J. (1991) The costs and benefits of bone marrow transplantation. *The New Zealand Medical Journal*, **104**, 303–305.

Beresford, B. (1995) *Expert Opinions: a national survey of parents caring for a severely disabled child*. Bristol: The Policy Press.

Beutler, E. & Sullivan, K. (1994) Bone marrow for sickle cell disease *in* Forman, S., Blume, K. & Oski, F. eds. *Bone Marrow Transplantation*. Boston: Blackwell.

Brochstein, J. (1992) Bone marrow transplantation for genetic disorders. *Oncology*, **6**(3), 51–66.

Brown, H. & Kelly, M. (1976) Stages of bone marrow transplantation: a psychiatric perspective. *Psychosomatic Medicine*, **38**(6), 439–446.

Brown, J. & Ritchie, J. (1990) Nurses perceptions of parents and nurses roles in caring for hospitalised children. *Children's Health Care*, **19**, 28–36.

Buchsel, P.C. & Whedon, M.B. (1995) *Bone Marrow Transplantation: administrative and clinical strategies*. Boston/London: Jones and Bartlett.

Carney, B. (1987) Bone marrow transplantation: nurses and physicians perceptions of informed consent. *Cancer Nursing*, **10**, 252–259.

Chauvenet, A.R. & Smith, N.M. (1988) Referral of paediatric oncology patients for bone marrow transplantation and the process of informed consent. *Medical and Pediatric Oncology*, **16**, 40–44.

Cleary, I. (1986) Parental involvement in the lives of children in hospital. *Archives of Disease in Childhood*, **61**, 769–787.

Crook, S. & Hopkins, M. (1996) How nurse education can inform clinical practice in meeting the needs of parents of children with Hurlers syndrome undergoing bone marrow transplant. *Bone Marrow Transplantation*, **17**, 154.

Delany, L. (1996) Altruism by proxy; volunteering children for bone marrow donation. *British Medical Journal*, **312**, 240–243.

Deméocq, F., Kanold, J., Chassagne, J. *et al.* (1994) Successful blood stem cell collection and transplant in children weighing less than 25 kilograms. *Bone Marrow Transplantation*, **13**, 43–50.

Dermatis, H. & Lesko, L.M. (1990) Psychological distress in parents consenting to a child's bone marrow transplant. *Bone Marrow Transplantation*, **6**, 411–417.

Department of Health (1989) *An Introduction to the Children Act 1989*. London: HMSO.

Department of Health (1995) *Calman Report. A policy framework for commissioning cancer services*. London: Department of Health.

Department of Health (1996) *The Patient's Charter Services for Children and Young People.* London: HMSO.

De Santas, K. & Cowan, M. (1992) Bone marrow transplantation. *Current Opinion in Paediatrics,* **4**, 92–101.

Dickenson, D. & Johnson, M. (1993) *Death, Dying and Bereavement.* London: Sage.

Dimond, B. (1995) *Legal Aspects Of Nursing,* 2nd edn. Hemel Hempstead: Prentice Hall.

DiSalvo, W. (1996) Principled centred empowerment: a prescription for the future in BMT. *Bone Marrow Transplantation,* **17**, 161.

Downs, S. (1994) Ethical issues in bone marrow transplantation. *Seminars in Oncology Nursing,* **10**(1), 58–63.

Doyle, B. (1987) 'I wish you were dead.' *Nursing Times,* **83**(45), 44–46.

Dyer, C. (1995) Girl with leukaemia will be treated. *British Medical Journal,* **13**, 687.

Ellis, P. (1992) A child's right to die; who should decide? *British Journal of Nursing,* **1**, 406–408.

Emery, J.L. (1990) Attitudes of parents and paediatricians to a baby's death. *Journal of Social Medicine,* **83**, 423–424.

Esbensen, B.A. (1996) Curative and palliative care – the ethical BMT nursing conflict and dilemma. *European Bone Marrow Transplant Nurses Journal,* **2**, 7–11.

Fallowfield, L. (1993) *The Quality Of Life. The missing measurement in health care.* London: Souvenir Press.

Foley, G.V., Fochtman, D. & Mooney, K.H. (1993) *Nursing Care of the Child with Cancer,* 2nd edn. Philadelphia: Saunders.

Ford, R. & Ballard, B. (1988) Acute complications after bone marrow transplant. *Seminars in Oncology Nursing,* **4**, 15–24.

Forman, S.J., Blume, K.G. & Oski, F. eds. (1994) *Bone Marrow Transplantation.* Boston: Blackwell.

Fradd, E. (1987) A child alone. *Nursing Times,* **83**(42), 16–17.

Futterman, A.D. & Wellisch, K.D. (1990) Psychodynamic themes of bone marrow transplant. *Hematology/Oncology Clinics of North America,* **4**, 179–180.

Garbett, R. (1996) Editors comments. *Nursing Times,* **92**(44), 38.

Gibson, C.H. (1995) The process of empowerment in mothers of chronically ill children. *Journal of Advanced Nursing,* **21**, 1201–1210.

Gibson, F. (1989) Parental involvement in bone marrow transplant. *Paediatric Nursing,* Oct., 21–22.

Gluckman, E. (1996) Cord blood transplant in Europe. *Bone Marrow Transplantation,* **17**, 146.

Heiney, S.P., Neuberg, R.W., Myers, D. & Bergman, L.H. (1994) The aftermath of BMT for parents of pediatric patients: a post traumatic stress disorder. *Oncology Nurses Forum,* **21**, 843–847.

Hostrup, H. (1996) Investigating the family's experience of the nursing care of children undergoing autologous BMT. *European Bone Marrow Transplant Nurses Group Journal,* **2**, 19–23.

ISHAGE & EBMT (1997) *Proposed Standards for Blood and Marrow Progenitor Cell Collection Processing and Transplantation.* Oslo: ISHAGE Europe & EBMT.

Kent, G. (1996) Volunteering children for bone marrow donation. *British Medical Journal,* **313**, 49.

Kinrade, L.C. (1987) Pediatric bone marrow transplantation sibling donors. *Cancer Nursing,* **10**(2), 77–81.

Kiss, A. (1996) Psychosocial aspects of bone marrow transplantation: the team side. *Bone Marrow Transplantation,* **1**(17), 48.

Korgaonkar, D. & Tribe, D. (1993) Children and consent to medical treatment. *British Journal of Nursing,* **2**(7), 383–384.

Kurtzberg, J. (1995) Umbilical cord blood, an alternative source of haematopoetic stem cells for bone marrow reconstitution in unrelated donor transplants. *Blood,* **86**, 290.

Lansdown, R. & Goldman, A. (1988) The psychological care of children with malignant disease. *Journal of Child Psychology and Psychiatry,* 555–567.

Lasagna, L. (1983) The professional patient dialogue. *Hastings Center Report,* **13**, 9–11.

Lawrance, T.A. (1997) Do Parents of Children Undergoing Allogenic Bone Marrow Transplantation Receive the Correct Information Pre-Admission to Enable them to Give Informed Consent on Behalf of their Child? Unpublished research proposal. Birmingham: University of Central England.

Lee, M.L., Cohen, S.E., Stuber, M.L. & Nader, K. (1994) Parent–child interactions with pediatric bone marrow transplant patients. *Journal of Psychosocial Oncology,* **12**(4), 43–60.

Lesko, L.M. (1994) Bone marrow transplantation: support of the patient and his/her family. *Support Care Cancer,* **2**, 35–49.

Lesko, L.M. & Dermatis, H. (1989) Patients, parents, and oncologists perception of informed consent for bone marrow transplantation. *Medical and Pediatric Oncology*, **17**, 181–187.

Lesko, L.M., Kern, J. & Hawkins, D.R. (1984) Psychological aspects of patients in germ free isolation: a review of child, adult and patient management literature. *Medical and Pediatric Oncology*, **12**, 43–49.

Leukaemia Research Fund (1997) *Bone Marrow and Stem Cell Transplantation*. London: Leukaemia Research Fund.

Lichter, I. (1984) 'Communication' in Doyle, D. ed. *Palliative Care: The Management Of Far Advanced Illness*. Kent: Croom Helm.

McCarthy, J. (1996) Choice/ dilemma: who decides? *Practice Nursing*, **7**(5), 17–18.

McConville, B.J., Steichen-Asch, P., Harris, R. et al. (1990) Pediatric bone marrow transplants: psychological aspects. *Canadian Journal of Psychiatry*, **35**, 769–775.

McDonagh, K. & Nienhuis, A. (1993) The thalassaemias *in* Nathan, D. & Oski, F. eds. *Haematology of Childhood and Infants*, 4th edn. Philadelphia: Saunders.

Mahaffey, P.J. (1996) Making decisions with children. *British Medical Journal*, **313**, 49.

Mallet, J. (1996) Sense of direction. *Nursing Times*, **92**(4), 38–40.

Maslach, C. (1979) The Burnout Syndrome and Patient Care *in* Garfield, C. ed. *Stress and Survival*. St Louis: Mosby.

Medical Research Council (1997) *Working Party On Acute Myeloid Leukaemia Trial 12* (AML 12). London: Medical Research Council.

Melvers, S. (1991) *Obtaining the Views of Users of the Health Service*. London: Kings Fund.

Molasiotis, A., Boughton, B.J. & Van Den Akker, O.B.A. (1994) Psychological morbidity, burnout and job satisfaction in nursing and medical staff who work in BMT units. In *Bone Marrow Transplantation EBMT 1994*, abstract of presentation, p. 259.

Moore, M.A.S. (1993) *Ex vivo* expansion and gene therapy using cord blood CD34+ cells. *Journal of Haematology*, **2**, 221.

Moore, I.M. Glasser, M.E. & Ablin, A.R. (1987) The late psychosocial consequences of childhood cancer. *Journal of Pediatric Nursing*, **3**(3), 150–158.

Olin, H.S. (1982) A proposed model to teach medical students the care of the dying patient. *Journal of Medical Education*, **47**, 564–567.

Outhwaite, H. (1998) The European Bone Marrow Transplant and Allied Professions (UK) Group. *Bone Marrow Transplantation*, **21**(supplement 1), 244.

Parkes, E. (1977) The dying child and family *in* Steiner, P.D. ed. *Psychological Problems of the Child and his Family*. Toronto: Macmillan.

Parr, M.D., Messino, M.J. & McIntyre, W. (1991) Allogenic BMT: procedures and complications. *American Journal of Hospital Psychiatry*, **48**, 127–137.

Pass, M.D. & Pass, C.M. (1987) Anticipatory guidance for parents of hospitalised children. *Journal of Pediatric Nursing*, **2**, 250–258.

Peck, H. (1992) 'Please don't tell him the truth.' *Paediatric Nursing*, March, 12–14.

Peterson, F.B. (1996) Cost effectiveness of blood and marrow transplantation – how far can we go without touching ethical borders. *Bone Marrow Transplantation*, **17**(1), 149.

Pfefferbaum, B., Lindamood, M. & Wiley, F. (1977) Pediatric BMT: psychosocial aspects. *American Journal of Psychiatry*, **134**, 1299–1301.

Phipps, S. & DeCuir-Whalley, S.D. (1990) Adherence issues in pediatric BMT. *Journal of Pediatric Psychology*, **15**, 459–475.

Pinkerton, R., Cushing, P. & Sepion, B. (1994) *Childhood Cancer Management. A practical handbook*. London: Chapman Hall.

Prows, C.A. & McCain, G.C. (1997) Parental consent for bone marrow transplantation in the case of genetic disorders. *Journal of the Society of Pediatric Nurses*, **2**, 9–18.

Rees, G.J.G. (1985) Cost effectiveness in oncology. *Lancet*, **ii**, 1405–1407.

Rennick, J. (1986) Re-establishing the parental role in a paediatric intensive care unit. *Journal of Pediatric Nursing*, **1**, 40–44.

Rudman, M. (1996) Learn to share care. *Nursing Times*, **92**(44), 42.

Ruggiero, M.R. (1988) The donor in bone marrow transplantation. *Seminars in Oncology Nursing*, **4**(1), 9–14.

Russell, N.H. (1996) The place of blood stem cells in allogenic transplantation. *British Journal of Haematology*, **93**, 747–753.

Selwyn, S. (1980) Protective isolation: what are our priorities? *Journal of Hospital Infection*, **1**, 5–9.

Shedd, P. (1991) Nursing staff stresses and ethical dilemmas in caring for bone marrow transplant patients *in* Whedon, M.B. ed.

Bone Marrow Transplantation: principles, practice and nursing insights. Boston: Jones and Bartlett.

Shelley, P. (1992) Finding out what people want. *Cascade*, July, 4–5.

Singer, D.A. & Donnely, M.B. (1990) Informed consent for BMT: identification of relevant information needs by referring physician. *Bone Marrow Transplantation*, **6**, 431–437.

Soutter, J., Bond, S. & Craft, A. (1994) *Families of Misfortune Proposed strategy in the Northern Region for the Care of Children with Life Threatening Illness and their Families.* Newcastle: The Northern Regional Health Authority.

Takaue, Y., Kawano, Y., Abe, T., Okamoto, Y. *et al.* (1995) Collection and transplantation of peripheral stem cells in very small children weighing less than 20 kilograms. *Blood*, **86**, 372–380.

Tesno, B. (1995) A comprehensive pediatric BMT documentation tool. *Oncology Nurses Forum*, **22**, 841–843.

Thomas, D.E. (1983) Bone marrow transplantation: a life saving applied art. *Journal of the American Medical Association*, **249**, 2528–2536.

Tomlinson, T. (1986) The physicians influence on patients choice. *Theoretical Medicine*, **7**, 106.

Turner, T. (1993) Children should be involved in decisions on treatment. *Nursing Times*, **89**(43), 8.

UKCC (1996a) *Guidelines for Professional Practice.* London: UKCC.

UKCC (1996b) *PREPP – The Scope of Advanced Practice.* London: UKCC.

UKCCSG (1996) *Recommendations of Care Post Bone Marrow Transplant.* Bristol: UKCCSG.

Vianello, R. & Lucamante, M. (1988) Children's understanding of death according to parents and paediatricians. *Journal of Generic Psychology*, **14**, 305–316.

Wagner, J.E., Kernan, N.A. & Steinbuch, M. (1995) Allogenic sibling umbilical cord blood transplantation in children with malignant and non malignant disease. *Lancet*, **346**, 214–219.

Walker, F., Roethkes, S., Sandman, V., Clark, K. & Martin, G. (1994) A guide to peripheral cell transplants for patients and families. *Oncology Nurses Forum*, **21**, 587–591.

Whedon, M.B. ed. (1991) *Bone*

Marrow Transplantation: principles, practice and nursing insights. Boston: Jones & Bartlett.

While, A., Citrone, C. & Cornish, J. (1996) *A Study of the Needs and Provision for Families Caring for Children with Life-limiting Incurable Disorders.* London: Kings College, Department of Nursing Studies.

White, A.M. (1994) Parental concerns following a child's discharge from a BMT unit. *Journal of Pediatric Oncology Nursing*, **11**(3), 93–101.

Whittaker, J.A. (1995) Guidelines for the provision of facilities for the care of adult patients with haematological malignancy including leukaemia, lymphoma and severe bone marrow failure. *Clinical Laboratory Haematology*, **17**, 310.

Wiles, R. (1996) Quality questions. *Nursing Times*, **92**(44), 38.

Wiley, F. & House, K. (1988) Bone marrow transplantation in children. *Seminars in Oncology Nursing*, **4**, 31–40.

Zabora, J.R., Smith, E.D., Baker, F., Wingarow, J.R. & Curbow, B. (1992) The family: the other side of bone marrow transplantation. *Journal of Psychosocial Oncology*, **10**(1), 35–46.

Further reading

Buchsel, P.C. & Whedon, M.B. (1995) *Bone Marrow Transplantation: administrative and clinical strategies.* Boston: Jones and Bartlett.

Forman, S.J., Blume, K.G. & Thomas, E.D (eds) (1994) *Bone Marrow Transplantation.* London: Blackwell Scientific Publishers.

Whedon, M.B. (ed.) (1991) *Bone Marrow Transplantation. Principles, practice and nursing insights.* Boston: Jones and Bartlett.

Resources

Anthony Nolan Bone Marrow
Trust
Royal Free Hospital
London
NW3 4YR

British Bone Marrow Register
Bristol Transfusion Centre

Southmead Road
Bristol,
BS10 2nd

European Bone Marrow
Transplantation Nurses Group
(UK Group)
Haematology Department
University College Hospital
Grafton Way

London
WC1 6AU

Royal College of Nursing
Paediatric BMT Special Interest
Group
Royal College of Nursing
20 Cavendish Square
London
W1M OAB.

Discharge – a planned event

9

ANITA COX

Introduction

This chapter will look at the need for careful planning and good communication between the members of the multidisciplinary team when considering an individual's discharge from hospital. The importance of having a discharge planning co-ordinator will be illustrated and the benefits of having specific documentation for a discharge will be identified with some examples given. The basic concept is that discharge planning will help the individual and their family progress towards a return to health (Rorden and Taft, 1990) – physical problems should be addressed but thought should also be given to the fact that although the family is to be reunited, 'normality' has now altered and there will be certain adaptations within the family unit in order to cope with the newly diagnosed child, the child recovering from bone marrow transplantation or the child who is terminally ill. The need for individualism is paramount in order to keep the discharge event 'family centred', but the general principles will be highlighted in this chapter in an attempt to encourage you to appreciate the importance of a smooth and planned discharge and how you as a specialist practitioner can avoid the scenario described above.

Case study 9.1 highlights just a few of the issues involved in discharge planning – it also shows how disastrous a discharge from hospital can be if careful planning and organisation are not emphasised. In this case, the family were not well prepared for taking their son home, they had minimal information, no community liaison and were given no time to consider any concerns they may have had about going home. Discharge from hospital for the individual and their family can be as equally distressing as admission to hospital, yet the emphasis tends to be on pre-admission preparation (Glen, 1982) and the lack of available literature relating to discharge indicates that it is not treated with the same importance as admission.

Key points
- Definitions of discharge planning
- Emphasising the need for a planned event
- Co-ordination of the discharge – who and why?
- Information giving – benefits and pitfalls
- Documentation
- Focus on four different discharges
- Short term
- Long term
- BMT discharge
- Palliative care

Case study 9.1*

Sam is a 3-year-old little boy who has been recently diagnosed with acute lymphoblastic leukaemia (ALL). He has commenced his induction treatment and a medical decision has been made for Sam to be discharged home and to continue the remainder of his induction phase at his local hospital, which is only 10 minutes from his home. Sam's mother is keen to take her son home that evening as her husband will be able to take them all in his car when he comes to visit. The alternative is to try and arrange hospital transport for the next day, although this cannot be guaranteed due to the lateness in the day of the decision for discharge. The medical team have taken the responsibility to inform the local hospital that Sam will be attending the general paediatric ward for his L-asparaginase and possible antibiotics during his neutropenic phase, and are happy for the family to go home. An emergency admission on another ward means that no medical staff are available to see Sam's parents before they leave the ward.

The nursing staff on the ward are busy when Sam's father arrives and it is only when the family are about to leave that a team member has a chance to ask if the family are happy to go home and whether they want to ask any questions before they leave. Sam's mother asks for the direct telephone number to the ward and inquires about when Sam should be given his oral medication next. These pieces of information are written onto a piece of paper which Sam's mother places into her handbag. The family then collect their belongings and hurriedly leave the ward, obviously keen to get on their journey home.

Efforts are made to contact the relevant community teams, but as it is after 6 p.m. messages can only be left on answering machines and reminders are left in the ward's communication book for the community teams to be followed up the next day.

There is a telephone call at 3 am the next morning – Sam's mother has suddenly realised she is at home with her son who has been recently diagnosed with cancer and she is scared that something will happen to Sam while he is at home. The night staff do not know Sam and his mother but reassurance is given as much as possible and Sam's mother is told to ring again if she wants to. Later on the same day, Sam's mother is on the telephone again, this time she is at the local hospital and nobody seems to know anything about them. At the same time the registrar of the ward is being bleeped by the doctors at the local hospital asking who Sam is and what treatment he needs. No one has spoken to the local hospital.

* Case studies 9.1–9.6 all relate to variations of the same case – 3-year-old Sam with ALL.

Definitions of discharge planning

Discharge planning is a process of steps (or phases) with an immediate goal to anticipate changes in individual care needs, and a long-term goal to ensure the continuity of health care. Rorden and

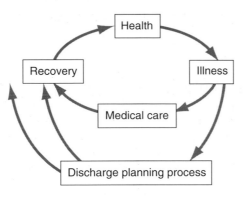

Figure 9.1 Discharge planning process (reproduced with permission from Rorden & Taft, 1990)

Taft (1990) believe that the discharge planning process should parallel and remain supportive of an individual's progress through a continuum of care (Figure 9.1). As Figure 9.1 shows, once an individual becomes ill and medical intervention is necessary, the discharge planning process should begin and continue until the individual is recovered and no longer requires medical input. In the case where a child is suffering from cancer, this period may last years before no further treatment is required, but each discharge from hospital is important for the family involved. The sooner that community teams and local hospitals are involved in an individual's case, the easier it is to plan for discharge.

Takacs (1991, skill 5 p. 19) defines discharge planning as:

> …an organized process whereby the nurse evaluates, in collaboration with the child and family, readiness for discharge from the acute setting, care needed after hospitalization and necessary resources for continuity of care. Discharge planning also encompasses investigating and securing resources to provide a smooth transition to another facility or home.

Hamilton and Vessey (1992) parallel the discharge planning process with the nursing process and consider it to be made up of four phases:

- assessment
- planning
- implementation
- evaluation.

The evaluation is crucial, as without feedback there is no real way of knowing how effective the discharge event has been. This is relatively simple when a child is to return to the ward or clinic but when an individual and their family are to be discharged for the 'final time' – probably the most important discharge – how

What evaluations were missing between the nursing and medical staff and Sam's family in Case study 9.1?

will you evaluate your discharge then? Some ideas will be offered later in the chapter.

Common groundrules

Common groundrules do emerge from the literature on discharge planning and they act as a good basis for principles to consider while discharging individuals from hospital to home (or to a local hospital):

- Discharge planning begins with early assessment of the individual and family care needs.
- Discharge planning includes concern for the individual's well being.
- The individual and family/caregivers are involved in the planning process.
- There is collaboration and co-ordination among all health care professionals involved.
- Confusion and overlapping are prevented as far as possible.
- The primary or named nurse should be the central co-ordinating individual.

If discharge is not planned then the scenario illustrated in Case study 9.1 with Sam and his family could well occur. One person is left to deal with the individual and their family at the time of discharge, having only enough time to discuss the bare minimum facts, leaving the family no time for discussion or allowing them to air their concerns. Families are usually keen to leave hospital as soon as possible so it is your, the practitioner's, responsibility to ensure that the families in your care are supported and that the transition to home care is successful.

The multidisciplinary team input

How many multidisciplinary team members come to visit a patient who has already been discharged?

Incorporating other members of the multidisciplinary team into the discharge plan requires organisation and once discharge is being discussed, appropriate team members should be approached and their specific input into the discharge process should be identified. The experience of each health care professional plays a vital part in an individual's care while an inpatient and they can also contribute to a smooth discharge – as long as they are aware that an individual is being discharged.

Of course it would be impossible to inform every member of a multidisciplinary team of each patient who was discharged, but it is an idea to keep those people informed who have regular contact with specific individuals and their families. For example, the dietitian may have had a lot of input with a particular family, suggesting various ways of getting the child to eat or drink or suggesting supplements which the child may like. If a dietitian finds out that efforts made to provide suitable dietary input for a child who has been discharged a few days earlier are no longer needed, the dietitian may not be too impressed. Also, if the family has built up a decent rapport with a particular dietitian, it would be beneficial to ask the dietitian to speak to the family about going home and how to continue building up their child with ingredients that the family may have at home.

Physiotherapists can also provide excellent ideas for individuals going home. If a child has been in hospital for some time, they will have lost muscle tone and will not be as strong as before their admission. Obviously the child may not feel like playing or taking any exercise when they do go home, but the frustration they will feel when they want to play but are not strong enough to do so will make things far harder for the family at home. The physiotherapist will be able to suggest exercises which may encourage the child to begin using muscles again which are usually fun to do as well. Again if the physiotherapist has had input during the individual's admission to hospital, their input prior to discharge will be far more beneficial as the family will know the physiotherapist and therefore be more responsive to them.

Social workers are another group of very important people who can help to aid the transition from hospital to home. Many families have great concerns when the time for discharge arrives and are worried that they will not be able to cope when left at home alone. White (1994) highlights some of these concerns felt particularly by families who have left the bone marrow transplant environment – concerns which can easily be applied to any family in the oncology setting. The financial aspects of caring for a sick child were identified as being problematical and the specialist to help with such concerns is the social worker. Families should routinely have access to a social worker who can help them with appropriate benefits or equipment to ease the stress of having a sick child. The social worker can also play a valuable role in being a support mechanism for families. It is not always easy for some people to talk to nurses about their concerns or problems – they feel that they are taking up valuable time or they feel uncomfortable discussing private problems with team members who they will have to face on a daily basis. The social worker can be a vital member of the multidisciplinary team and one who the families feel able to talk to, thereby helping the families work through some of the concerns they may be having about their pending discharge, encouraging them to believe they will cope at home without the support given to them within the clinical environment.

Paediatric oncology outreach nurses who are based within the hospital setting (e.g., CLIC nurses, Macmillan nurses and clinical nurse specialists) play a vital part in the discharge planning process. These tend to be the individuals who have the best knowledge of the local hospital and community services that discharged children will have contact with and therefore will be a special link person between the hospital, home and community for the discharged families. By arranging for these outreach practitioners to meet families during their treatment, preferably on first admission, relationships can be developed enabling the families to trust the outreach nurses once they leave the specialist hospital. Knowing that there is a service provided for families outside

Case study 9.2

As Sam and his family were discharged quicker than anticipated on his last admission, no member of the outreach team from the specialist centre had a chance to meet the family. Communication with the local hospital had been lacking on Sam's discharge, so greater care needed to be taken on his next admission to ensure that a similar situation does not occur again.

Sam is admitted for his intensification block which begins with the insertion of a central venous access device. Sam receives his chemotherapy uneventfully and is prepared for discharge with more care this time. The nurse looking after Sam for the days before he is due to go home ensures that his local hospital is kept up to date with his progress and the nursing staff are aware of when he may be needing treatment from them for his neutropenic episode. The outreach team are contacted and messages are left to inform them that Sam is an inpatient on the ward. The outreach nurse who is to be linked with Sam and his family is unable to visit the family prior to their discharge but asks for a message to be passed on that the family will be visited at home within the next week. Prior to their discharge, Sam's mother is told that she will be receiving a telephone call from the outreach team member to arrange a home visit and she is also reassured that the local hospital have been contacted and told of Sam's discharge.

Once again Sam's mother rings the ward later when the family have gone home and is obviously upset. Having spoken to another parent prior to leaving the ward, Sam's mother believes that the outreach nurse is going to give her bad news as only children who are going to die are visited by these nurses. No one seems to have explained to Sam and his mother the role of the outreach team and so once again the family have been discharged feeling confused and upset.

Why do you think it is important to introduce these specialists as soon as possible to newly diagnosed children and their families?

of but with links to the specialist centre is great reassurance to parents of children discharged from oncology wards.

Co-ordinating the discharge

Having identified the need for a planned event involving all the appropriate members of the multidisciplinary team, it seems clear that co-ordination is vital. The one individual who is in the best position to co-ordinate all the multidisciplinary team members while having a good rapport with the family is the nurse. The literature available agrees that the nurse should assume the role of discharge planner, and specifically a nurse who has taken responsibility for the child on the ward who arranges the discharge (Brack *et al.*, 1988; Wong, 1991; Rorden and Taft, 1990; Thornes, 1993). As the primary or named nurse should have the most continuing contact with the patient and family, they are more likely to have a relationship of trust within which reassurance and support can be given effectively and efficiently. By having a unique close contact with individuals and their families, the role of the named or primary nurse in discharge planning is imperative in order that the individual needs of the family system are accounted for.

Discharge can produce many anxieties in the individual and their family – anxieties which may not necessarily be verbalised. If the nurse who is co-ordinating the discharge of an individual does not know a family very well, they will be unable to pick up on non-verbal cues of anxiety. The close contact the named or primary nurse has with the individual and the family gives the ideal opportunity to notice signs of stress or anxiety in the family setting, especially those anxieties brought on by a pending discharge.

What non-verbal cues would lead you to suspect that a family were stressed?

Having built up a relationship of trust and understanding (Hancock, 1992), the family will hopefully feel comfortable enough with the named nurse to be able to discuss any concerns they may be having. Additionally the nurse should be able to identify both verbal and non-verbal cues should the family be experiencing anxieties related to the discharge from the protected clinical environment.

The nurse co-ordinating the discharge should also be able to identify which multidisciplinary team members are appropriate for a family to see prior to their discharge. Returning to one of the groundrules highlighted earlier under common groundrules: 'The individual and family/caregivers are involved in the planning process'.

A family's input is vital as they know what help or assistance

Case study 9.3 (alternative to Case study 9.2)

Sam is to be discharged following his first intensification which he has had uneventfully. The day before Sam is due to go home, his allocated nurse takes time to sit down and talk to Sam and his mother about his remaining treatment and about how the family feels about going home with a central line to care for now. Sam's mother is concerned that she will be too protective over Sam – not letting him do anything active as he may tug his line – but she realises the importance of allowing Sam to be as normal as possible. Time is taken to give reassurance and tips are given as to the best ways of protecting Sam's new line. Sam's mother ends up feeling more confident when the practical issues of how to secure the line if it splits or is pulled out are repeated with her. However there is still concern that something will happen at Sam's playgroup which mum is hoping he will continue to attend when well. The nurse explains about the outreach nurses and how they can help by visiting Sam's playgroup to talk to the staff at the playgroup. Sam's mother goes very pale and silent. Usually a chatty and friendly person, a change has obviously occurred. Initially, Sam's mother insists that nothing is wrong and that she just wants to go home and get on with normal life. However further gentle probing shows that Sam's mother thinks that the outreach nurses just deal with dying children as other parents have told her this. Thankfully, this situation is dealt with prior to discharge and Sam and his mother are relieved to know that they are to be visited at home by a member of the specialist centre in the near future.

they really need in order to cope with the change from specialist centre to local hospital or home. Discharge planning is not an activity that is done to or for the patient, the patient (and the family) should have active involvement. There is no point in carefully organising a discharge based on what you think the needs of the family are if the family unit has not been involved and consulted. Families will probably know which team members they wish to see prior to them going home, although newly diagnosed families may need suggestions put to them so that they are aware of which disciplines are available for them to gain help from.

Information giving – benefits and pitfalls

In order for individuals and their families to be well prepared for discharge, a great deal of information needs to be given. To begin with, the nurse needs to draw on all her communication skills in order to build up a clear picture of how the discharge event is perceived by the family. Once this is established, you will then be able to provide the individual and the family with the correct amount of information for them to be able to understand. This is the planning stage of discharge planning as already mentioned by Hamilton and Vessey (1992). It must also be taken into consideration that families will be excited as well as worried about their child's discharge, so their usual level of competence and understanding may be altered. Information may well need to be repeated or clarified before it is finally remembered and understood.

Individuals and families depend on nurses for information, the acquisition of which can reduce uncertainty, and it is seen as one of the most basic forms of coping (Ohanian, 1989). Well-informed patients and their families are more likely to comply with the plan of care and therefore achieve a favourable adaptation to the change in environment (from hospital to home). As the nurse it is your responsibility to ensure that you are giving information which is language appropriate for the child's age and parents' intelligence.

Individual personalities also affect learning capabilities and a person's ability to control events; for example, Rotter (1966), who discusses the differences between an internal and external locus of control:

- Internal locus – individuals tend to believe that their own behaviour is the most important influence on events in their lives. They believe that one 'make's one's own luck'.
- External locus – individuals believe that their own behaviour has little impact on events in their lives. Outside forces such as God, luck or fate are seen by them as more important.

The locus of control can be pictured as a continuum, with each individual having a specific place on it depending on their beliefs (Figure 9.1). The more internally focused an individual is, the more they will be interested in participating in their own (or their child's) care. Conflict may arise between the named or primary nurse and family at the time of discharge if a vast difference in this locus occurs. Individuals who choose careers within the health field typically have an internal orientation towards health beliefs; if a patient and/or their family tend towards the opposite end of the belief continuum then the nurse must take care that the family can cope with the amount of control and participation they are being given.

Individuals with more internal locus will find it easier to take responsibility for their child's care on discharge, but consideration must be given to the fact that all individuals are different and that their needs may be constantly changing.

How many attempts did it take you to remember something for a school exam that you were worried about?

Documentation

?

What would you consider appropriate to be included in a discharge document for your ward?

Having thought about how important it is to plan a child's discharge in advance and with help from the various members of the multidisciplinary team, the question must arise as to what should happen to all this information and co-ordination? It is also important for other nurses who are also involved in a particular child's care to understand what has been organised already. The simplest and most obvious way to share the information and planning is through documentation. Many wards and units have very comprehensive admission packages where checklists allow any individual caring for a child to be able to see what and when the child and their families have been told about their admission to hospital. However, despite the fact that, as already identified, discharge can be as traumatic as admission to hospital, documents used for discharge are not as widely available. Through the use of well-designed documents covering all related aspects of discharge, more families will be better prepared for leaving the hospital environment, be it for a week or more.

Some examples of discharge documents are given in Figures 9.2–9.4.

The literature reviewed shows a lack of documentation is often the weakest aspect of the discharge planning process (Gikow *et al.*, 1985; Rorden and Taft, 1990; Thornes, 1993). All aspects of discharge planning should be documented and checked by the named nurse (or the nurse co-ordinating the discharge), and discharge checklists should ensure that every aspect of the discharge plan is communicated to the child, their family and also the community team who will be taking over the child's care post discharge. By using checklists, it is easy for anyone taking over the discharge planning of a child to see what has been done already and what is outstanding (assuming of course that the planning so far has been documented!)

Using an appropriate discharge planner also helps to organise and co-ordinate the discharge process. By highlighting the aspects of discharge which need attention, each child should have a well-organised and documented discharge.

As part of co-ordinating a child's discharge, the named nurse plays an important part in documenting specific areas that the child and family may find stressful. Having already identified that the named nurse will hopefully know a family well enough to be able to assess how the family is feeling about discharge, it is also useful to have any major concerns documented. One suggestion would be for the named nurse to have an informal 'interview' with the family prior to discharge. This would ensure that a specific time had been set aside for a family to talk through any worries

Case study 9.4

Sam is to be discharged following his second course of high-dose methotrexate (HDMTX). He and his family are getting used to their visits to the hospital, but Sam's mother does get anxious when she is going home after a block of treatment. Sam has shown a slight delay in excreting his methotrexate on this admission so it is decided that a repeat glomerular filtration rate (GFR) should be taken prior to Sam's last HDMTX. Sam's named nurse commenced his discharge planner on admission but she is now off sick so the discharge checklist is consulted by Sam's allocated nurse for the day to see what is left to organise. The nurse contacts Sam's local hospital to arrange for a GFR, but is told that the hospital cannot do the test. The test is therefore booked at the day care unit in the specialist centre, although this means a long journey for Sam and his family. A message is left for the local community team for them to visit Sam at home to carry out a routine blood count and the team is also informed about his pending GFR.

The nurse approaches Sam's mum and, assuming that she has already been informed of the GFR, explains that a visit to the specialist centre is booked for the following week. Sam's mum is very cross that she has to make an extra trip and insists on seeing a member of the medical team before the family goes home. The senior house officer comes to see Sam's mum, before the nurse is able to contact him, and explains the need for Sam's repeat GFR and informs her that the local hospital are expecting her and Sam for the test and when the appointment has been made. Sam's mum is naturally very confused – she has just been told two different pieces of information about the same situation. The doctor is able to clear up the confusion and speaks to the nurse to find out how the situation arose. When contacting the local hospital again, the nurse was informed that another nurse had already liaised with the community team in order to ensure that Sam would be able to have the test closer to home. It became apparent that the named nurse had made the arrangements but had not documented the plans on Sam's discharge planner.

and concerns they may be feeling. (Such 'interviews' will probably be of most relevance when a child is being discharged from inpatient treatment, but these will be discussed in more detail in the specific parts of the chapter.)

It is very rare for parents to outrightly share their problems with the nursing staff – frequently they will view us as too busy to stop and talk. However, if time is put aside for the purpose of ironing out any concerns, the families will appreciate being able to talk through their going home and what it will mean – for them and also for the rest of the family. If any particular concerns are aired and discussed, if such information is documented then this will help any other nurse who may be discharging the child and family on another occasion.

Having set time aside for discussion, this may be a suitable time to evaluate the discharge planning process and is occasionally a good way to find out any problems that families may have encountered on their last discharge. If the last discharge was very upsetting for a family then obviously they will be concerned that any subsequent discharges will be equally upsetting to them. By evaluating the discharge process, you will be able to identify the areas of discharge which may need more time and consideration in order to ease the transition form hospital to home for the family. If there is no evaluation then you will not know whether children and their families are being adequately prepared for discharge or not. Telephone calls are another simple way to evaluate a family's discharge and are also a good way to reassure the family. However if this idea is to be implemented, then the family should give their consent prior to them going home – some families are keen to forget hospitals as much as possible during their periods of 'normality' at home.

Having highlighted the need for documentation of discharge planning, it is also important to ensure that individual variations are taken into consideration during the planning process. Such aspects as a family's culture, first language and motivation can dramatically affect the amount of time needed to plan a discharge and also how easily a family will be able to adjust to the move from the clinical environment back to home life again. The named nurse will invariably have more of an insight into a family's overall typical lifestyle and therefore will be able to anticipate problems that may arise when the family is discharged and prepare the family for such problems. A discharge planner needs to have ample space for flexibility and specific information or organisation needed for certain families. No two families will need the same input for their discharge, so individualising the planning process is imperative. Obviously some aspects will be the same for each family being discharged, for example contacting the local hospital and/or community team, but not all aspects will apply to each family going home.

?

Are the discharge documents being completed well or are they too long for people to fill out with all the relevant information? All documentation can be reviewed and renewed and by evaluating each family's experience of going home, your discharge planning can be altered accordingly.

Focus on different discharges

The following sections will look at specific discharges, emphasising the need for variations in the preparation and planning phase. Firstly, the discharge of a child who will be returning for more treatment will be looked at, followed secondly by a more 'long-term' discharge in that the child identified has finished their inpatient treatment. Thirdly, a child being discharged after bone marrow transplantation will be highlighted and the specific needs of this patient addressed. Finally, a child who is being discharged from the hospital environment to the palliative setting at home will be looked at and the issues that can arise during the transition identified.

Short-term discharge

This occurs when a child has been in hospital for diagnosis or treatment and the family are to spend some time at home before being admitted again for further treatment. As already identified in the scenario with Sam earlier in the chapter, families can easily be discharged without really appreciating all that has happened after diagnosis. This discharge, after the initial diagnosis and treatment, can perhaps be seen as one of the most crucial, as it is the time when a family is trying to understand what it is going to be like with a child who has a life-threatening illness when they do not know all the facts yet. This is a time when they are most vulnerable and probably the most scared. The child and the family will have been given a fair amount of information which may or may not have been remembered, but once outside the clinical setting, panic can easily set in very quickly. Perhaps one of the most important facts to get across is that the family can ring the ward at any time of day or night. Often just knowing that there would be someone available to speak to if needed is enough for a lot of parents.

The short-term discharge can mean that a child and family are going home for anything from a few days to a few weeks. The length of time at home obviously affects how much equipment families need to go home with (where relevant) and usually how much organisation is needed as well.

By working through a discharge document such as the one shown in Figure 9.2, all aspects of a discharge should be covered. The family needs to be prepared for any community input they are likely to receive and it is usually preferable for a name to be given to the family and an appointment made for each visit. Many families with a child with cancer find it hard to leave the specialist centre and return to their local or shared-care hospital but if the importance of this is emphasised at the beginning of a child's treatment then the road will hopefully be fairly smooth. The closer the links are between the family and their community and local hospitals, the easier it is for communication to take place between the professionals – it is very difficult trying to arrange for a community nurse to visit a child after all their treatment when there has been no contact since initial admission.

One way to ease the link between two hospitals and the community (as most of the children will have this set up) is to keep up-to-date records for each professional to have access to.

Case study 9.5 (alternative to Case study 9.1)

Sam is a 3-year-old boy who has been recently diagnosed with ALL. He has commenced his induction treatment and a medical decision has been made for Sam to be discharged home and to continue the remainder of his induction phase at his local hospital which is 10 minutes from his home. Sam's mother is keen to take her son home that evening as her husband will be able to take them all in his car when he comes to visit. The nurse looking after Sam explains that there will be some arrangements to be made before the family can go home and are advised to wait an extra 24 hours before going home. Although not overjoyed at this suggestion, Sam's mum admits that she is worried about going home and so would like a little bit more time to get used to the idea.

Sam's discharge checklist has already been started so the nurse checks what is left to organise and makes some notes in the communication book for the following day's staff. She leaves a message for Sam's community nurse, explaining who he is and what he will need while at home, leaving the ward number and the name of Sam's named nurse for further contact.

During the night, Sam's mum does not sleep well and seems distressed, although she is not keen to talk to any of the night staff who pass this information over to the staff on the morning shift. Once Sam and his mum are up and about, the named nurse approaches them and asks if they are looking forward to going home. Sam's mum begins to cry and says she is scared that she will do something wrong or not notice if Sam is not well. The named nurse spends some time with Sam and his mum reassuring her that she will be able to cope and asking her what she will be looking out for and why – emphasising that she is aware of what to look out for in her son and therefore able to care outside the 'protective' environment of the ward.

Sam's mum appreciates the time spent with her and is much calmer about going home. Later on the same day, Sam's mum asks about her son's next block of treatment, making sure that she has understood what is to happen on their next admission to hospital which includes the insertion of a central venous access device. The local hospital are contacted about Sam attending the paediatric ward for his L-asparaginase and possible antibiotics during his neutropenic phase and the community have also been in contact with the ward staff. Sam and his mum are discharged in the evening feeling prepared and happy to be going home, knowing that the local services are expecting them the next day and that they can contact the specialist centre if necessary.

Shared care booklets can work very well but these are dependent on the professionals remembering to fill out details of treatment, blood results and any changes in protocols, as well as the families remembering to carry the booklets with them when they attend hospital.

For families who have been receiving treatment for a few

Great Ormond Street Hospital for Children NHS Trust
ADMISSION AND DISCHARGE PLAN

Ward: Giraffe/Lion/Robin/......................

Name:...   Hospital Number:...............................

Date of birth:...   Cost code:...

....

Date of admission:...............................   Named nurse:......................................

Consultant:...

Assessment

Planned date of discharge:...

Co-ordinator:...

Action	Date	Outcome	Signature
1. Named nurse discharge interview			
2. Nurse specialist (IV) Other			
3. Symptom care team			
4. Hospital social worker			
5. Dietician			
6. Equipment/supplies			
7. TTO's and drug information			
8. Other			
9. Community nurse team			
10. Health visitor/GP			
11. Other			
12. Transport Escort			
13. Further appointment/admission			
14. Ensure update of continuity of care folder			

Figure 9.2 Admission and discharge document (reproduced with permission from the Hospital for Sick Children, Great Ormond Street, London)

months, they will be more used to the hospital routine of admission and discharge but care should always be taken with every child who is going home after treatment. Some families have built up very close links with their community nurses or local hospitals and are quite happy to arrange their own out patient

■ How many parents ring your ward to say they have run out of oral drugs at home?

■ If a well-negotiated and organised discharge had been carried out, this should rarely happen, when in fact it is a problem that does occur time after time.

appointments to fit in with the rest of their family life, but they still need advice and guidance from you, the nurse, about when they need blood tests or check-ups. Through negotiation with families, you will be able to identify how much input they require from you to arrange their care outside the specialist centre.

The discharge planning process can be seen to be accumulative for the child with cancer and their families, as after each admission they have more knowledge and understanding of the illness and treatment they are receiving. Once the family have realised that they can actually care for their child at home with support from health professionals, discharge from hospital should not be so traumatic. Of course instances do occur where local hospitals may not have the expertise of the specialist centre, which leaves the parents feeling insecure and worried for their child's well being. Such situations need addressing carefully in order that the family are not left to feel out of control of their child's care and also that any problem areas are highlighted and corrected in a constructive manner. The local (or satellite) hospitals should also feel as though they are part of the team who is caring for a child and their family so they should receive training and support from the specialist centre, even when they appear to do no right in the eyes of the parents.

Long-term discharge

This aspect of discharge is applied to those children who have finished their inpatient treatment and will now be followed up on an outpatient basis. For at least 6 months, these families will have been part of the ward team with many admissions for chemotherapy, radiotherapy and/or surgery. Friends will have been made with other families and a network of support may have been established with parents and also with the ward staff. Although there will be a great sense of relief that a course of treatment has been completed, there will also be a sense of loss in that friends and acquaintances made during the time spent in hospital will no longer be part of a family's routine.

The amount of time that a family is to spend attending an outpatient clinic may well reflect the amount of input needed at the time of inpatient discharge. For example, a child with ALL will have a lot of contact as an outpatient due to their bone marrow aspirates and lumbar punctures, whereas a child with acute myeloid leukaemia (AML) will have far less contact as their treatment is mostly carried out as an inpatient without the long-term treatment of the ALL children.

The regular hospital contact for the child with ALL will act as a support for the family, as they will be seeing a senior doctor on a fairly regular basis. The child with AML, who will have hospital contact, may need more preparation for discharge as the family will receive less support and have less of an opportunity to ask questions that may be worrying them.

Because of the amount of information that needs to be covered if a discharge is to be successful, an adequate amount of time needs to be set aside for the information to be given the child and their family. If all the information and advice is given in one go, it is unlikely that any more than a portion of it will be remembered and retained. Spreading the information over a longer period of time and backing up the verbal advice with written information will increase the amount of retention and lead to a more successful discharge from the clinical unit. If one person is dealing with a family's discharge, then they will know what they have already discussed and what remains to be addressed and also what areas the family are concerned about. By acknowledging that discharge from hospital can be frightening, the family will feel able to open up and discuss their concerns and worries. Considerable time and effort is required to care for someone outside the clinical area, especially when a home and family still need time and attention too. This needs to be recognised and addressed – just as you, as a nurse, anticipate the initial needs of patients who are acutely ill and hospitalised, so must you anticipate and recognise the needs of the patient and family going home (Oberst *et al.*, 1989). As a named nurse, you will have built up a trusting relationship with a family and should be able to identify the needs of the family and address these issues during the discharge phase.

When would you begin discharge for a child with AML?

Returning to family normality after a long period of hospitalisation or disruption through regular hospital admissions can be very problematical but is rarely considered by families being discharged. The thought of having the whole family back together again and returning to a normal routine is in the forefront of parents, minds and the prospect of any problems will not be considered. However, it can be an enormous shock when the family is re-united to find that the siblings squabble, the parents are unsure how to act and their whole system of family dynamics seems to have altered beyond belief.

If Sam and his family had been prepared for the problems that they are experiencing in Case study 9.6, then they would have been able to cope much better. Although not wanting to scare a family into dreading the final discharge, they need preparing for the fact that the family will need time to adjust to being a proper family again. While a child has been in hospital, all the normal family roles have been put on hold and it takes time for all the family members to come to terms with living together again. Siblings may feel left out if their brother or sister gets lots of

Who would you consider to be the most appropriate person to intervene in this situation?

Case study 9.6

Sam is discharged home following his second intensification. The family are looking forward to getting back to a normal routine again and are excited that the majority of Sam's treatment is now over. Sam has had lots of problems with infections and so has spent a lot of time in his local hospital as well as the specialist centre. Sam and his family know the staff in both hospitals relatively well, but consequently Sam has spent very little time at home and he is keen to return to his own home and toys. Sam's mum has been resident with her son during his hospital admissions and her husband has remained at home caring for their 6-year-old daughter, Jessica, while trying to keep working too.

When Sam comes home the family have a small party with themselves and a few close friends who have helped the family during Sam's inpatient treatment. All are relieved that the family can now begin to get their routine back to normal again.

Over the next few days Sam and Jessica play together but Jessica wants to use all the toys and destroys anything that Sam builds or makes. Sam's mum tells them to use their own toys but Jessica now thinks that all the toys are hers as she has been using them most of the time while Sam was in hospital. Eventually, Jessica is sent to her room until she can learn to share her toys and as she storms to her room, she announces that she wishes Sam had stayed in hospital forever. Sam begins to cry and doesn't understand why his sister is shouting at him. Sam's mum rings her husband at work for a bit of support but is told that he is too busy to speak and that she must sort the problem out herself.

Sam's parents find it very difficult to live together again, having spent so much time apart. Sam's dad has got used to coping with working, looking after Jessica and running the family home as well. Now his wife is back at home, he finds it very difficult to re-establish his role in the home – he feels his wife is trying to be superwoman to make up for the time she wasn't at home but is leaving him feeling inadequate and useless.

Sam's mum is trying to prove that she is able to run the home again but is constantly worried that Sam will relapse and cannot concentrate on anything else. She feels guilty that her husband was left to cope with so much at home and is now trying to make up for her absence. The couple are not having any real relationship and are having difficulty in talking about anything that doesn't involve the children. The family feel as though they are falling apart and feel very isolated and do not know which way to turn next.

attention and presents when they come home and they may get less attention than their sibling. Being naughty is a good way of getting people to take notice of you and it is a good trick that most children learn when they are being ignored. If parents are aware that situations like those in the scenario can occur when a family goes home properly, they will be able to consider ways to

> ☞ **Case study 9.6 (continued)**
>
> Sam and his family continue to have problems and Sam's mum is worrying more and more that the family will fall apart. A routine telephone call from a member of the outreach team at the specialist centre ends with Sam's mum in floods of tears and the outreach nurse arranges to visit the family the next day.
>
> Sam's mum explains her concerns about her son relapsing and how hard the family is finding living together again. The outreach nurse takes time to explain to Sam's mum that the problems she has been experiencing can occur following long spells in hospital and reassures her that life will return to normal eventually. Sam's mum feels relieved that there is some light at the end of the tunnel and asks the outreach nurse to come again the following week.
>
> Sam's mum spends time that evening talking to her husband and the family begin to learn how to live together again in harmony, using the outreach nurse as a telephone link for further advice and help.

overcome the problems and not consider themselves as being useless and unable to cope when before their child was ill, family life was routine and 'normal'.

Discharge post bone marrow transplantation

There are many stresses associated with bone marrow transplantation (BMT), including the life-threatening nature of the procedure, prolonged hospitalisation in a protected environment and the required compliance in the various daily routines (Phipps *et al.*, 1994). However distressing the time within the isolation unit has been, most families still remain apprehensive about leaving the clinical area – the prospect of caring for a child outside the protected environment, knowing that immunosuppression is still a potential hazard, can overwhelm many parents (Wiley and House, 1988). Comprehensive care for marrow transplantation patients and their families is based on an understanding of both the physiological and psychosocial aspects of transplantation, which should be taken into account when planning the child and family for discharge (Haberman, 1988). The BMT experience does not end with discharge from the clinical environment, but this in itself is an important milestone (White, 1994), and at the time of discharge the physical, psychological and emotional impact of the transplantation on the family needs very careful addressing.

Phipps *et al.* (1994) highlight the fact that the high level of nursing care required for BMT patients along with the intensity of the setting, tends to promote the development of close nurse–patient relationships. This unique close contact allows the named or primary nurse to focus on the patient as a member of a family system – an important issue to remember when a child is to rejoin their family unit outside the BMT clinical environment. However, the intensity of such relationships can also be problematical, as the level of security and dependency that a family gains from the clinical area may hinder them in their perceived ability to cope after discharge.

One specific way to avoid such anxieties is to maintain the family 'roles' during the transplant period, as far as possible. Through negotiation at the beginning of the BMT, parents should feel able to retain their parenting role while their child is in hospital and also feel valued in their contribution to their child's care (Casey and Mobbs, 1988). Children and their parents will still have the security of the close nurse–patient relationship, but they will not be so dependent as they are maintaining a degree of control, resulting in an easier transition back to the family life known pre transplant. Parents will feel more confident in coping at home if it is pointed out to them that they have retained their vital parenting role to their sick child while they have been in hospital.

A BMT unit by its very nature promotes a patient's regression and infantilisation (Brack *et al.*, 1988), so discussing ways of promoting normalisation prior to discharge is vital. The whole family are shifting from one set of guidelines/routines to another when leaving the BMT unit after many weeks of occupation. This alone causes much confusion and needs to be addressed within the discharge planning process. White (1994) explored parental concerns following their child's discharge from BMT units and six major themes emerged (see Box 9.1). By having a greater understanding of the concerns that families may have post BMT, you are in a better position to prepare them for the transitional period from being comfortable in hospital, to being comfortable at home again.

Pot-Mees (1989) recognises the potentially stressful experience of the adjustment process after discharge from a BMT unit and advocates specific information which should be communicated to the family. Typical behaviour reactions shown by children after discharge should be discussed and the child and family should be prepared for a period of reintegration and adjustment. By identifying potential problem areas, and taking time to discuss them, families will be prepared for changes in their family life outside the clinical area. Preparation will lessen the anxiety caused by leaving the BMT unit and the child and parents will feel more confident in their abilities to cope with their new freedom.

As the child and family begin to prepare for discharge, they may have feelings of separation anxiety, along with the anticipated loss of readily available medical and nursing personnel (Haberman,

Box 9.1

Six major themes of the post-BMT experience (reproduced from White 1994, p 96)

The return home
Glad to be discharged; family relief and joy
Separation/isolation but support from other families
Fears/relief at returning to 'own' hospital

Working with this
Financially; loss of wages a concern
Emotionally; faith, coping techniques
New supportive relationships

The new norm
Continuing the adjustment/back to school/social life
Feelings of decreased fear but vigilant attitude

Changing relationships
Fathers performing in mother's domain
Mothers functioning as single parents
Sibling antagonism; extended family

Learning the rules
Discharge planning comprehensive but anxiety-producing
Patient and family with new tasks
Infection precautions – new guidelines = confusion

The uncertain future
What next? Thoughts of relapse/failure
Separate normality from abnormal
Potential long-term side effects.

1988). As the nurse planning for discharge, you will need to be aware that depressive moods may emerge as families grieve the loss of their prolonged relationship with members of staff who have cared for them, and also that the end of treatment has finally come – BMT being the final step for many children with malignancies. The nurse needs to draw on all available communication skills in order to build up a clear picture of how the discharge event is perceived by the child and family and then negotiate the discharge planning accordingly.

Most families on discharge from BMT will need varying degrees of educating about infection precautions and continuation of clean diets and will also need direction and teaching in the administration of oral medication. There is a lot of information to be given at a time when anxiety will be high, so it is important to regularly evaluate how much information is being retained by the family. By allowing parents to take over most of their child's care prior to the discharge, you will not only be evaluating how efficient your discharge planning has been; you will also be giving the family a chance to feel confident in caring for their child properly.

As for discharges following a course of chemotherapy, there is a great need for documentation to ensure that all aspects of

Bone Marrow Transplant Unit -
DISCHARGE PLAN

Name:...   Number:...

Date of discharge:...

No: Skill:	Information:	Comp? Yes/No	Comment........Sig:
1. Medication	a. Drugs labelled correctly b. Drugs given to parents c. Parents able to administrate drugs safely d. Aware of cyclosporin side effects?		
2. Hygiene	a. Instruction on shower /bathing given b. Clothing/laundry		
3. Skin care	a. Condition of child's skin on discharge discussed b. Aspects of skin GVHD and skin pigmentation discussed c. Parent can recognise skin deterioration e.g. redness, itching, rashes d. Sun/skin protection		
4. Gut GVHD	a. Parents understand about gut GVHD & diarrhoea		
5. Clean diet	a. Parents have seen dietician b. Special diet supplied c. Parents aware of food to be avoided (BMT guidelines)		
6. Central venous line care	a. Parents seen by IV team i. Central venous line (CVL) exit site care discussed ii. Safe flushing of CVL iii. Care of CVL bungs and clamps iv. All equipment given for CVL care v. Blue clamps given		
7. Temperature	a. Parent able to check temperature. b. Thermometer available at home?		

Figure 9.3 Bone marrow transplant unit – discharge plan (reproduced with permission from the Hospital for Sick Children, Great Ormond Street, London)

Bone Marrow Transplant Unit -
DISCHARGE PLAN (Cont'd)

Figure 9.3   *(cont'd)*

No: Skill:	Information:	Comp? Yes/No	Comment.......Sig:
	c. Parents understand the implication of a high temperature and know that they must contact the hospital if the child's temperature is above 38C d. Masking effect of paracetamol on temperature explained to parents		
8. Infection and infectious disease	a. Parents have an understanding of risks of contact with infectious disease, (e.g. measles, chicken pox, shingles, cold sores) and know to contact Robin ward immediately b. No contact with persons who have had live polio (i.e. oral) vaccination in previous 6 weeks c. Parents know how to prevent infections, e.g. avoid crowds, building dust d. Parents know that their child can not receive any immunisations until 1 year post BMT		
9. Discharge correspondence	a. Discharge letter completed and sent b. Informed of discharge: i. GP ii. Community nurse iii. Symptom care team iv. Health visitor v. Shared care hospital c. OPA made (parents aware not to give Cyclosporin on morning of OPA) d. Transport booked e. Seen by BMT coordinator		

the planning process are covered and that it is easy for individuals to see how far discharge planning has progressed. A similar planner to the one shown would be suitable to cover all the important aspects highlighted in the previous passage (Figure 9.3). Discharge planning requires many skills from those involved and as the nurse planning the discharge, you will need to be aware of the implications and problems that can occur post BMT if you are to prepare families properly for the move back to their home environment.

One very important aspect of the discharge process following BMT is communicating with the community health workers who will be involved in a child's care. Although transplants are becoming more common, there are still a lot of medical and nursing practitioners who will not have had contact with a child post transplant. In order to ease the discomfort these individuals may feel due to the exposure to a new situation, they should be given enough information for them to understand what procedure has taken place and what their role is in the recovery period post-BMT. A discharge summary is used in the author's own workplace (Figure 9.4) which covers the various potential problem areas that the community teams should be monitoring. By giving this information to people who have not been involved in the acute phase, it will help build up a rapport between the specialist centre and the community services caring for the child and family after transplantation. By giving a contact name (usually the named/ primary nurse) the process is more personal and the communication links will be easier to continue.

Discharge to palliative care

There have always been some children who do not respond to conventional treatment or who relapse on treatment, indicating a very aggressive disease type. Once it is obvious that there is no proper cure for these children, alternative arrangements have to be made. Very few children actually die in hospital now – most families prefer to take their child home to have some time together as a family in their own familiar environment. The discharge to the home setting when there is no further treatment available to the child is a very delicate one and can cause a lot of upset if not handled with care and consideration for the family's feelings. Not only does the nurse have to cope with the family who are coming to terms with the fact that their child is terminally ill, but also the fact that the overall emphasis has changed from a fighting one to a supportive one. This can be particularly difficult when the environment remains the same.

When the time arrives for a child to be discharged for palliative care, it is imperative that adequate care and support are available in the community for the family. The family must not be left feeling abandoned or isolated, a situation which may happen if a thorough and comprehensive discharge is not carried out. Home care teams (such as CLIC, Macmillan or outreach nurses) can be a valuable link between hospital and home, so it is vital that

GREAT ORMOND STREET HOSPITAL FOR CHILDREN NHS TRUST
Great Ormond Street, London WC1N 3JH   0171 405 9200

NURSING discharge summary for ....

Date: ....   G.O.S. Hospital no: ....

Date of birth: ....   Diagnosis: ....

had a   matched unrelated bone marrow transplant
               sibling bone marrow transplant
               peripheral stem cell transplant
               umbilical cord blood transplant
               maternal/paternal transplant
               other ....   on ....

               and is .... engrafted

The conditioning prior to the transplant involved the following:

               Bulsulphan   Cyclophosphamide
               Campath   Melphalan
               Total/partial body irradiation   Thiotepa
               Other ....

On discharge he/she continues with the following drugs:

Drug	Dose	Route	Frequency
Cyclosporin			
Acyclovir			
Septrin/pentamidine next due:			
Penicillin			
Folinic acid			
Sandoglobulin next due:			
Fluoride ion			
Potassium chloride			
Magnesium glycerophosphate			
Itraconazole/fluconazole			
Others:			

Prior to   platelets   blood   Sandoglobulin
a premedication of IV Piriton .... and IV hydrocortisone .... is needed.

He/she is also 'allergic' to ....
               ....
               ....

During the first week home twice weekly (Monday and Friday) blood counts, U/Es, LFTs/magnesium are needed.

Please call the outpatient BMT team .... or .... on
0171 405 9200 bleep 575, with the results and they will also liaise with you re further blood sampling.

She/he has a double lumen Hickman line in situ which is dressed with
Opsite 3000   Mepore   Tegaderm

The parent(s) is/are able to: change the dressing
                                 heplok the lines   } weekly
                                 take blood samples

He/she is still at risk of developing:
  • Graft and host disease (GvHD)
    of the skin – resulting in skin rashes
    of the gut – resulting in increased frequency and passing liquid green stools
    of the liver – resulting in raised liver function tests and jaundice
  • Cyclosporin toxicity
    – resulting in headaches, nausea, vomiting, tremor, high blood pressure
  • Effects of an immature immune system
    – resulting in raised temperatures and to avoid being in contact with chickenpox, measles,
    shingles – please contact Robin ward if contact is made

As .... is still severely immune suppressed should she/he have any problem she/he should
be seen on .... ward. Anticipated problems may include pyrexia, line infection, chickenpox,
shingles. If admitted he/she will need an isolation room, mix with own siblings only and cared for by
staff who are infection free.

A brief summary of issues discussed with the parents:

Figure 9.4 Discharge summary letter (reproduced with permission from the Hospital for Sick Children, Great Ormond Street, London)

Case study 9.7

Lauren is 6 years old and has recently been treated for a relapse of her leukaemia. Unfortunately, Lauren has failed to achieve remission and her family have decided to take their daughter home without further aggressive treatment. Lauren is still receiving antibiotics for a central line infection and her parents have asked for these to continue until the course is finished. Lauren's parents are obviously very upset at the news of their daughter's relapse and have been keeping themselves shut in their cubicle since they heard the news. Despite being offered a discussion with a consultant, the family have not asked for any meeting to be arranged. The nursing staff feel that the family are not accepting the prognosis for Lauren and that Lauren is receiving treatment which is not suitable for a child in the terminal phase. There is concern that Lauren will remain on the ward until she dies, something which the family have always expressed concern over – they had been adamant that Lauren should be at home if she was going to die.

It is the middle of a week before a long bank holiday weekend and Lauren becomes very unwell overnight. There is grave concern that she may die quite quickly and it is felt appropriate to offer the family the opportunity to take their daughter home within the next few days. Organising community services for the long weekend will prove problematical if the wheels are not set in motion soon. The registrar asks to see Lauren's parents privately and explains that Lauren may deteriorate quickly and that now might be the time to make formal plans to take her home. Lauren's father is very angry and accuses the doctor and nurse present of being uncaring and penny-pinching. When asked what he means, he shouts that he knows his daughter is using up a lot of money and resources and that there is a child who will live who is waiting to jump into Lauren's bed when the ward can finally get rid of her. The registrar takes time to explain to Lauren's father that no one is trying to get rid of Lauren or her family but that the medical and nursing staff are aware of the family's feelings on their child dying in hospital. Lauren's father breaks down in tears and apologises, saying that both he and his wife know that their daughter is going to die but that they are too scared to think about taking her home. Lauren's mother suddenly speaks and talks about how they imagine her dying at home quickly and without them having time to say goodbye and that by keeping her in hospital keeps the inevitable further away. The registrar explains how the local community services are utilised in situations such as Lauren's and mum realises that there will be support while the family is at home and they will not be left 'to get on with things themselves' as they thought. It is suggested that the family go home for at least one day over the long weekend, depending on Lauren's condition, to see how they cope. Lauren's bed will be kept for her until the family feel they are able to remain at home for good, with the support of the local hospital and primary health care team who will take over Lauren's care for the specialist centre. This stepping-stone approach to discharge allows Lauren's family to decide when they go home for good and how much time they spend at home prior to the final discharge. The family appear relieved that their feelings have been addressed, and the situation discussed with a plan built for the next few days, which allows everyone involved to know what is happening.

families are introduced to these individuals as soon as possible so that they can identify who will be the main co-ordinator of the child's care when they have been discharged home. District nurses and local hospital community teams also play important roles in the care of the child with terminal disease but these people can only help if they know about the child's circumstances. Discharging children and their families for terminal care can be a traumatic experience for those people who have been involved in the child's care. In some instances, there is very little time to prepare a family for going home and the majority of the responsibility falls to the community team members. However, when there is time to help the family begin to cope with their child's discharge to palliative care, being a named nurse who has a close relationship with the family, you will have an important part to play in the discharge process. Families may be spending periodic times at home so you will be able to assess how the family is feeling about being at home alone with their child, providing of course that you know the family well enough to be able to pick up on verbal and non-verbal cues of concern or stress.

As more children are dying in their own homes, nurses within the hospital setting are having less exposure to children in the terminal phase and therefore less ability to cope with the family of the child. Community teams have built up expertise in dealing with these situations and can be a great support to ward staff who may be feeling inadequately skilled to deal with terminal care on the ward. Senior members of staff can be a vital resource and support in circumstances where junior staff are trying to cope with a family who's child is going home to die. For continuity of care, the named nurse will want to remain looking after the family but this nurse may feel lacking in appropriate skills; the senior nurse/nurse-in-charge will play an important role in supporting the junior or less experienced staff members while allowing them to continue caring for their allocated family. Having been supervised through the period where the family is prepared for going home in the palliative situation, the junior member of staff will learn from the experience and feel more comfortable in similar situations in the future.

An open forum after a child has died is sometimes a good way for people to air their feelings and views about the situation and can be a learning experience. However, a facilitator should head such a forum as individuals' opinions can differ and emotions may cause disagreements and people will be left feeling worse than before the meeting. Staff need reassurance that they have performed well in these circumstances and there should always be support available for those involved with the palliative care family, both during the inpatient care and also afterwards.

?

As a senior member of staff supervising a junior staff member discharging a family home for the child's palliative care, identify what steps you would take after the discharge to ensure your colleague benefits the most from the experience.

Conclusion

Comprehensive discharge planning for children with cancer and their families is imperative and is the responsibility of all members of the multidisciplinary team. However, there needs to be a central co-ordinating individual in order to ensure that all aspects are covered and the family is fully prepared for life outside the clinical environment. The need for formal documentation of discharge planning is vital in the process for the family's smooth transition to home after periods of time spent in the clinical environment. In summary, the common groundrules will be reviewed.

Discharge planning:

- begins with early assessment of the patient and family care needs
- includes concern for the patient's well being
- process involves the patient and family/caregivers
- involves co-ordination and collaboration among all health care professionals
- avoids confusion and overlapping as far as possible
- has a central co-ordinating individual who is usually the primary or named nurse.

Additionally, discharge planning is not:

- an activity that is done to or for the patient/family without their active involvement
- limiting concern to the physical well being only of the patient
- the responsibility of the discharge planning specialist alone, e.g. the named or primary nurse only.

Imagine yourself being discharged home from hospital with your own child and ensure that you would be happy and contented with the amount of advice and preparation that you are giving to the child and family.

Each family being discharged will have their own unique needs in order to achieve a stress-free transfer from hospital to home and back again or from specialist centre to shared care hospital. The nurse co-ordinating the discharge is responsible for identifying these specific needs and acting accordingly. Each discharge should begin as soon as a patient is admitted and there is no substitute for keeping regular contact with shared care hospitals or community services who will be caring for the child and family outside of the specialist centre. It is always easier to have named individuals to speak to rather than being passed from one person to another, until you find an individual who knows the patient in question. Also, by identifying an individual who the families will have contact with when they are at home, the family will feel more confident that someone knows who they are and that they will be able to seek advice and support when needed at home.

The four different types of discharge identified in this chapter each carry their own importance and should all be carried out with a family's individual needs taken into consideration. By improving discharge planning, families will feel more confident in their own ability to cope with their chronically ill child at home. This will mean that the family are more relaxed about coming into hospital for treatment which will then mean you, as a specialist nurse, benefit more from a satisfied and well-prepared child and family.

?

- Consider the discharge planning process in your ward/unit – does it include the main points highlighted in the chapter?
- Evaluate your existing discharge planning documentation or develop a planner if one does not exist already.
- Compare the different types of discharge – is a different planner required for each one? If so, develop one.
- Do junior staff feel experienced enough to discharge a family effectively? Organise teaching sessions to give them some ideas and help.
- Identify ways to evaluate the discharge planning process in your ward/unit.

References

Brack, G., Clare, H. & Blix, S. (1988) The psychological aspects of bone marrow transplantation; a staff's perspective. *Cancer Nursing*, **12**, 221–229.

Casey, A. & Mobbs, S. (1988) Partnership in practice. *Nursing Times*, **84**(44), 67–68.

Glen, S. (1982) Hospital admission through the parents' eyes. *Nursing Times*, **78**(31), 1321–1325.

Gikaw, F., Anderson, E., Bigelow, L., Bossi, L., Hanferd, J. & Kissieluis, J. (1985) The continuing care nurse. *Nursing Outlook*, **33**(4), 195–197.

Hamilton, B. & Vessey, J. (1992) Pediatric discharge planning. *Pediatric Nursing*, **18**, 475–478.

Hancock, C. (1992) The named nurse in perspective. *Nursing Standard*, **7** (1), 39–42.

Haserman (1988) Psychological aspects of bone narrow transplantation. *Seminars in Oncology Nursing*, **4**(1), 31–40.

Oberst, M. Thomas, S., Gass, K. & Ward, S. (1989) Caregiving demands and appraisal of stress among family caregivers. *Cancer Nursing*, **12**, 209–215.

Ohanian, N. (1989) Informational needs of children and adults with cancer. *Journal of Pediatric Oncology Nursing*, **6**(3), 94–97.

Phipps, S., Hinds, P.S., Channell, S. & Bell, G.L. (1994) Measurement of behavioural, affective and somatic responses to pediatric bone marrow transplantation; development of the BASES scale. *Journal of Pediatric Oncology Nursing*, **11**(3), 109–117.

Pot-Mees, C. (1989) *The Psychological Effects of Bone Marrow Tranplantation in Children*. Amsterdam: Elsevier.

Rorden, J. & Taft, E. (1990) *Discharge Planning Guide for Nurses*, p. 23. Philadelphia: WB Saunders Company.

Rotter, J.B. (1966) Generalized expectancies for internal versus external control of reinforcement. *Psychological Monographs: General and Applied*, **80**, 11–28.

Takacs, D. (1991) Unit 1. Skill 5. Planning discharge *in* Smith, D. ed. *Comprehensive Child and Family Nursing Skills*, pp. 19–21. Missouri, USA: Mosby Yearbook.

Thornes, R. (1993) *Bridging the Gaps – caring for children in the health service* (CCHS). London: Action for Sick Children.

White, A. (1994) Parental concerns following a child's discharge from a bone marrow transplant unit. *Journal of Pediatric Oncology Nursing,* **11**(3), 93–101.

Wiley, L. & House, K. (1988) Bone marrow transplants in children. *Seminars in Oncology Nursing,* **4**(1), 31–40.

Wong, D. (1991) Transition from hospital to home for children with complex medical care. *Journal of Pediatric Oncology Nursing,* **8**(1), 3–9.

Care in the community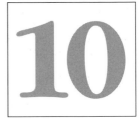

ANNE HARRIS AND SALLY CURNICK

Introduction

The aim of this chapter is to explore the support required to enable children undergoing treatment for malignant disease to be successfully maintained within their own community. Much research had demonstrated the far-reaching psychological affects of the hospitalisation of young children (Bowlby, 1953: Robertson, 1958: Butler, 1986), therefore, wherever possible, support should be made available to enable sick children to be cared for within their own community. The dictionary definition of community is 'a body of people in the same locality' which gives a clue to the role of the community worker – supportive intervention should be available to everyone with whom the child and family have contact, but it should always be on a needs-led basis. The Children Act of 1989 states that professionals should be acting in partnership with the child and the parents, with the needs and rights of the child being of paramount importance. With this in mind it is necessary to explore the various aspects of community living that may require intervention to facilitate the smooth passage of the child from hospital to home.

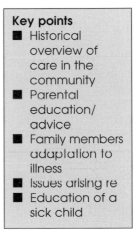

Key points
- Historical overview of care in the community
- Parental education/advice
- Family members adaptation to illness
- Issues arising re
- Education of a sick child

Historical overview

The changing face of treatment for a child with malignancy has meant that although the majority of newly diagnosed children will receive initial therapy in one of the 22 UK Children's Cancer Study Group (CCSG) centres, many will return to their local hospital for 'shared care' with the regional centre. While this has many benefits for the child and family, it has resource implications for district general hospitals.

The gap in community paediatric provision was initially noticed in the early 1970s in both Southampton and Nottingham, these centres employed generic community paediatric nurses attached to the hospital but working exclusively in the community. This

appeared to set a trend and other districts followed suit, establishing similar services to meet the expressed need in their local
area.

With the development of the UKCCSG regional centres, the
concept of shared care evolved. The South West was the first
region to fully establish shared care, radiating from the regional
centre in Bristol. Initially specialist paediatric oncology nurses
were employed to focus specifically on palliative care, however
by the mid 1980s it was recognised that optimum family support
would be achieved by involving community nurses throughout
the treatment process.

Throughout the 1990s this service spread country wide and
there are now approximately 50 posts. Initially the majority were
funded by national voluntary organisations, but funding for many
is now the responsibility of the local health authority.

Establishing partnerships of care

As has been discussed in Chapter 9, considerable preparation
should have been undertaken prior to the initial discharge into
the community. Each family should have been given the opportunity to discuss their anxieties about leaving the secure knowl-
edge-filled environment of the hospital, and returning to an
environment in which they may feel vulnerable and lacking the
necessary skills to care adequately for their sick child.

Current trends and treatment mean that the initial admission to
hospital is now likely to be of a much shorter duration than in
previous years, therefore the child and family are being expected
to cope with a change in family functioning and the resultant
problems at a time when literature indicates (Judd, 1989) that they
are likely to be in the denial stage of coping with the illness. In
order to reinforce teaching that was started in the ward situation,
the family should be provided with comprehensive written material covering the key points relating to their child's health needs.
These parent-held records should include:

- care of venous access
- oral hygiene
- skin care
- dietary advice
- advice regarding neutropenia
- disease-specific information
- relevant contact numbers.

It is important that the child and family have met a link person
while still hospital based, however it should be noted that the role

of this person often does not have any particular relevance for the individual family until they are community based. Muir (1993) argues that community children's nurses should ensure that services identified to meet the needs of children should be developed in a collaborative and integrated way – with this in mind it is important that the child and family view the community- and hospital-based staff as working together in partnership with the family.

Although the family of a child undergoing treatment are often actively encouraged to contact the hospital for advice or treatment, it should be remembered that once the child has been discharged to the community, the main responsibility for care reverts to the primary health care team. As has been discussed in the previous chapter detailing partnership in care, to offer optimum levels of care to the family, strong partnerships should be forged between the hospital- and community-based teams. The family need to feel secure that both members of this partnership are working in the best interests of their child. To promote this idea, both teams must demonstrate that they are working in co-operation and with a free exchange of relevant information. Therefore, prior to discharge, contact between the hospital and primary care teams should be made and a visit arranged to meet the following aims:

- Exchange of information – disease-related and relevant family history.
- Allocation of roles to avoid either swamping or abandoning the family.

This meeting should also allow an opportunity to discuss the impact of diagnosis on the family and wider community, including the primary health care team who are likely to have a supportive role to other members of the community dealing with the illness (Figure 10.1). Ewles and Simnett (1992) identified six dimensions of health:

- physical
- mental
- social
- emotional
- spiritual
- societal.

This meeting should acknowledge that the diagnosis of cancer will impact on each of these six dimensions and thought must be given to addressing them for every member of the family. General practitioners (GPs) can be an invaluable source of support and knowledge of individual family dynamics and available local resources.

While ward-based staff usually view discharge as a positive step, the impact on the family should not be minimised. In what way could you work towards increasing a family's confidence prior to discharge?

Figure 10.1 Liaison
meeting with the GP
(reproduced with
permission)

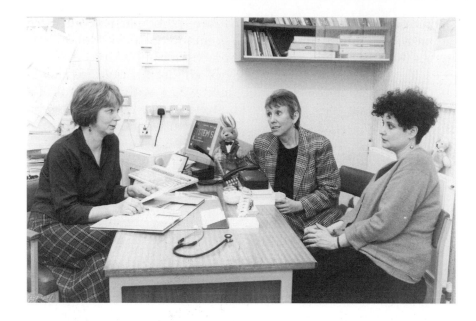

In order to facilitate such support, the GP needs to be in receipt of up-to-date information regarding the disease and also current treatment. It should be acknowledged that treatment for malignant disease changes rapidly; many GPs may not feel confident in their knowledge base without input from the hospital team.

It is also necessary to ensure that regular discharge summaries are sent to the primary health care team to ensure that they are kept up to date throughout the treatment process. Parents need to feel secure in the knowledge that their GP is aware of the current situation regarding their child's illness and treatment.

Education

Education remains crucially important to the child's prospects. This is increasingly so as medical advances have made recovery possible from a number of previously life-threatening conditions. Without effective education the child's personal happiness, life and career chances as adults may be irretrievably disadvantaged (Department of Health, 1994).

As the emphasis during treatment is to maintain as normal a life as possible, the need for continuing education should have been explained during admission. The child would have had contact with the hospital-based teachers, who in turn should have made contact with the child's mainstream school. While this contact will centre around the child's education and current progress, a separate contact to raise psychosocial issues is necessary. With the permission of the child and the family, a visit to the school should be offered to meet with the teacher and relevant staff initially, and then a further visit may be arranged to visit the child's peer group (Figure 10.2). Topics covered in the initial meeting with staff should include:

- Disease-relevant information.
- Side effects of treatment: altered body image, hair loss, fatigue, immunosuppression, physical limitations.

This meeting should also cover the importance of reintegrating

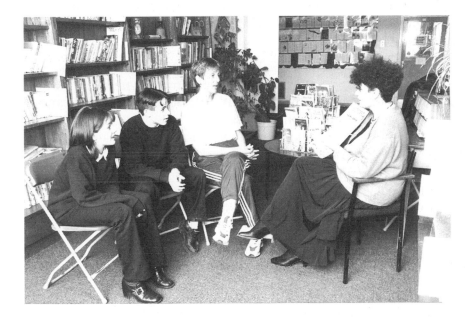

Figure 10.2 Meeting with the head of year at school and two peers (reproduced with permission)

Case study 10.1

Susan, a 14-year-old girl having treatment for a large spinal tumour, was anxious to return to school. Although a visit to discuss the implications of her treatment was offered, the school did not consider it was necessary and felt they could manage her return (to school). Despite assurances that any difficulties she encountered would be met in a sympathetic manner, the school had not acknowledged the practical difficulties that would arise from her lack of mobility. The school she attended was a large secondary school built over a widespread site. Susan could not manage to get from lesson to lesson within the small time allowed, as a result she received a 40-minute detention every time she was late for a lesson, this was, in part, due to the fact that not every member of the staff knew about her illness and the limitations that it caused. Had a meeting taken place, there would have been an opportunity to disseminate information.

the child as fully as possible. The purpose of school should be to enable the child to mix back in with the 'healthy' peer group as an equal participant, the child should not be singled out for unnecessary praise or attention which will further reinforce any feelings of difference.

It is our experience that neglecting this particular liaison role can lead to specific problems in returning to the community. As long-term survival is the likely outcome for the majority of children with malignant disease, it is of vital importance this disruption to schooling is kept as minimal as possible.

> Cancer challenges the adolescent's sense of self-esteem, leading to feelings of loss of control at a time of life when self image is pivotal to normal development (Lewis, 1996).

As an adolescent, Susan in Case study 10.1 was very conscious of her altered body image. The developmental tasks of adolescents are complex enough without dealing with the implications of a potentially life-limiting illness.

As teachers need to have clear information to enable them to deal with the situation, the child's peer group should also have the opportunity to ask questions and have basic honest information given to them.

Given that cancer is often viewed as a taboo subject and one that is shrouded in myth and half truths, it is important that various areas are fully explored with the young people:

- The *exact* nature of the disease and treatment.
- That the cause is not known but that the 'fault' does not lie with the sick child.
- That cancer is not catching.

Given your knowledge of the research surrounding the developmental tasks of adolescents how would you prepare Sharon's peer group for her eventual return to school?

Case study 10.1 (continued)

As Susan was returning to school having lost her hair, she was particularly anxious to avoid scrutiny. Although some teachers did not comment on the fact that she wore a cap pulled right down over her face, others insisted that it was removed – once members of the wider pupil group became aware of the fact she was 'different', she became the subject of ridicule and mild bullying. Consequently Susan elected not to return to school although the teaching staff were anxious to help her and were then happy to meet with hospital-based staff to address the issues that had been raised, the damage to her fragile self confidence had been done. Despite strong support from a close knit group of well informed peers, she chose not to return to school until the end of her treatment.

- That cancer is rare and that any ill health that the listener may have is unlikely to be cancer.
- That treatment is being given to aim for cure.

Young people should be prepared for the likely appearance of the sick child, hair loss, weight loss or gain, and the existence of any permanent venous access should be explained. The reasons for these should also be explained and the fact that they are not permanent.

If the session is open to questions, the most likely question will be 'is the sick child going to die?' – within a mixed child and adult group this always causes concern among the adults, who can find discussions surrounding death uncomfortable; however, if the question is raised it should be dealt with as honestly as possible given the information available. Conversely, problems can arise if a young person receiving treatment for cancer returns to school looking and acting as 'normal'.

Perhaps the most important function of the hospital or community team in respect of supporting the child's education is to offer regular support and contact to the school staff in their day-to-day dealings with the child. The teaching and support staff are experts in dealing with school life and while they will require the information necessary to deal with a child's illness they will be able to assess its effect on their environment.

In order to ensure optimum holistic care for the child it is necessary for everyone involved in aspects of the child's life to collaborate and recognise each other's role and area of expertise.

Bullying

There will always be situations when, despite the previous mentioned groundwork, the child returning to school will be the focus

Case study 10.2

Johann is 15 years old and undergoing treatment for a resistant disease. All her therapy is on an outpatient basis, causing very minimal time away from school. Both she and her peer group have found difficulty in knowing how to cope with the knowledge of her illness. Johann finds herself removed from the frivolity of normal adolescence; her peer group find it hard to remember that she is ill. Within the school environment, two teachers who attended a meeting to pass on information have been helpful and supportive, however within a large school complex, a pupil who is not obviously unwell is treated as part of the main school. This highlights the complexity of adolescence, they want to be treated as part of a group but to have acknowledgement of their special needs.

of bullying. Although this situation needs to be quickly addressed and resolved, careful consideration to its reasons is needed. Prior experience of the child within the school must be taken into consideration, it may be that the focus of bullying is not directly related to the child's illness but previously unresolved issues within the classroom situation. The school staff should be encouraged to implement their pre-existing anti-bullying strategies and follow through procedures without focusing on the child's illness.

School refusal

Children who are diagnosed with cancer come with a vast range of previous history. Not all children with cancer will have had a good educational experience and will therefore have different problems in returning to school.

Children who persistently school refuse prior to the diagnosis of their illness will require very different support and multi-agency intervention to try to secure adequate education. In these situations there should be a multidisciplinary meeting, to include the child and parents, to produce a planned structured return to school. In these instances, failure to integrate to school is less likely to be related to the child's illness and the family experience, and continued school refusal is more appropriately dealt with by the education welfare service than the hospital or community staff.

Case study 10.3

Lance was a 14-year-old boy diagnosed with an untreatable abdominal tumour. At the time of diagnosis his life expectancy was known to be short, he was aware of this and started to make various plans in order to tie up what he viewed as loose ends. It was important for him to go to school to be with his peer group, however at the time of his diagnosis he was indefinitely excluded from school because of his recurrent antisocial behaviour.

With considerable persuasion and given the unusual circumstances, the school staff were prepared to waive the exclusion order as long as Lance remained on daily report. He was made aware that any misdemeanour would reinforce the exclusion order immediately.

In order to maintain school discipline, his year group was told why he was returning to school, they were also made aware that the reasons for the exclusion order remained in force and that his behaviour, and his immediate peer group, would be closely monitored.

Once Lance knew that it was possible for him to return to school, the desire to do so became less strong and in practice he returned only for a couple of days to make his peace with staff and friends.

Home tuition

Although reintegration into school is the main aim, it must be acknowledged that at certain times during the child's treatment school attendance will not be possible. During these periods the hospital education services will, with medical support, be able to arrange home tuition to enable the child to have some educational input at home. Local education authorities retain the discretion, desirably in consultation with parents and the medical professionals, to provide home tuition if it is in the best interests of the child.

The home tutor can act as a link between the child and the child's mainstream school and can help towards the reintegration process. Home tuition is a very valuable structure to the day and gives some normality to the child's life. Although of a much shorter duration than a normal school day, the one-to-one focus often means that the child will make up ground lost through ill health and will often keep up with the work that peers are doing in mainstream schooling. Depending on the stage of the child's education, it is possible to arrange for the child to sit state examinations or assessments in examination conditions. To be able to offer this facility and to encourage the child to work towards their pre-arranged goals is a big psychological boost for the child in helping them view their illness and perspective.

The co-operation between education and health service staff is vital and needs to take into account a child's wellbeing to achieve the greatest possible benefit for the child's education and health (Department for Education, 1994).

Day-to-day care

The main focus of care has to be to enable the family to live as normal a life as possible within the confines of treatment. A balance must be achieved that will leave the family feeling supported but not swamped by the child's illness.

Belson (1981) also suggests that home care is important to:

- Avoid the disruption of repeated outpatient attendance.
- Provide support and encouragement to parents in the care of their child.

If implemented sensitively, these two guidelines should enable the family to adapt to their altered circumstances. The effect of discharge cannot be minimised, the family are returning to a community which does not have full knowledge of their child's condition and is likely to have many preconceived fears and beliefs about cancer. The family are in a situation in which they are coping with the emotions of their friends and family and having to support them. Parents will very often give two distinct scenarios, they will either be swamped by people who are tearful and distressed and uncertain as to how to cope, or they are avoided by friends who feel so overwhelmed by the situation that avoidance seems the only way to manage.

Following an initial discharge, contact should be made by a member of the community team within 48 hours. A telephone call is often all that is required to reinforce the family that advice and support are available should the need arise. During this telephone call, arrangements for a home visit should be made. It should be remembered that while in hospital the family are likely to be conforming to what they perceive to be the acceptable norm. It is unusual for families to feel in control in the ward situation, and any judgements made regarding their understanding of and coping with their child's illness may well require re-assessment when they are seen in their own environment. To visit a family at home infers entering their domain and the professional needs to accept the family norm. While in their own environment, the child and family are more in control of the situation and can dictate the pace of events. It is not uncommon for some families to feel very clear that they want no involvement from the hospital in the community. The parents often identify home as a 'safe' place for the child and do not wish to see that compromised by visits from hospital staff to take blood or carry out procedures. It must be remembered that the family has the right to choose or refuse this intervention. It can be difficult for hospital staff to accept that families do not want any direct contact, however their wishes should be respected.

The experience of having a sick child is very disempowering to parents who will often seek to regain control in which ever way they can. Equally the sick child can become distressed by procedures at home and in an attempt to minimise their distress parents may refuse visits. Children who do not have central venus access and who rely on finger prick to gather capillary blood samples often become distressed by invasion of the home safety, and parents may prefer painful procedures to be associated with the hospital.

As the time at home increases, the child and parents are likely to grow in confidence and rely less on direct contact with the hospital in terms of making day-to-day decisions. However they should be aware that there is an open channel of communication.

It is often when the family are first at home that the implications of the diagnosis begin to dawn on individual family members and they may need support in dealing with these.

The child who has become the identified patient will often,

at this stage, not feel sick and will struggle to deal with the label that has been given to them and the restrictions that it places on their lives. As has been discussed in Chapter 4, the young person will struggle to cope with how unfair they perceive the situation to be as they view their peer group continuing in day-to-day life. This can often lead to struggles within the family as the young person feels overprotected by their parents and challenges the boundaries that are being imposed. The parents of the sick child will often appreciate the need to treat the child as before with no extra restriction on their activities, but find it difficult to manage in practice when they are trying to protect them from perceived harm.

Every family will take a differing length of time to accommodate the sick child in the new role. Treatment will affect each child differently and the family need time to deal with the side effects of therapy. Previously well behaved children can demonstrate mood swings that are out of character and can challenge any family norms.

The feelings of guilt and blame that surround the diagnosis of malignant disease are well documented in Chapter 3; however families often do not expect these feelings to be long lasting or to impinge on everyday life. It is quite common, however, for families to find these emotions behind much of their everyday functioning. As the course of their child's illness is uncertain, families will often search for reasons and many relationships often undergo periods of extreme stress as parents find differing ways of coping with the situation.

Children who are undergoing pulsed chemotherapy are often very well during their time at home and are taken into hospital at the peak of their condition to have treatment – younger children can perceive this as a punishment, they are well at home and then taken back into hospital to be 'made sick' again. In these situations a sick child can direct considerable anger at parents who they hold responsible for this. Parents who are struggling to deal with their own emotions can find an unprompted attack on their parenting skills hard to cope with, and will then direct their feelings of hurt and guilt towards another family member. Without help to stop this cycle of behaviour, each family member can become polarised and antagonistic to the rest of the family.

Within the family the sick child can become adept at spotting the power that they have and unless supported in their attempts, the family can find it difficult to maintain previous boundaries of acceptable behaviour. The sick child can also become very skilled in manipulating events around the treatment.

Given that the main focus of care has to be to ensure that the experience of malignant disease does not have a permanent damaging effect on family dynamics – although the family should

Case study 10.4

Stephen is an 8-year-old boy undergoing treatment for a leukaemia. His mother finds administering his medication virtually impossible – Stephen employs three main tactics:

- He reduces himself to tears and becomes hysterical at the mention of any tablets.
- He flatly refuses to take them, threatening considerable aggression if coerced.
- He assures his mother that he has taken them but empties them into the waste disposal unit where she will later discover them.

This leads to considerable family disruption. His mother is aware of the importance of these drugs and finds his refusal to cooperate bewildering. She finds that she is shouting at him and this increases her feelings of guilt about the whole situation, or finds that she is bribing him, which she considers undermines her parenting role. His father has more success in administering the drugs, which she also finds undermining. In discussion with Stephen, he claims to be aware of the importance of taking the drugs but uses this as his only control within the situation.

be aware that some change will be inevitable – there are situations in which a referral to more structured support services should be considered. The use of psychology and child and adolescent psychiatric services can be invaluable in enabling a family to deal with the problems they are experiencing within the framework of multidisciplinary care. It is to be hoped that the family will view the involvement of further professionals as complementary to the care their child is already receiving, as opposed to highlighting their particular difficulties.

Referrals should be considered for families with pre-existing functional difficulties at the time of diagnosis, for those who manifest acutely disturbed behaviour during the treatment process. The family, as always, should be viewed as a whole and consideration should be given to each family member and their coping mechanisms. As has been discussed in Chapter 7, all individuals will operate different coping mechanisms, the majority of which will be healthy; the professionals should always be wary of challenging a pre-existing mechanism within a family.

Siblings

It has long been acknowledged that the sibling of a child with a potentially life-threatening illness will have considerable difficulties in adjusting to their altered position within the family (Eiser, 1990, 1993). Special consideration should therefore be given to their needs:

- Feelings of guilt and self blame are not uncommon.
- Resentment of the sick child and the attention they receive.
- Relief that the illness has not affected them, coupled with the fear that it might in the future.
- Overwhelming obligation to be nice.

As with a sick child, a common parental reaction is to protect the healthy sibling by not involving them in the initial illness experience. While the professional needs to realise that this is in part a coping mechanism, in that the parent may not have the emotional energy to meet the needs of their healthy children, in the long term this is not acceptable and will need to be addressed to prevent permanent family disfunction.

Siblings should be given age-appropriate explanation about the illness and its treatment and, more importantly, the opportunity to ask questions. All information should be given at a pace dictated by the child and it should be remembered that the child will ask if they feel that they would be given an honest answer to what they want to know (Stallard *et al.*, 1997). Along with an explanation of the illness, the siblings should be given the same reassurances as the parents, while the cause of the illness is unknown, the medical staff can be categoric in their assurance that the sibling is in no way to blame. This reassurance will often need to be repeated over a prolonged period. Children tend to view themselves as the centre of the universe and believe in cause and effect, they frequently believe that they have caused the illness either by arguing with their sick sibling or by failing to protect them in some undetermined way. As children are often reluctant to talk in front of their parents, either fearing that they will upset them or feeling under pressure to be good, it can be valuable to offer them time alone with a member of medical or nursing staff to discuss issues that are of concern to them.

While acknowledging that parents may have difficulty in helping their healthy children deal with the situation, it is important the nursing staff remind parents of the need to keep them involved.

Alternatively, parents may be preoccupied with the ill child, resulting in their failure to recognise the needs of their healthy siblings. (Havermans and Eiser, 1994).

This should be particularly borne in mind while dealing with families who have been referred to the regional unit for initial diagnosis of treatment, the sick child is likely to be accompanied by both parents who will be reluctant or unable to leave the hospital to deal with their other children. The experience of the other children should be considered, they are likely to have been sent to stay with friends or relatives with minimal explanation, they will be aware that their sibling is ill although they may have had no inkling of this prior to departure, they will also be aware that their parents are upset and can be left in a period of limbo with no further information. The children need the opportunity to make sense of what is happening; parents should be encouraged to arrange for their healthy children to visit as soon after transfer as is practical. This allows them to form an impression of where their parents are staying and, more importantly, of how their brother or sister is. While stressing to the parents the importance of sibling involvement, the nursing staff should also take time to find out about the siblings and keep them involved in conversations. Nathan, the 7-year-old brother of a younger child on treatment, once remarked that he didn't like going to the ward as 'all the nurses know my brother and my mum and dad, but no-one even knows my name'.

Siblings may also experience extreme feelings of jealousy directed towards the sick child, which can be very difficult for the child to cope with or even understand. They are aware that their sibling is ill and while they would not wish that experience, they resent the extra parental time and attention given to the sick child and the gifts that are inevitably showered on them. They are aware that these emotions are unacceptable to their parents and need to be helped to find a means of expressing them in a safe environment. The child needs to know that they are not alone in having these feelings and that they are not to be punished or viewed badly by professionals involved with the family for expressing them.

On return to the family home, siblings who have had time away from their parents may well resent re-imposed discipline in the family norm, and will act out against parental instruction. Parents should be advised that while they need to understand the reasons behind this behaviour, they should not radically alter their pre-held family rules. As with the sick child, siblings need to feel secure within the family and need to have boundaries for their behaviour. Conversely, siblings will often resent any parental attempt to compensate them for the situation and can be very disparaging towards any adult who in their eyes do not fully understand their experiences in the family situation.

Within the experience of treatment for disease, siblings are likely to have both positive and negative feelings arising from altered family dynamics. Some feelings that arise can be viewed as both positive and negative; in particular they may view time away from their parents in a dual light, which can illustrate the ambivalent experience of siblings, and they may need some help to make sense of their emotions.

If one accepts that the siblings of a child with cancer are likely to have difficulty in adjusting to the disruption in family life, it is necessary to consider intervention techniques to help them. Children will adapt if they, in keeping with the sick child, are involved in what is happening within the family; however, some will require additional support.

In addition to liaison with the sick child's school, it is important that contact is also made with the sibling's school. This contact allows for an exchange of information and also for advice on how to help the relevant child within the school. Siblings are often under considerable pressure to conform within their home environment, and as a result will act out in an environment which they perceive to be safe. In order to be able to support a child, teachers need information regarding the treatment process and likely outcome. From this information they will be able to form a plan of support for the child that does not identify them as having special needs.

There should also be an opportunity to inform the child's peer group of the situation. Within the school, this will offer extra support and is likely to facilitate good communication. It is desirable that the child feels as included in the illness experience as the sick child – to visit their school is to demonstrate the concern that the hospital feels for their wellbeing.

In order to minimise the experience of isolation that siblings have, it is recognised as beneficial to consider their inclusion in a support group. This offers them the opportunity to express emotions that they find difficult to express at home and also to identify with other children in the same situation. As with all group meetings, a code of confidentiality should be enforced,

---

☛   Case study 10.5

Paul, the 7-year-old sibling of a 9-year-old boy receiving treatment for a large spinal tumour, expressed the belief that he was directly responsible for his brother's illness. He felt responsible for the resulting family dysfunction and concluded that the only way to make amends was to attempt suicide. He was clear about the mode, place and time that he intended to attempt self harm, and had he carried it out, he would have undoubtedly been successful. It would have been unethical to keep his distress confidential within the group, however it required considerable negotiation on the part of the facilitators to gain his agreement to obtain expert help.

What other scenarios would you consider it necessary to report out within the group setting and to whom would you report your concerns?

in that all group members should be told that the content of the group will not be discussed by the facilitators with their parents. The only possible exception to this must be the disclosure of anything that would adversely influence the child's safety.

As with parents who are often reluctant to acknowledge the stress they feel, siblings can find it difficult to share their fears as they are reluctant to increase parental worry. This means that active intervention is required. The group setting will often allow children to legitimise their fears about the illness and treatment and will often give them a forum in which they can gain information and dispel their fantasies. It also allows the facilitators an opportunity to gain a greater insight into the child's understanding.

It is important to recognise the benefit to siblings of being away from their parents, thus allowing them the freedom and permission to voice questions that they consider their parents would view as unacceptable.

The involvement of the sick child's siblings must feature as a necessary part of family support and should be viewed as an important role of the community staff.

However, some siblings will manifest particular problems in dealing with the implications of diagnosis. Within families who may have pre-existing functional difficulties, an extra difficulty such as maladapted behaviour of the healthy children can prove to be an intolerable stress. It must be acknowledged that group support is not appropriate for all children, while some may require very minimal support, others will require one-to-one intervention to help them come to terms with and cope with their sibling's illness.

One-to-one intervention should be on a planned short-term basis and should be structured to allow the child time and space to work through the difficult feelings they are experiencing. It may be that it is acceptable to the child for someone already involved with the family to be the source of one-to-one work, however this should be explored with the child who may have a strong need to have a neutral professional identified.

One-to-one work should be aimed at helping the sibling to view their family as a system and that the illness as something that has disrupted the normal functioning of this system. Within this, children can be helped to see how roles are allocated but often altered within a family. The use of books such as *When Someone has a Very Serious Illness* (Heegaard, 1991) can enable children to verbalise and acknowledge feelings that may be too deep rooted to be easily dealt with. In this way, the aim is to help siblings cope with the changes to their life while living through the treatment experience.

Grandparents

Grandparents are frequently deeply affected (Faulkner, Peace and O'Keeffe, 1995) when the diagnosis is made. They often mirror the emotions expressed by the parents such as disbelief and anger, but also often an overwhelming sense of the injustice of the situation. The fact that they may perceive themselves as having had their life, and remaining healthy, proves unacceptable in the face of the diagnosis of a potentially life-threatening illness in a child. It should be borne in mind that it is likely that grand-parents have a more outdated and negative view of the long-term outlook for children with malignant disease, and may need considerable time with the medical staff to understand current treatment trends.

Grandparents can often be torn between concern for their sick grandchild and a very real concern for their own child. They will often express feelings of extreme helplessness while trying to deal with these emotions.

It is often grandparents who take on many of the practical tasks of helping the family to run smoothly during the disruption caused by treatment, they often adopt care of the other children, either by going to live in the family home or by agreeing to have children to stay. The increased strain put on grandparents who may be elderly should not be minimised.

As with other family members, grandparents can be reluctant to express their feelings for fear of further upsetting their children; they can also perceive it as their role to be strong for their child. It is an essential role for the professional to ensure that grand-parents are given the opportunity to ask questions and to express their emotions away from the rest of the family.

The role of the community nurse

The extension of the children's nurse role into the community is not a new phenomenom, and children's nurses acknowledge that this service must be delivered by appropriately trained and qualified experts. Children are now being discharged with signifi-cantly more complex problems (Fradd, 1994). Their care must not be devolved to generic (adult-trained) community nurses. They do not possess specialist paediatric knowledge and experience. 'PCNs are highly skilled, competent nurses who care deeply about the care of children.' (Hennessey, 1993).

The main role of the community nurse is to smooth the tran-sition between hospital and home (Fradd, 1992). The Community Children's Nurse can provide practical support and advice to

Figure 10.3 Taking a routine blood test at home (reproduced with permission)

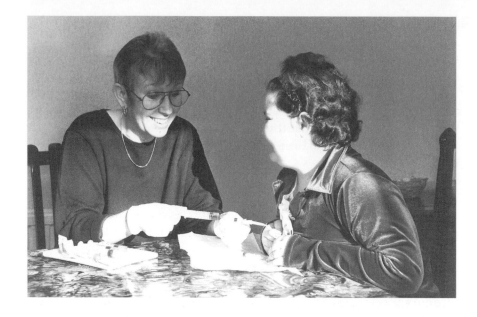

parents in their own home and help bridge the gap between hospital and community staff (Fradd, 1992; Glasper and Tucker, 1993). In the way outlined above, the community nurse acts as a support for the family throughout the treatment phase. By undertaking various nursing procedures at home, the nurse becomes a familiar face to the child, which means that the relationship can be maintained on a low key basis but can easily be increased if the situation alters (Figure 10.3). Benner (Bishop, Anderson and McCulloch, 1994) states that the nurse–patient relationship must be based on mutual trust and genuine caring. In paediatric nursing this relationship extends beyond the child to include the whole family. Furthermore, it is imperative that there is recognition of family strengths and individuality and respect of different methods of coping. As the relationship between the family and the community nurse develops, so the idea of working in partnership should develop. The community nurse is ideally placed to ensure that all involved parties work together to co-ordinate optimum care for the child.

Another facet of the role of the community nurse is education and support of health care professionals within the community. As a professional working full time within the field of paediatric oncology they are able to offer practical up-to-date information about current treatment trends.

The role of the social worker

The specialist social worker is an important member of the

paediatric oncology team and can bring specialist skills to establishing good relationships. They are often perceived as a member of the team who is not medical or nursing and can become the recipient of fears and confidences.

Donally-Wood (1988) cites social work involvement with families as having three main aims: supporting crisis, assessment, and prevention of identified problems or the minimising of their effects. He also states that involvement can be concentrated around specific times in the course of the child's disease. He identifies key times at initial diagnosis, maintenance, relapse, cessation of active therapy, terminal phase, death and bereavement.

The social worker can help families adapt to altered family functioning and with the practical difficulties that can present following a return to the community. They are in a position to negotiate with parents' employers, and can act as an advocate for both parents and children.

It is acknowledged that having a child with a chronic or life-threatening illness can put a strain on family finances. The social worker therefore can advise the family on possible statutory benefits available, as well as sources of financial support from voluntary organisations.

Many social workers employed within paediatric oncology units are funded by Sargent Cancer Care for Children, an organisation that will give direct financial assistance to families with children with any form of cancer.

References

Belson, P. (1981) Alternative to hospital care. *Nursing*, **23**, 1015–1016.

Bishop, J. Anderson, A. & McCulloch, J. (1994) Hospital-at-home: a critical analysis. *Paediatric Nursing*, **6**(6), 12–15.

Bowlby, J. (1953) *Child Care and the Growth of Love*. Harmondsworth: Pelican.

Butler, N. R. (1986) *From Birth to Five*. Oxford: Pergamon.

Department of Education (1994) *The Education of Sick Children*. Circular No. 19/94, DH LAC (94) 10, NHSE HSG (94) 24, p. 13. London: HMSO.

Department of Health (1994) *The Education of Sick Children*. NHS Executive Circular No. 12/94 London: HMSO.

Donally-Wood D. (1988) Oncology social work *in* Oakhill, A. ed. *Supportive Care of the Child with Cancer*, pp. 180–191. Bristol: Wright.

Eiser C. (1990) *Chronic Childhood Disease – an introduction to psychological theory and research*. Cambridge: University Press.

Eiser, C. (1993) *Growing Up with a Chronic Disease: the impact on children and their families*. Jessica Kingsley: London.

Ewles, L. & Simnett, I. (1992) *Promoting Health: a practical guide*. London: Scutari Press.

Faulkner, A. Peace, G. &

O'Keeffe, C. (1995) *When a Child has Cancer*. London: Chapman & Hall.

Fradd, E. (1992) Working with the specialists. *Community Outlook*, June, 29–30.

Fradd, E. (1994) Whose responsibility? *Nursing Times*, **90**(6), 34–36.

Glasper, E. A. & Tucker, A. (1993) *Advances in Child Health Nursing*. Oxford: Scutari Press.

Havermans, T. & Eiser, C. (1994) Siblings of children with cancer. *Child Care, Health and Development*, **20**, 309–322.

Heegaard, M. (1991) *When Someone has a Very Serious Illness*. Minneapolis, MN: Woodland Press.

Hennessey, D. (1993) Purchasing community nursing care. *Paediatric Nursing*, **5**, 10–12.

Judd, D. (1989) *Give Sorrow Words: working with a dying child*, London: Free Association Books.

Lewis, I. (1996) Cancer in adolescence. *British Medical Bulletin*, **52**, 887–897.

Muir, J. (1993) Integrating services in community child care. *Nursing Standard*, **8**(7), 32–35.

Robertson, J. (1958) *Young Children in Hospital*. London: Tavistock.

Stallard, P. Mastioyannopoulu, K. Lewis, M. and Leuton, S. (1997) The siblings of children with life threatening conditions. *Child Psychology and Psychiatry Review*, **2**(1), 26–32.

Survivorship and rehabilitation

MOIRA BRADWELL AND JEANETTE HAWKINS

The way we care for the child determines the cure; the cure should not determine the care. (van Eys, 1991)

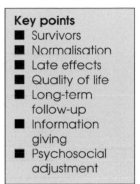

Key points
- Survivors
- Normalisation
- Late effects
- Quality of life
- Long-term follow-up
- Information giving
- Psychosocial adjustment

Introduction

The rehabilitation of children with cancer begins at diagnosis in much the same way as discharge planning starts at admission. In all that we do today there must be a consideration of its implications for the child's future. We want them to survive and we want them to survive with a quality to life that is acceptable to them – to have adjusted to the consequences of their treatment – to be able to get on with their lives – to be rehabilitated (Hawkins, 1990).

This chapter is separated into four sections to explain fully all the issues involved for cancer survivors and the people who care for them. Firstly, we have to consider who exactly are the survivors, are we just looking at physically cured children? Secondly, having established our definition, we move on to exploring the issues that affect the normalisation process of the 'cancer experience'. This section is followed by an exploration of the psychosocial effects identified in some survivors, especially when the normalisation process fails or when adjustment difficulties occur. This will include some physical late effects which have direct implications for social opportunity. Our final section considers how we, as nurses, can work towards supporting survivors to achieve successful rehabilitation, adjusted to the consequences of their treatment. Throughout the chapter those children and families who have found the cancer experience to have been a positive one, and who can offer some guidelines on positive approaches of care, will be considered.

Who are the survivors?

Defining the survivors

Many lay people and indeed health professionals would define children 'cured' from cancer as those who have had 5 years' disease-free remission. It is often only at this point that patients and their families allow themselves to hope that the disease will never return. Is this the only way we should consider 'cured' children, simply by looking at those patients who are 5 years off treatment, or as Lozowski (1993) postulates, do patients become potential survivors from the time of diagnosis? There are also groups of children who have survived with their cancer for many years, following a repeated pattern of remission and relapse. In this chapter we have taken survivorship to include all children diagnosed with cancer as potential survivors, and for this reason we will explore the issues of survivorship and rehabilitation from the child's diagnosis.

Survivorship and cure

There is, of course a correlation, between survivorship and cure. As you will come to understand not all those children who survive the cancer journey will be cured in the holistic sense of the word. In our own experience, and throughout the literature on late effects, it has become obvious that we need to look beyond the absence of disease in our definition of cure. The cured child has at least three components of their life which will have been affected in some way by the cancer, biological, psychological and social. There needs to be cure in all these components of life for the child to be 'truly cured' (van Eys, 1991). Each of these aspects have, associated with them, the overriding consideration of quality of life for the child and adult survivor. Information on the need for a more holistic cure has become more available to us, through improvements in protocols, better survival rates and a greater increase in monitoring outcomes of a physical, social and psychological nature (Chang, 1991; Lozowksi, 1993; Robison, 1993; Koocher, 1985). The quoted figures for overall cure rates in Britain today are 65–70%, varying within specific diagnoses (Cancer Research Campaign, 1990). The impact is such that by the year 2000, one in a thousand 20 year olds will have survived childhood cancer (Morris-Jones and Craft, 1990). It has therefore become apparent, from qualitative studies into late psychosocial effects, that the treatment of a child with cancer cannot focus on the disease as a purely biological phenomenon. We are therefore aiming for a child who is not only cured physically, but 'for one who can relate to his peers and who is on a par in development, maturity, achievements and aspirations' (van Eys, 1991).

Adjusting to the cancer experience

As earlier chapters will have shown the cancer experience is devastating, and will result in the child and family never being the same again, whether this is seen as either a positive or negative outcome (van Eys, 1991). For those who have managed to survive the experience in a positive way, the evidence suggests that they were able to 'normalise' the experience: 'Life, the business of the child, must be ongoing, not in spite of the cancer, but with the cancer' (van Eys, 1991).

It is obvious also that we cannot separate the physical effects of what is happening to the child from the psychological trauma alongside it. In just the same way we cannot separate the child from the family. In order for the child to accept the cancer, parents have to be given support and guidance in dealing with both the physical and psychological consequences of the child's treatment.

The impact of diagnosis and treatment is perceived as being different for the parents than the children. Parents will often mistakenly think that although their children may have child-like feelings, with enough information and explanation they can be made to understand and reason like adults. van Eys (1991) suggests the opposite is true and that children will often experience the same feelings as adults, for example: 'loneliness, abandonment, disintegration, loss of control, and having anger just like adults'. van Eys also states that, 'no number of adult-given facts or information will alter that'.

If then the cancer is the cause of these feelings, it would seem essential that the cancer be acknowledged and accepted as a reality of life and dealt with in the best possible way, thus producing the concept of normalisation at an early stage. This means that despite the disruption in all aspects of family life, families must continue living their life in a way that is meaningful to them and gives them some satisfaction. Even though children may spend up to several months at a time in and out of hospital, we now know that if they continue to have the contact, love and support of their family and friends, are able to have the opportunity to play and learn, they will have the potential to continue to develop and mature (Bowlby, 1953). However, we have to be realistic and acknowledge that hospitalisation, excessive vomiting, pain, altered body image, etc. are hardly normal experiences and we are not advocating that anyone should treat them as such, or that having cancer and treatment is necessarily a positive experience. The impact of this on the child cannot always be minimised, but much better that the child is allowed to express any dislikes and distress felt about what is happening to him. What we are suggesting is that if the child and family are able to accept the reality of these experiences, even though they are unpleasant, they will find a new normality, that creates a more mentally healthy atmosphere. One of our parents gave us an insight into their experience of learning to adjust:

Our first Christmas during treatment was particularly difficult. In the way that this sort of disease and treatment progresses, our lives were lived on a knife-edge of admissions and discharges. On this occasion, we were discharged at the last moment and few of the usual comfortable Christmas arrangements had been made. Each of us was struggling to find our new place in the restored family unit. Tempers flared, and harsh words were exchanged – followed by all of us shedding tears. One of the younger children wailed 'I hate this cancer, when will our lives be normal again?' In the midst of comforting and reassuring, I realized there would have to be a 'new normal'.

When the unpleasant aspects of the diagnosis and treatment are ignored or denied the mental health of the child and family are affected. On many occasions we have seen families who embark upon the treatment of their child's disease with the view that this is a phase in their lives that has to interrupt everything else. These families put many of their usual activities and routines on hold, treating the cancer experience as 'time out'. They unfortunately assume that as soon as the treatment is finished they will be able to pick up where they left off and everything will return to normal. Sadly, this return to a previous normal is far from the actual outcome, due to changes both within themselves and in the community around them that they have detached themselves from.

The alternative to this 'time out' approach are those families who manage to integrate all the new routines, the new experiences, the new circle of friends, the new reality, into their existing lifestyle. For example, the following quote from a parent gives us an example of how important, but also how difficult maintaining friendships can be for them:

I did work at keeping relationships going during the treatment – I now realize how hard that must have been on other people sometimes, but generally they were wonderfully supportive of me and the rest of the family. Inevitably, whilst we were immersed in the battle with the disease it was all too easy to let go of long-standing relationships. However, almost without exception, friends were most supportive and only too glad to begin to rebuild our relationships, by being pro-active with letters and cards along the way, especially in the early days.

These families are adapting to their changing environment and, following the theory of Charles Darwin (1859), adaptation is the key to survival and evolution. Of course the balance of things changes between the old lifestyle and the new during the periods of intensive treatment, but as long as the old links still exist there is the opportunity to return to the old lifestyle, enriched, or maybe just wiser, but at least with a mental state that has not lost touch with reality and with a social network that is still intact. For those of you who are new to oncology, you may still be trying to understand how some families do appear to cope amazingly well with this shattering experience, who still laugh and enjoy life, alongside having a very sick child. Lozowski (1993) refers to the 'juxtaposition of feeling positive as a result of a life tragedy'. She quotes a comment from a long-term survivor who said:

> Survivors as well as current childhood cancer patients have created a phenomenon which remains inexplicable to those who may not understand the strange compatibility between cancer and optimism.

Psychosocial assessment in cancer survivors

Before we begin to explore the real issues of survivorship and rehabilitation in our next three sections of the chapter, we will broadly discuss some of the literature available in this field. It is important to look at who has studied the survivors we are discussing, why is adjustment and normalisation considered to be of such importance, and what are the difficulties in assessing psychosocial effects in children for researchers?

The pioneers of late psychosocial effects of cancer treatment around the early 1980s have paved the way in our understanding of survivorship and rehabilitation. Koocher and O'Malley (1981) are widely regarded as the first to embark on studying this previously uncharted territory. Prior to this, the focus of the 1960s and 1970s was in improving the outlook for paediatric cancer patients. In the 1960s, for example, the success rate for childhood acute lymphoblastic leukaemia (ALL) was in the region of 30% survival at 3 years (Sposto & Hammond, 1985). The establishment of the United Kingdom Children's Cancer Study Group (UKCCSG) in 1977 improved the organisation of childhood cancer studies. Treatment trials and protocols were established and many new chemotherapeutic agents were introduced, together with the advent of multimodal therapy (that is, chemotherapy, radiation and surgery). Thus, the outlook for childhood cancer sufferers improved dramatically, and survival rates began to increase. However, the approach, at that time is perhaps highlighted in the following quote, 'If someone lived long enough to develop long-term complications, we would jump for joy and treat the complications' (Karon, 1973). Many of the late effects of treatment seen today are being monitored in survivors who received far less intensive regimens than children today. So what then does the future hold for children treated in the 1980s and 1990s with multiagent intensive regimens?

With respect to the late effects of treatment, much of the literature in the 1980s was dominated by our psychologically aware colleagues across the Atlantic. American literature dominates the reviews, and in part this is due to the size of the country and number of specialist paediatric oncology centres, but there also appears to be a slight reflection that in the UK we as nurses are only just beginning to wake up to the reality of the psychosocial consequences of treatment ourselves. Studies and literature are becoming more available in the UK in the 1990s, and it is certain that this is a development that will continue to grow. Despite the predominance of American literature, the information produced has relevance for the UK given that we are on a par politically, socially and financially, and that our cultures are similar, both having a predominantly white western culture, with large populations of ethnic cultures from around the world. Our health service provision has different origins but our paediatric oncology services are developing in parallel, with many links between both countries from sharing study results and experiences, to friendships that have arisen from work exchanges and meeting regularly at conferences.

There are difficulties in assessing psychosocial issues in children, some are obviously related to age and development, but others are less apparent at first glance. Studies appear to fall into two main categories: those that study the child's state of health, for example, actual measurement of cognitive deficit and IQ, and those that look at quality of life issues, such as emotional stability, self esteem and job opportunities. Immediately the difficulties become clearer. How do you accurately assess self esteem in a child who has a cognitive deficit as a result of treatment the child has received? What are the attributes that make up quality of life? Are these quality attributes the same for everyone, of every age? Do we look at the quality of life that the child desires, or their parents, and are they always compatible? Do we assess the child's psychological state before we start treatment? If not, how can we be sure of the actual effects of the treatment? Similarly, do we know the psychosocial issues within the family that will have an effect on the child in addition to the treatment's effects? Although this at present is a list of questions with no attempt at the answers, some of the answers will develop within the chapter, whereas others will remain questions. It is, however, important that you bear such points in mind as you consider our own thoughts and experiences, and our presentation of available literature. A further issue raised by Barr, Furlong and Dawson (1993) is that when assessing children psychologically there also needs to be a consideration of the distinction between capacity and performance, i.e. what the child can actually do, and what they choose to do. The route of the effect also needs to be established, in that a child may not reach their anticipated educational potential, not because of the effects of cranial irradiation, not because of a brain tumour or surgery, not because they were particularly lazy or disinterested, but because the child did not have access to schooling during treatment and was unable to reintegrate fully into school when treatment was completed.

When the child is unable to express for themselves their thoughts and feelings, either due to age, developmental level or cognitive impairment, an alternative is to use teacher, parent, nurse and doctor appraisal in psychosocial studies. The danger with appraisal from an observer is that the information is potentially very subjective. Unless the appraiser is particularly skilled there may be error in what is observed and how the behaviour is interpreted. One study by Moore, Glasser and Ablin (1987) found a difference in the perception of social and emotional problems reported by teachers and parents, parents believing their children to have less problems than reported by their child's teacher. Eiser and Jenney (1996) also found that parents were not always the most reliable source of information, but that 'most agreement was between nurse ratings and behavioural observations'. Parents own anxiety is thought to be one cause for disparity in their reports, but it is still worth using parental reports for certain information.

Issues affecting the successful normalisation process of the cancer experience

It would be all too easy to make grand and bold statements about how children and families should behave to ensure that their progress through the cancer experience is smooth and uncomplicated, that will guarantee both they and their children come through the experience holistically cured. But of course life is not like that. We can approach anything in our lives with the best of intentions and the most positive of attitude, only to discover that something totally unexpected is about to knock us sideways, and all our best intentions dissolve as we have to put all our energy into dealing with the new crisis, completely neglecting the recommended route we were originally planning to take. Overriding every issue that we will discuss in the next section is the acknowledgment that every child and every family are different, all bringing with them their unique life experiences affecting how they will respond to the new experiences they are likely to encounter. The following discussions all relate to factors which have been found to inhibit the normalisation process, thus preventing the child to be truly cured, as defined in our first section.

Medical intervention and duration of treatment

One of the biggest factors that will affect a child and family psychologically is the effect of the medical intervention on the child. The duration of treatment for different diseases varies and there is much evidence to support the fact that the duration of therapy, the number of side effects and the treatment of high-risk category patients affects the psychosocial outcome for a child (Moore *et al.*, 1987; Barr *et al.*, 1993). Taking the treatment for acute lymphoblastic leukaemia (ALL) as an example, two similar boys, with similar prognostic factors at the start of treatment, are illustrated in Case study 11.1.

Many of our survivors have vastly different experiences of their treatment which has affected their psychological health. Much of the research supports the fact that the intensity and duration of a child's treatment has a direct effect on the prevalence of psychosocial late effects (Barr *et al.*, 1993; Eiser & Jenney, 1996).

Case study 11.1

One child with ALL received the induction block, the intensification blocks and moved onto maintenance treatment with very little in the way of side effects, having had few admissions for pyrexia and neutropenia, and returning home after the usual forecasted number of days following each in patient block of treatment. The other boy, Richard, stumbled at the first hurdle and had a particularly tough time at induction, suffering with effects of tumour lysis syndrome which required several days of intensive care support. Having barely recovered from this episode he went on to develop steroid-induced diabetes. Each admission for treatment was prolonged by infection and he was frequently unable to be discharged home before becoming neutropenic and developing a further infection. The family often only had a couple of days at home during the early stages of his treatment. As Richard moved on to the high-dose methotrexate blocks, he suddenly had a convulsion linked to the intrathecal therapy. Eventually things settled down for Richard and he thankfully experienced an unproblematical maintenance phase of the treatment. For these two families the experiences were very different. Richard's family became so used to him developing every known side effect, at each step of the way, that when he came off treatment they had heightened anxiety that he would relapse or develop late effects. Every future viral infection was viewed with suspicion by the family and they required numerous visits to clinic for reassurance.

It is often the physical short-term effects of the treatment that have longstanding psychological effects, for example excessive vomiting, alopecia and weight changes. In some instances it is possible for a child to be deeply traumatised by medical intervention, particularly in the case of venepuncture. We have sadly seen a change in character of many children who have indeed suffered throughout their treatment. Where a child may once have been lively and sociable, they become markedly quieter, reduce eye contact, hold their heads down and look as if they have chosen to lock themselves in to protect themselves from any further harm. We cannot continue to cure childhood cancer and leave children as scarred as this. Although, as you will see in our last section and in earlier chapters, there is much we can do to prevent such terrible trauma, yet, there are also new developments in treatment, such as bone marrow transplantation, that present greater challenges to our ability to protect children from severe psychological trauma as they become long-term survivors.

A further factor in intensity of treatment is relapse. As treatment develops and cure rates improve, there are consequently a greater number of children who are at risk of relapse. For those children whose disease does return, they then have to embark upon another usually more intense protocol. We have become so used to curing children in the 1990s that if anyone, be it nurse, parent, or doctor, suggests that perhaps we should not retreat this relapse, there is an outcry that we are somehow letting the child down. Some extraordinary ethical issues have arisen in recent years, both locally within our own unit and more widely afield in the national press, for example 'Child B' (Garbett, 1996); van Eys (1991) picks up this point by saying:

> The boundary between success and failure of medical intervention is frequently equated with the choice between life and death. The mind-set of the caregivers becomes life at all cost. Almost any medical intervention can be considered if it offers even a slight possibility of life.

As we have said before, we are already seeing late psychosocial sequelae among survivors treated 10–20 years ago who were treated on far less intense regimens than those being used and contemplated now, so what does the future hold for the current generation of survivors? Even if we could predict the extent of such late effects, would we suspend treatment in certain cases if the morbidity was seen to be too great? Do we need to readjust our perspective of cure, so that it includes psychological and social cure, when we are faced with progressive disease decisions? Case Study 11.2 illustrates the dilemmas involved when deciding on the extent of treatment to be used.

Case study 11.2

Several years ago, Mark underwent audiometry testing to detect hearing loss as a consequence of his cisplatin treatment. Although his mother was aware of the late effects of this drug and knew why the test was carried out, an issue arose when the decision was made to reduce the dose of cisplatin in the following course. However, Mark's mother became distressed by this decision, knowing the poor prognosis of his disease, she felt that his treatment was being compromised. Her natural instinct as a mother was to save him at all costs and stated she would prefer a 'deaf child to a dead child!'

Age at diagnosis

Almost hand in hand with intensity and duration of treatment, it is well documented that the age of the child at diagnosis and during treatment also affects the long-term outcome of psycho-social issues. Children are affected in different ways according to their age. Very young children find hospitalisation and interrupted caretaking difficult to cope with because they are unable to understand the reasons (Eiser and Jenney, 1996). They will pick up anxiety in their carers and be aware for a while that circumstances have changed. They are particularly susceptible to trauma from painful procedures because they cannot rationalise that the pain is short lived, nor understand why it is happening. However, they generally have fewer late psychosocial effects because they have the benefit of being more able to forget the experience. They can reintegrate into school much more easily, with longer opportunity to catch up with any non-physical developmental delays, are not burdened by the fear of death or the awareness of altered body image in our society, and to a certain extent because they are not old enough to realise any different, they are much more able to normalise the experience, and adjust to the change in routine. There is well-documented evidence, however, that the younger the child is when they receive cranial irradiation the more likely they are to have resulting cognitive deficits (Mostow, Byrne and Connelly, 1991; Barr *et al.*, 1993).

The older child has far greater difficulty adjusting to the treatment because they recognise the abnormality of the situation. Moore *et al.* (1987) suggest that difficulties experienced by older children are reflective of the fact that 'the mastery of developmental tasks of school aged children and adolescents is more likely to be disrupted by cancer and it's therapy'. Earlier chapters will have discussed the effects of treatment in detail, but we need to remember that older children who have adjustment difficulties at the time of treatment are far more likely to carry those difficulties with them into survivorship.

Fostering dependence

The issue of dependence and overprotection is one which affects many aspects of the survivor's life. Parental overprotection will be discussed in more detail when re-integration to school, employment opportunities, marriage and long-term follow-up, are considered. It should be stated here that overprotection and limiting a child's normal development because of the disease will lead to the child becoming dependent on others and not achieving their optimum potential in independence:

> Overindulgent and overprotective parents foster regression and undermine the child's effort at mastery and autonomy (Chang, 1991).

In the same way that parents can overprotect their child and foster dependence, it is possible for the hospital environment and all its members to do the same. Jan van Eys discusses the dangers involved for families when health care workers encourage dependence from families to satisfy their own needs, because the gratification they receive by families is so rewarding.

> Such individuals can be very destructive to the child and family, by making the child and family dependent in ways that preclude normal progress towards adjustment and independence. Those health care workers, be they physicians, nurses, social workers, or psychologists are often seen as the most dedicated, devoted, untiring, and involved members of the team. It is hard to challenge that behaviour. (van Eys, 1991)

Indeed within our own department we began to detect a changing pattern in nurses' involvement with families after discharge from hospital. There has been an increase in the amount of home visits and telephone contact to families made by ward nurses over the last 5 years, particularly in their off-duty hours. When questioned, these nurses felt that there was no harm in continuing a 'friendly' relationship with families once treatment was complete. Thus, there appeared to be emerging an era of overinvolvement by some nurses, which as the evidence suggests plays a part in fostering a dependence on hospital staff. What happens when the nurse stops visiting or telephoning, does the family feel the nurse does not care any more? Furthermore, does the nurse discuss treatment issues during this 'out of hours contact' and where are the responsibilities of that individual. Do the families see the nurse as a professional or a friend? There are many moral and ethical issues raised by this point (Fitzmaurice, 1996).

Failures in the multidisciplinary team – the biological approach

Through working in a large paediatric oncology centre, we have good experiences of working with a functional multidisciplinary team. The weekly psychosocial ward round is attended by medical and nursing staff, social workers, dietitians, Macmillan nurses, ward pharmacist, psychologist and school teacher. Some of the literature suggests that this has not always been the case in paediatric oncology care. Historically the approach to care was very medically orientated, leading to many psychosocial issues for the child being overlooked. Some of the adults we are now reviewing have been victims of this approach and were not, for example, offered skilled psychological support. There has been greater recognition in recent years that the medical team are not the experts in every aspect of care:

> It is important to give coequal voice to all sets in the care of the child – medical, nursing and mental health – to avoid the danger of amateur solutions and decisions based merely on feelings. (van Eys, 1991).

School attendance and isolation

In conjunction with the disruption to family life, for children with cancer, treatment can also bring major disruption to their social and educational life. Much of a child's social life will revolve around school. Activities in school, friendships and extracurricular activities are all important to the social and educational development of the child. Weeks/months of hospitalisation and immuno-suppression, where the child is unable to attend school, can produce a socially isolated child.

Adolescents in particular can feel socially isolated. Lack of self esteem and altered body image will often play a major part in adolescents' reluctance to attend school or face their peer group in any setting. Difficulty with peer relationships and achieving a positive self concept may continue to be problematical throughout the disease trajectory and may manifest itself as a truly late psychosocial effect (Moore et al., 1987).

However, difficulty with body image may not always be a problem. It is both heartening and encouraging to meet an adolescent with a more positive approach, and an example is given in Case study 11.3.

For most of the children and indeed the parents, school attendance has to be actively encouraged. Home tuition is offered to most of the children for the first 3–5 months when treatment is at its most intensive and almost continuous hospital attendance both as an inpatient and outpatient is at its height. However, as soon

> **Case study 11.3**
>
> Liz a 16-year-old, at the time when her rhabdomyosarcoma was diagnosed, had a mop of short dark hair. You can imagine our surprise when having taken up the offer of a free wig service, she turned up for her clinic appointments sporting a full head of waist-length blond ringlets! Not only that, but despite her bleak moments of nausea and vomiting, however ill she felt when attending for treatment, she never failed to wear make-up and her 'special wig'. She said it made her 'feel great' regardless of what else was happening to her. Sadly this attitude appears to be in the minority.

as possible with medical consent, children will be actively encouraged to return to school. This in itself proves a challenge for nurses and the hospital teaching staff, in providing a suitable reintegration programme for the children. Firstly, parents themselves have to be encouraged that this is the right step for their child. It was certainly not uncommon in our experience to remember the time when children would often have home tuition for the duration of their treatment, because the parents were too afraid to let the children attend school. They worry particularly about their children's susceptibility to infections and the risks of 'teasing' because of their physical appearance. One mother who did try and take her 3 year old into nursery school, was met in the playground by other parents actively pulling their own children away as if they would 'catch the cancer'. Fortunately, as society becomes more aware and confident in both understanding and discussing issues around cancer, this kind of attitude will be stamped out.

Parents' natural protectiveness to their sick child has long-term consequences which can lead to increased dependence on parents, social immaturity, poor self image, decreased confidence and fear of failure (Moore *et al.*, 1987). If survivors of cancer are to be encouraged to reach their full potential, educational issues are paramount in their progress through the cancer experience.

There is much in the literature relating to areas of medical research looking into the late effects of treatment on the cognitive ability of the child treated for cancer, with particular reference to the effects of cranial irradiation and intrathecal methotrexate (Brouwers and Poplack, 1990; Hoppe-Hirsch, Renier and Lelloch-Tubiana, 1990; Brown, Madan-Swain and Lambert 1992). In research it is recognised that children can be impaired intellectually as a consequence of their treatment. Deasy-Spinetta (1993) states in her article 'School issues and the child with cancer' that:

The challenge of the 1990's and beyond is to refine the

advances of the 1980's and make school intervention efforts an integral part of psychosocial care in all pediatric haematology/oncology centres.

Mental health and coping before diagnosis

Unfortunately, many will begin their child's treatment already burdened with psychosocial problems. Several years ago a young boy of 14 years of age was diagnosed with acute lymphoblastic leukemia within 6 months of his 19-year-old brother having been tragically killed in a motor bike accident. Clearly, for the family their coping abilities were compromised at that vulnerable time in their life. We can think of several other families who had deaths of close relatives, just prior to, during or just after treatment. Other families have had a parent who themselves had a chronic illness or even cancer, and we have a few families for whom we are treating more than one of their children. For some of our other families ongoing marital problems, recent divorce and separation put additional stress on the family:

> Concurrent stresses put families at risk for poor coping ... When other stresses make demands on time, energy, and family resources, the child's care and treatment may be ignored or inadequately addressed by the family. (Kupst, 1993)

Having focused on parents who are already burdened with psychosocial problems at diagnosis, there are also children who have had particularly stressful lives, in particular a child who had spent most of his young life in frequently changing foster care, and another who had suffered abuse. Such children need particularly sensitive care, and communication with all disciplines previously involved with them should be maintained. Kupst suggests that 'the adequacy of coping tends to run in families, that is parents' and children's coping are strongly related'.

As nurses we should be aware that families' additional needs will influence how we care for them. It will be so much more difficult for families with additional stresses to adjust to this enormous burden of a child with cancer and normalise the experience.

Myths about the cancer experience

Throughout our nursing career we are sometimes privileged to attend a lecture which really opens up a new concept for us, often identifying for us things that we have vaguely been aware of but not spent much time considering. After hearing such a lecture our perspective remains permanently changed. Professor John Spinetta, a psychologist from San Diego University, USA, speaking about the myths of surviving childhood cancer at a late effects conference in Manchester in 1993 provided such an experience. Some of these myths are interspersed into the text to highlight salient points, but others are included here. These myths provide another dimension of factors that influence the normalisation process of the cancer experience.

Survivors of childhood cancer are true heroes

People may often comment to cancer survivors that having survived cancer nothing else in life could be as bad. The survivor is expected to cope with everything that comes their way and may find it impossible to live up to the expectations of others. Being a hero becomes a burden and family and friends treat the survivor as someone special who they should all live up to.

Children with cancer grow with the experience

Some children will gain positive things from the experience, but as already mentioned some will not. Spinetta points out that the survivor may still be unhappy with life. Coming through cancer does not mean that life will never again churn out any nasty experiences.

We must protect our children from pain and harm

Spinetta rejects this myth, in as much as we cannot protect children from every pain and harm. He advocates that we should 'hold their hand, walk them through it and teach them how to deal with it'. Otherwise, he believes we end up with adults who have difficulty coping.

Psychosocial effects

The following section begins to explore how the cancer experience actually affects survivors. For some this will be positive, for some it will be negative, and for most there will be combination of feelings and reactions which may change in intensity at different periods in their life.

Incidence of late psychosocial effects

There appears to be a degree of consistency among various studies that although psychosocial late effects can range from mild to severe, the incidence of true psychopathology is rare. Those studies which consider quality of life attributes as a measure of psychosocial adjustment, broadly, find that it is very rare for an individual to be negatively affected across the whole spectrum of quality of life issues (Barr *et al.*, 1993).

Before moving on to discussing how survivors may have the

quality of their lives affected, first it is necessary to establish what is meant by quality of life. Although individuals may have a unique definition of what constitutes quality of life for them, there are recognised themes that are generally held to influence this quality. These are:

- peer relationships
- school and work opportunity
- impaired sensation, mobility and communication
- ability to perform self care
- independent living
- self esteem
- cognition
- freedom from pain
- fertility
- marriage status
- emotional state.

(Chang, 1991; Barr *et al.*, 1993; Eiser and Jenney, 1996)

Eiser and Jenney (1996) in their article 'Measuring symptomatic benefit and quality of life in paediatric oncology' quote Mulhern, who says that in quality of life issues, 'It is important to make at least three broad distinctions between physical function, psychological function and self-satisfaction'. Nurses working in the field of paediatric oncology need to be aware of these quality of life attributes throughout their contact with the child and family.

Chang (1991) states that 'it is conceivable that survivors may not be at a greater risk for serious psycho-pathology than the general population. They may, however, be more vulnerable to intermittent and minor adjustment difficulties.' The incidence of psychiatric disturbance in the general population is 15% and Zeltzer (1993) reports that the incidence is no higher in long-term survivors. Zeltzer's article reviews the literature on psychosocial aspects of cancer in adolescents and young adults and cites a study which reported the incidence of suicide attempts, running away and psychiatric hospitalisation was no different between survivors and sibling controls. They did report a higher incidence of periods of mild depression among survivors which was worse among males. There are two further mental health issues that can affect cancer survivors; excessive denial and obsession. Both of these mental states highlight that the normalisation process has gone astray for these children/families. van Eys (1991) reports that excessive denial is unsustainable and that during a future period of intense stress the child or family will have to suddenly face the reality of either the present situation or that which has gone before. Similarly when survivors are intensely obsessed by the cancer it directly affects their perspective of reality and they are unable to move on to return to normality, being stuck in the drama of the cancer experience.

The Damocles syndrome

Much of the literature relating to psychosocial late effects refers to the work of Koocher and O'Malley (1981) on the 'Damocles syndrome'. Damocles was a member of the court of the monarch Dionysius. Dionysius made Damocles sit and eat a feast of 'unparalleled splendour'. As Damocles looked up he saw a sword hanging above his head held only by a hair. This was all part of the monarch's tyranny, but it illustrated to Damocles how precarious life was. Koocher and O'Malley, and indeed many writers since, have used this phrase to describe how survivors feel, particularly when they come off treatment. 'The fear of recurrence is very real to cancer survivors' (Mullan, 1984). Cancer survivors describe their feelings as 'living in limbo' (Chang, 1991) and in a study by Moore *et al.* (1987) one boy said of his parents, 'Whenever I get sick, I know they are always thinking, is it happening again?' One of our mothers explains how these fears creep into her daily life some 15 years after her son's diagnosis:

> I would be lying if I said we have no concerns for the future. Fortunately, my son now enjoys excellent health, but a small part of me dreads what it might be if he is ever unwell. As puberty approaches there are new and different issues that will need to be worked through. Just occasionally, my heart skips a beat when they pop into my mind, but I know we will find our way through those issues together if the need arises.

At a conference on the 'Late Effects of Cancer Treatment in 1993, Dr A Meadows stated that 5–15% of survivors will develop a new neoplasm within 10–20 years of initial diagnosis; a 10% greater risk of developing a malignancy than the general population. (Meadows, 1989). If cancer survivors take health risks as well, the risk is even greater due to the synergistic effect of the risk behaviour and the potential existing compromise of some of their organs from chemotherapy or radiotherapy (Fraumeni, 1975; D'Angio, 1982).

Academic achievement, career, employment and income

Children who survive their cancer will at some point themselves begin to think about their own future prospects with regards to a career and/or employment. If reintegration into school has not been successful, or indeed if the child has significant cognitive difficulties directly due to their treatment, then academic achievement is likely to be poor. Hays (1993) points out in his research conducted with a group of American survivors that:

> Although the percentage of survivors graduating from high school usually has been approximately the same as that of control subjects, the proportion of these survivors who are college graduates has been significantly less.

Hays' research also demonstrates that during the treatment phase possibly 1 or 2 years may be lost in the child's education. Difficulty with schooling may then lead onto difficulty in attaining vocational skills and employment. Long-term survivors with physical disabilities may need rehabilitation and retraining. Children with special needs caused by severe cognitive and physical disabilities will need on-going assessment and the support of all community services in caring for their long-term needs, particularly when their own parents/carers need the facilities of respite care.

Employment can also been difficult for the adult survivor, as employers may demonstrate significant discrimination against them. Koocher and O'Malley (1981) draw the conclusion that this is because the employer has a fear of repeated absenteeism. Such ignorance may still be apparent today in the 1990s. Entry into the uniformed services is also a problem for the survivor. Hays (1993) in his research shows the experience of several centres in the USA that a significant 10–20% of long-term survivors have been denied entry into the armed forces. Together with issues of unemployment the survivor may also be faced with the prospects of having difficulty in obtaining life insurance, and consequently a mortgage.

Home life and marriage

Earlier we discussed issues around fostering a dependence on parents and home life for the child with cancer. The protectiveness of the parents is sometimes overwhelming for the child. This will often continue far beyond the cessation of treatment and into the long-term follow-up period and survivorship. Peer relationships can be drastically interrupted by the demands of the disease and treatment process, and will be even more severe when this occurs in conjunction with overprotection by parents. Lansky, List and Ritter-Sterr (1985) state that many of these young adults describe their mother as their 'best friend' and will often live at home much longer than their peer group. Parents have great difficulty in 'letting go'. One young survivor of Hodgkin's disease who was 18 years old had managed to 'fly the nest' and was living with her boyfriend. She attended her outpatient appointment with him for the first time. Within a short time of arriving in clinic her mother telephoned, absolutely distraught that she could choose to bring her boyfriend to clinic and not her! This mother had great difficulty in coming to terms with not directly receiving the medical information about her daughter and being directly involved as she had been used to. Young children may not recognise this dependence themselves until they reach their adolescent years, when an attempt is then made to obtain their independence as this young girl had done.

Physical disability and disfigurement occurring in survivors may also contribute to the dependence on parents and the survivor's inability to establish meaningful relationships. Research carried out by Koocher and O'Malley (1981) reported less than 50% of the 60 survivors married at the time of the interview. However this may have been accounted for by the relatively young age of the survivor group in comparison to the national population. Other studies have also reported that cancer survivors are less likely to marry, especially men treated for brain tumours (Byrne, Lewis and Halamek, 1989). The authors propose the reasons for a difference in marriage rates for men related to social expectations for men to be the primary wage earners, and that job opportunities and earning potential were affected more in men with cognitive impairments, particularly in terms of their own self esteem.

Anxieties regarding infertility may contribute to the survivors' apprehension in developing long-term relationships. Again Zeltzer identifies a difference between males and females in their eagerness to discover their fertility status, males wanting to know less. Females were also found to be more concerned about the health of their offspring than males. How many of our survivors have been fully informed of their potential infertility? It is our experience that many young adults attending the follow-up clinic may not be aware of this distressing late effect of treatment, particularly for children treated several years ago when the emphasis on information giving was left entirely to the parents of that child. This situation arose several years ago in our long-term-follow up clinic when a young man of 19 having had treatment for Hodgkin's disease proudly brought his fiancee with him. It quickly became apparent that this young man had no idea that there was a possibility that he could be infertile. His parents had not discussed this issue with him at all, even though they had been informed of the potential late effects of his treatment. This situation suddenly posed a dilemma and a stressful situation for all concerned.

Family and siblings

The long-term impact of having a child with cancer can break up families and induce significant behaviour problems in siblings (Morris-Jones and Craft, 1990). This is a fairly strong statement and shows just how much damage can spread from the illness of one family member to impact on those closest to them. Earlier chapters will have discussed the impact of treatment on family and siblings, but the manifestation of this impact on the future of the family should be briefly mentioned. Because this chapter has placed so much emphasis on normalisation, the following quote relating to families during treatment is worth adding:

> Siblings of a sick child have been shown to fare better emotionally if they remain part of the household and experience the family's reality. (Cincotta, 1993)

Fertility and offspring

As previously highlighted, most children and adolescents with cancer now survive, therefore issues regarding the late effects of therapy on fertility and the health of offspring are increasingly important. Direct irradiation to the gonads in either sex usually causes infertility. Alkylating agents, for example, cyclophosphamide, widely used today in many of the treatment protocols, are also known to potentially cause infertility. In a study carried out in 1991 by Levy and Stillman, their research showed that the effects of chemotherapy differs in boys and girls, and that the use of ankylating agents resulted in a 50% reduction in fertility among the male survivors but had only a minimal effect on female survivors. It would seem, therefore, that the ovary is better able to withstand the effects of chemotherapy than the testes. Many girls who survive will therefore be able to conceive. Many babies have now been born to mothers and indeed fathers who had cancer as children, and fortunately there seems to be no increased risk of congenital abnormalities or of cancer in the offspring (Morris-Jones and Craft, 1990).

In our experience, successful sperm banking from adolescent males occurs rarely. Firstly, the boy has to be capable, both emotionally and developmentally, of producing a specimen. Secondly, to expect a young male to be able to produce a specimen at such a stressful time before starting treatment, adds to the poor success rate of this service. Occasionally, the question of egg collection (which involves 'ovarian slicing') from pubescent females arises, but we have no experience of this. Our medical colleagues inform us that there are ethical issues surrounding replacing the ovarian slice after treatment, i.e. potentially giving rise to reintroducing the original disease.

It is worth considering at this point the responsibilities of all who are involved in the long-term care of cancer survivors with regard to their potential offspring. As the numbers of survivors increase and the follow-up programme extends, it would seem important and essential to study these offspring and to collect information, so that clinical counselling and advice can be given to survivors and their partners with regard to the possible risks of untoward outcomes of pregnancy.

It is natural to conclude that survivors of cancer may fear that their offspring may develop cancer, or at least, that they may have an 'unhealthy child' (Nicholson and Byrne, 1993). Survivors may fear for their own health should a pregnancy occur. This is not without just cause, particularly for survivors who had anthracycline therapy, as pregnancy is known to cause some degree of cardiorespiratory stress.

In research carried out by Nicholson and Byrne (1993), in the analysis of their statistics, they conclude that 'The lack of excess cancer risk in the offspring is a valid result'. However, they also state that the average age of the offspring was only 11 years, so they could not 'adequately address cancer in the offspring during adolescence or early adulthood'.

It would seem essential then that opportunities be given for survivors to discuss their anxieties and concerns regarding fertility and offspring, and that as health professionals we should be offering advice and counselling. At present, qualified counselling is offered to all survivors who are known to have inherited tumours, retinoblastoma being the most common.

Positive effects: Evidence of successful normalisation and rehabilitation

Despite our many references to problems faced by cancer survivors, there is also much evidence to suggest that some survivors adjust very well following the experience. In Zeltzer's literature review (1993), there is a report that 'most survivors were satisfied with their employment'. He goes on in his conclusion to say that 'given the opportunity, a majority of survivors had positive things to say about their childhood cancer experience, indicating that they had learned new things about themselves and how to enjoy and appreciate life to a fuller extent'.

Positive effects of the cancer experience will, of course, affect other family members. As we have shown many times before it is a *family experience*. Despite the difficulties siblings and parents face, the following quotes show that whole families can find aspects of the cancer experience positive:

> I do feel I can say that we have essentially left the experience behind us. We were all undoubtedly changed by it, but not all for the worse. In fact much of what has resulted has enriched our lives. (Both of our daughters now work in London hospitals in the area of Oncology)

I feel I should add that the other children have commented on how I have 'mellowed' so they have benefited too! It has been hard to let go of my natural cautiousness but I know we have all benefited from my change in perspective. My attitude of late has been much more one of encouraging us all to 'have a go' rather than doubting, and trying to discourage the more adventurous ideas!

How do we work towards supporting survivors to successful rehabilitation adjusted to the consequences of their treatment?

The often heroic efforts mustered by patients, their families, and the health-care team to treat the cancer successfully should not have to result in a cured disease but a psychosocially devastated survivor. (Zeltzer, 1993)

The final section of this chapter aims to make suggestions about the nursing care of children with cancer and their families with the aim to prevent having 'psychosocially devastated survivors'. By this stage we have discussed many of the influences in achieving this aim, which have included issues outside nursing, but in view of the fact that we work so closely in co-operation with other disciplines it has been necessary to do this. Our final section also includes suggestions which are beyond the boundaries of purely nursing, particularly some of the ethical debates about information giving, but given our influence within the multidisciplinary team it is important that nurses can negotiate and debate knowledgeably.

Box 11.1   Myth – Long term survivors will be able to put the experience behind them eventually

'Survivors should aim for a new life *without* forgetting. They must continue living and moving forward, but they should expect the experience to resurface from time to time.' (Spinetta, 1993)

Information giving to promote mental health

Monitoring long-term survivors in clinic not only involves physical health but also the mental health of the survivor. In order for effective communication to take place survivors need to be well informed of their disease. Everhart (1991) in her experience with the long-term follow-up programme in the Children's Medical Center, Dallas found that with a group of her survivors:

'their comments often indicate that their concepts of the

disease and its treatment are lodged at the cognitive development level they had reached at the time they were originally diagnosed and treated, even though they have progressed in their cognitive maturity in other respects.

It would seem important for the nurse caring for the survivors in the long-term follow-up clinic that, before embarking on quality of life issues and health-risk behaviours, discussions take place to illicit the degree of understanding survivors have about their original disease. Everhart (1991) suggests that even without concrete research evidence, there are obvious strong clinical reasons why the individual's level of understanding may be 'stuck' at the cognitive level they had achieved at the time of diagnosis and treatment. She suggests that 'The stresses of childhood cancer, as well as the gap between what children may be told and what they understand at typical stages in their cognitive development' are two such reasons. After the impact of the diagnosis and adjustment, children also may never need to re-examine or revisit these issues again, thus failing to have an ongoing dialogue about their cancer in line with their cognitive development. Short, comprehensive questionnaires asking basic questions may well be appropriately handed out in the long-term follow-up clinic, to serve as a baseline for information giving. For example:

- What type of cancer did you have?
- Where was your cancer located?

In the UK work has recently been carried out by the United Kingdom Children's Cancer Study Group (UKCCSG) Late Effects Group in designing and producing a booklet entitled *After Cure: Surviving Cancer: what does that mean for you?* (Blacklay, 1997) in order to improve the information given to long-term survivors. The aim of information giving at this stage is to promote a level of understanding that enables the survivor to have a clear healthy mind about all aspects of their disease, in the early stages and to understand the aims of long-term follow-up (Box 11.2).

Information giving, ethics and nurses' attitudes in relation to late effects

'The management of a child with cancer is always a balancing act, weighing the need for cure against the risk of late effects' (Ruccione, 1985 pp. 205–221). Many of our children pay a price; most would consider it worth paying, but as nurses we have a significant role to play in supporting our survivors and their families to adjust to the consequences of their treatment. We need to work closely with our medical partners, sharing the responsibility for managing this ever unfolding and developing aspect of

---

Box 11.2   Myth – Open communication is best regarding the cancer experience, including amongs friends and family; i.e. talking about it helps

This may not be necessarily true. Sometimes in life open verbal communication can be threatening. Spinetta states that people have a right to privacy including children. He believes that within families, non-verbal communication has always been successful and we do not need to insist that everything is put into words, so that everyone in the family is exposed by discussing their feelings about the cancer experience. Open discussion does not necessarily assist psychological health and adjustment. Spinetta advocates that we as professionals should make open communication available, but let families choose whether or not they need to use verbal communication for themselves. (Spinetta, 1993)

---

treatment. Although it is usually the child's consultant or registrar who first knows the diagnosis and treatment plan and begins discussions about treatment with parents, nurses do have a role in information giving.

Following an interview with medical staff the parents will usually seek out the nursing staff to clarify certain points, or to ask things they forgot to ask the doctor, or to ask for a further interview with the doctor. As a general rule our medical staff always ask a nurse to be present at interviews, so that we are able to fulfil this supportive role and are clear about what the doctor has said.

The role of advocate is very dominant within paediatrics and can easily lead the nursing staff to be in conflict with one party or another. They are, after all, trying to act in the best interests of the child and the family, while weighing up their physical versus their psychological best interests, and their short-versus their long-term best interests. Putting aside the difficulties involved with advocacy, experienced paediatric oncology nurses are in the best position to ensure that our children and families are well informed, 'to interpret the needs of their clients to others, and act as a go-between when other health care professionals appear, to the patient, to be unapproachable'. (Burnard and Chapman, 1992). We should have the knowledge and expertise to be able to communicate information to children and their families, whatever their age and cognitive level, and to check their understanding, to be able to explain the alternatives and ensure that they under-stand the implications of each particular course. Advocacy should be at the invitation of the child and family and it should not be assumed that just because nurses often have the role of advocate they are always the best person to advocate in every situation.

As Brown stated in Burnard and Chapman (1992): 'Advocacy is a means of transferring the power back to the patient'.

Another way to transfer power back to the patient/parent is through truthfulness and giving appropriate information. This belief is based upon an adaptation of the following statement (we should substitute patient for parent in some cases, due to the age or cognitive level of the child):

> Not telling does not keep information from the patient; it merely keeps him from sharing his burden and deprives him of the opportunity of getting accurate information instead of frightening misconceptions about his illness. Instead of participating in his care, he is debarred from contributing to his own management. It is the lack of control over his own life which is most damaging to his peace of mind and to his self-esteem. (Lichter, 1989 pp. 7–16).

We need to be realistic and address our responsibility towards families whose children are to face these unpredictable long-term effects of the treatment, which may both compromise health and incur a degree of suffering in later years. Information giving allows autonomous individuals to make decisions about their own lives, or for parents to make informed decisions about their children. It is worth noting that we may not always know exactly the effectiveness of various different types of chemotherapy, or be able to predict outcomes or late effects, but this is not a justifiable reason not to fully inform parents or autonomous adolescents when we suspect that there may be some risk of after effects. Informing parents and children about the possible consequences of treatment does not relieve us of the responsibility to minimise the risks, but rather the purpose is to forewarn families about the possibility and encourage them to help in the early detection of signs and symptoms.

There is a big debate within paediatric oncology about when is the right time to discuss late effects with families. As earlier chapters will have highlighted, parents are often in a state of shock at diagnosis, and in this state they are expected to learn about their child's condition, to learn about the immediate treatment, to learn about the short-term side effects, cope with the immediate threat to their child's life, watch their child suffer early side effects, take on the responsibility for starting to care for their child at home and continue being a caring responsible parent. This hardly seems an appropriate time to start discussing potential late effects, and yet if these effects are not discussed before the child receives any treatment how are the parents giving informed consent? It is truly agonising deciding when is a 'good' time to talk to parents and give them information that they will be able to take in.

Information giving should also be an ongoing process, assessing the family's ability to take in and understand the consequences of the treatment at all stages of the child's disease trajectory. However, nurses should bear in mind that parents' response to the information that is given can be variable. Case studies 11.4 and 11.5 are prime examples of this.

As the above scenarios illustrate, parents vary tremendously in their response to information giving. In an assignment for a diploma in nursing course, one of the authors identified four basic responses to information giving (Hawkins, 1994):

- There is the *ignorance is bliss* view – these parents hold the firm belief that what they don't know can't hurt them. They do not want to be presented with a plateful of worries that might never happen and don't want to know unless we are very certain of our facts. This parent tends just to ask to be told what will be happening today or in the very near future, which they 'need to know about'. This parent will often take

Case study 11.4

Helen was receiving an anthracycline infusion as part of her treatment for a Wilm's tumour. As the sister in the day unit was setting up the infusion she thought this would be a good opportunity to explore with the child's mother how much she understood about the long-term effects of anthracyclines and the reasons behind why the drug was infused over 4–6 hours. As the information was being given with regard to the long-term cardiotoxic effect of the drug, the mother became increasingly distressed and agitated. She then expressed her horror that we could even consider talking about 'problems in the future' when she had great difficulty herself in just dealing with the day-to-day issues of her daughter and the acute effects of the treatment. She did not want to hear at all at this stage problems her daughter may or may not encounter in the future.

Case study 11.5

On a separate occasion, under the same circumstances as in Case study 11.4, another little girl, Felicity, was also receiving an anthracycline infusion. This time as the mother heard the information with regard to the late cardiotoxic effect of the drug, she simply smiled and said 'I want to hear about things that may happen in the future, as it means you are thinking that my little girl *has* a future and that's what I want to believe'.

a back seat in communication and allow their partner to take everything on board.

- The *I'm not clever enough* view (often synonymous with Doctor knows best) – This parent feels that it is no use anyone trying to explain the condition, the treatment, the long words, because they won't understand it anyway. Once they have asked the basic question 'can you cure my child?' and received an answer that holds some hope, they claim to have total confidence in out expert knowledge and care and they trust us to do what's right. Such parents will often not give you the chance to explain anything, even from experienced staff who can simplify information and use supportive visual aids. This parent, however, does usually come round to being able to accept information, as their curiosity gets the better of them and they begin to talk to other parents with whom they can identify and who can demonstrate a good knowledge of what is happening to their child.
- A *bit at a time and I'll cope* view – this parent likes to be given information in small short bursts. They tend to take away the information, think it over, digest it, ask questions about it and fit it into their jig-saw until they have built up a global picture of the situation.
- The *tell me everything* view – this parent tends to be exceptionally anxious, often well educated and articulate. They want to know everything, immediately. They ask question after question and are often starting a new battery of questions while the bewildered nurse/doctor is still carefully explaining the last answer. This parent often confuses information because they have not given themselves enough time to understand what has been said. They often, also, pick up on relatively minor points or irrelevant information and ignore what is necessary at a precise moment in time to take on board.

Getting to know families well and learning how they respond to information is a key to success in empowering them with knowledge – the wrong approach can be disastrous and will often lead to conflict and confusion. Another consideration is that within a parental partnership each partner may have a different response to information giving and they may therefore need individual time.

Harris (1985 pp. 205–215) addresses this problem of the patient's will to receive information and in particular the view that patients have a '*right to remain in ignorance* if they so wish, or if, in the judgement of the doctor, full disclosure would somehow harm the patient'. This belief of an actual 'right' to remain in ignorance develops out of the concept of respect for persons and an obligation to respect individuals' wishes about themselves. Harris argues that although we may want to respect a patient's/ parents' wishes, they have no clear rights to have the information withheld: 'There are all sorts of unpleasant things in life that we might prefer not to know about, but it does not follow that anyone infringes our rights if they inform us'. Alternately Harris presents the view that [we] have 'a "positive duty" to disclose anything [we] know about others that might be relevant to any autonomous decision they might wish to make', although Harris also finds this an unsatisfactory argument as it advocates the telling of cruel home-truths in daily life. We do, however, feel that we have an obligation to disclose information that we know will be relevant to parents' decision-making process.

Lichter (1987) takes the refusal to accept information by patients/ parents a step further, in that he believes those who do express a wish not to be told are unaware of the distress that this decision will cause them by denying themselves the opportunity to discuss the fears they must surely have. He says that by the simple expression of a wish not to know, patients are expressing that they suspect there is something serious that they would rather not discover, and therefore it is just such patients who harbour fear and anxiety, who need the opportunity to discuss their feelings and be made aware of the 'good news' that there is help available.

Both Lichter and Harris uphold the belief that we ourselves would advocate, that given the right timing, honesty, empathetic support and caring, patients/parents are able to deal with bad news, or news about uncertainties in the future, which is the main consideration for our survivors. If the parents wish to be informed about the medical implications of their child's illness, then we have an obligation to tell them the truth and to include long-term side effects in that discussion. More to the point, this information should be given before any decisions the parents have to make, so that they remain autonomous.

Rees and Rees (1989 pp. 92–94) consider the philosophy of giving details of every possible outcome of late effects of cancer treatment in view of the high incidence of malpractice suits in America, and consider the implications for this country in which they quote Lord Justice Lawton:

> It is accepted that patients should be told about common or serious side effects, but not the rare ones…a recital to the patient of all the possible hazards of treatment is unnecessary in law, and, I assume, most undesirable in medicine. Legislation must not be allowed to inhibit sound and sensible practice.

Within the realms of this issue we need to make a closer examination of autonomy and in particular the autonomy of a child: 'Autonomy should not be forced on those who do not want it'. (Dunstan, 1986 pp. 1–9). Returning to the work of Harris, he forwards a strong argument in favour of promoting patient autonomy and does not see any significant change in this rule for children:

> ...children should be in control of their own destiny, including their own health care, in the same way as are any other people...To respect autonomy is to respect a person's decisions made in the light of their present character and priorities.

Harris is arguing here that although we know children change their minds frequently and therefore the decision they make today may change in time, this is not a good enough reason to exclude their opinion when discussing their health care. While on one hand we would agree with this statement, we would be cautious to suppose that this could be true when discussing the late effects of treatment with a child. Our caution is not in assuming that a child could not understand the late effects, if introduced at their cognitive level, but in that children have a much less realistic view of the future, living predominantly in the 'here and now', and therefore concerns in the future may have little realistic meaning for them. However, we do feel that discussions about late effects should include young children so that they become familiar with the issues and develop with them over the years, with the ultimate intention that as they move into adulthood and start to attend long-term follow-up clinics without their parents they will feel comfortable discussing their health care for themselves.

Of course the law and our culture recognise that we cannot expect children who are too young or too immature to make major decisions about their lives, and it is widely accepted that there are circumstances when we must make paternalistic decisions on their behalf. There are without doubt grey areas within the law relating to children and consent and principally this is a result of the very subjective nature of the decision of whether or not a child is competent. As the Medical Ethics Institute report (Medical Ethics Institute Working Group, 1986) states: the onus on the doctor would be heavy'. Competence is generally held as *'the ability of the particular individual to comprehend the nature and consequences of the proposed procedure'*. If indeed we find in a particular case that a minor is competent to give or withhold consent, then surely we are duty bound to give that child all the information necessary to make informed decisions, including the risks of late effects of treatment. The Medical Research Council do recognize a 'cut off point' of 12 years of age, below which no child is held to be capable of enough autonomy to give or withhold consent.

The burden of making paternalistic decisions for children, and in particular the cure versus risk of late effects decisions, by and large falls in the laps of their parents or legal guardians. As Harris points out we must not assume that all parents are competent to make those decisions. In cases where the child is exceptionally precious to the parent, for example a long-awaited only child, the parent may consent to putting the child through extraordinary treatment disregarding risks of imminent and late effects, for fear of losing their child, while not being able to realistically see the effect on that child, especially the psychosocial effect. There are numerous ethical considerations within paediatric oncology. One might, for example, wish to look at the rights of parents to subject another person to a life of unfulfilment and lost capacity, by consenting to any treatment at all (Wilde, 1989 pp. 45–50).

The Medical Ethics Institute Working Group report on Clinical Research on Children (1986) submits that:

> ...it may be necessary to give *more* information where the consent to be given is proxy consent ... it would follow that the doctor must give all that information which would allow the person consenting properly to exercise his responsibilities.

In the light of the earlier discussion about parental response to information giving, the task is not easy.

A very interesting study has been recently undertaken by our clinical nurse specialist, which looked at nurses' perceptions of their role in informing parents about the potential late effects of treatment for childhood cancer. (Woodhouse 1997). The study involved sending questionnaires to 20 paediatric oncology centres in Britain, via the ward manager, who was requested to select two members of nursing staff to complete the questionnaire. This was an accidental sample as the researcher had no control over the choice of respondents. A pilot study was conducted locally to test the questionnaire format.

The questionnaire firstly established details about nursing grade, oncology experience and the unit where the respondents worked (Figures 11.1–11.3). The second section established nurses' attitudes towards parents' rights to information about late effects, nurses' roles in information giving, type of information to be imparted and timing of information giving about late effects (Figures 11.4, 11.5). Further questions elicited information about the format of information (eg. written, verbal), who should be involved in information giving and whether or not there should be guidelines for nurses to assist in imparting information on late effects.

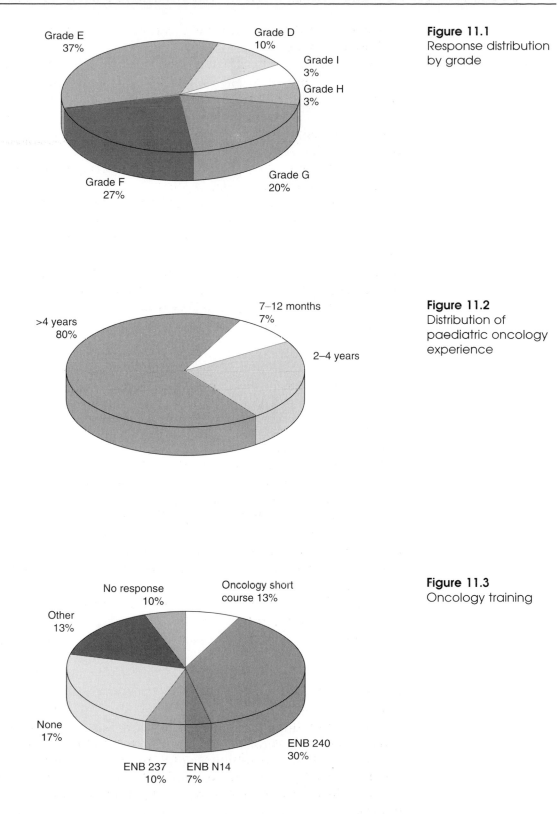

Figure 11.1
Response distribution
by grade

Figure 11.2
Distribution of
paediatric oncology
experience

Figure 11.3
Oncology training

Figure 11.4 Attitudes to specific categories of information

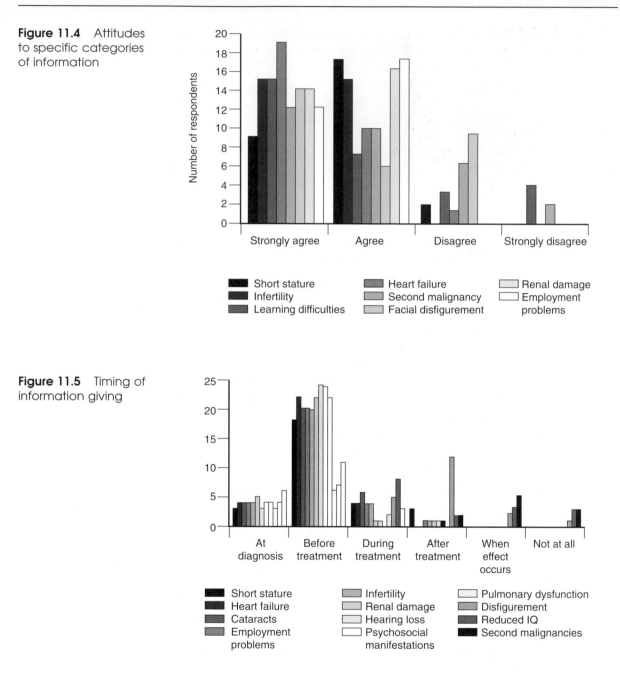

Figure 11.5 Timing of information giving

Some interesting issues were raised in this study. Only 13% of the nurses questioned felt that information giving about late effects was the responsibility mainly of the medical staff. While teaching on an ENB paediatric oncology course we encountered a nurse who said that her consultant 'would not be at all happy for nursing staff to give families information about late effects'.

In the study by Woodhouse (1997), however, 50% of respondents felt able to support information given by medical staff. All nurses in the study felt that it would be helpful to have guidelines for nurses on information giving in relation to late effects, either locally produced or through the Paediatric Oncology Nurses Forum (PONF) or jointly with the UKCCSG.

The results of this study prompted the author to produce written information for parents. The information is in the form of drug information sheets that are designed to fit into the parent/child personal held record (Hyne and Hully, 1993). Each drug sheet explains the action of the drug, appearance, how it's given, the early and late side effects and what to do if there are any problems. These were introduced in 1996 and appear to have been very well received by the parents. It would be interesting to follow up this research with further studies about the impact that this knowledge has had on the families' knowledge of late effects.

Re-integration into school

The population of children with cancer in any school district at any given time is small in comparison with the general school population. For many teachers a child with cancer is their first experience of dealing with a child with a life-threatening or chronic disease. Teachers need to be empowered by the medical team to assume a full partnership role in the reintegration of a child with cancer back into school. Deasy-Spinetta (1993)

Communication with the child's school as soon as possible is of paramount importance. Information should be of two sources:

- *Educational* – a two-way exchange of information from the child's teacher to the named liaison teacher within the hospital school, thus enabling similar educational programmes to be conducted even when the child is in hospital.
- *Medical* – with the parent's permission, the giving of relevant information regarding the child's illness and treatment, with direct reference to, for example, central venous lines, infections, and, in particular, contact with chickenpox and measles.

Visits to the school by the community oncology nurse specialist are also important. Face-to-face contacts with the child's teachers have proved, in our experience, to facilitate a smooth pathway for the child integrating into school. School teachers' study days held twice a year in our unit have also proved popular and effective. By adopting a positive approach with parents and encouraging teacher partnership, a successful integration programme can be developed.

As stated again by Deasy-Spinetta (1993):

Re-entry programmes are a cost-effective intervention when handled appropriately, they can prevent many future social and peer problems for the patient. They ensure continuity of education, which is the work of the child, and promote the continued acquisition of age appropriate adoptive behaviour skills.

Coming off treatment support, empowerment and survivor networks

The cessation of treatment would appear to be a positive event and certainly one to look forward to. However, it is becoming increasingly obvious that this is not always the case. In fact, on the contrary, this event can often lead to a crisis where families may need intervention strategies in order to facilitate their coping abilities. Initially the thought of up to 2 years of treatment with the often unpredictability of inpatient stays together with frequent attendances to the outpatient clinic seem such a daunting prospect at diagnosis; parents and children have little choice but to embark on this major disruption to their lives. However, as many of us working in the field of oncology are aware, the often long treatment phase will serve to forge strong relationships with members of the multidisciplinary team. Visits to clinic provide that much needed security as 'blood counts' are checked and children are seen and assessed at frequent intervals. When treatment comes to an end, many families feel this is a time to celebrate! Hair returns, often in a completely new format, and children will look forward to having central lines removed and that long-awaited dive into the swimming pool! But underneath all that, anxieties and fears develop for the family. In our experience many families comment that they suddenly lose their 'support network' and 'where is everyone now that we are off treatment?', even as an extreme, 'no one cares any more.' One mother sums up the mixture of feelings and new experiences that occur at the end of treatment:

When the treatment first ended, it was so hard not to have to go to hospital any more. It is strange how something that could be so intrusive was now longed for because of the reassurance it could give! In the same way, I could never have imagined I would lose touch with the friends I made in those days. During the treatment, the lives we lived on the ward, the other parents and myself, were lived in each others pockets. Much of the time we were experiencing incredible, intense emotion, and as a result, incredibly intense friendships were formed. As I look back, it is hard to believe they have passed; but of course, life has moved on for each of us, and our paths have separated. I found it hardest to come to terms with the fact that some of the parents, who had lost a child did not want me around because of the memories I carried with me. I ached to be able to help in some way and had to learn that staying away was the best support I could give them.

Little has been found in the literature with regard to identifying this as a crisis point for families, but we certainly see families experiencing something close to post-traumatic stress disorder, reporting 'flashbacks and nightmares'. Cincotta (1993), however, does state that:

> The exit from treatment rekindles feelings that may have been suppressed since the time of initial diagnosis and brings with it fear about the possibility of recurrence. Chemotherapy and clinic visits may have inadvertently served an emotionally comforting role. When the course of treatment is over and personal contact is less frequent, 'perceived protection' from cancer is lost and anxiety can be heightened.

For professionals this may also be a difficult time. On the one hand we want to share with the families their joy at coming off treatment, but on the other hand this may somewhat be tempered by the knowledge of other children whose disease has recurred after completing treatment. Issues again can be raised with regard to fostering the families' dependence on 'the team'. How often should families be contacted once they are off treatment? Should it be the role of the community oncology nurse specialist to initiate increased contact at home with the families at this point, or should we be empowering families to put their own coping mechanisms in place? Cincotta also suggests 'off-treatment' meetings similar to those that occur at diagnosis can be helpful to address concerns and prepare families for the future. Drop-in nurse-led, off-treatment clinics have also been suggested by our American colleagues as a way forward in recognising the support families may need at this time. For the survivors themselves coming off treatment is also a period of adjustment, as they must 'learn new skills to live beyond the diagnosis and treatment of malignancy – not an easy task for many who are not offered the level of support, teaching and rehabilitation that was available earlier in their illness.' (McCaffrey, 1991).

In Lozowski's work (1993) on the 'Views of childhood cancer survivors', out of 300 off-treatment cancer survivors interviewed 70% said they would like to meet other off-treatment cancer survivors. Clearly, long-term survivors of childhood cancer need to share their cancer experience with others in similar situations, not just during their diagnosis and treatment, but long into their disease-free years.

Developing the follow-up services

The purpose of follow-up for cancer survivors is twofold. Firstly it enables medical staff, nursing staff and researchers to collect data on the incidence and nature of late effects. The second purpose, and equally as important, is monitoring the health of the survivors. As knowledge of the long-term effects of cancer and its treatment increases, evidence is mounting that cancer survivors need to aim for a healthy lifestyle.

Health education is an essential role for oncology nurses working with cancer survivors. The development of nurse practitioners in this country is a role that is ideally suited to long term follow-up clinics. Nurses have a role in 'promoting new behaviours for enhancing the early detection of recurrent disease and reducing the risk factors for second malignancies' (Rose, 1989). This role also includes health education that simply promotes healthy living, which can have a direct effect on psychological well being. Both Gavin (1994) and Sullivan (1982) suggest that nurses are better placed than physicians to deliver health education, stating that nurses offer 'something special' that increases adherence and compliance.

The role of the nurse practitioner in the long-term follow-up clinic has been developed in oncology centres in the USA over the past 20 years. As far back as 1976 a paediatric nurse practitioner in oncology was developed by the oncology division at the Children's Hospital of Philadelphia, focusing on the development of nurse practitioner skills, such as history taking and physical assessment, and combining skills of the clinical nurse specialist such as those of educating and researching (Hobbie and Hollen, 1993).

This American model of combining the skills of the clinical nurse specialist and nurse practitioner would appear to be the way forward for nurses who wish to specialise in caring for survivors in the long-term follow-up period. Thus this developed advanced practice role would combine the function of direct care provider with the indirect care roles of change agent, community liaison and researcher.

Historically, follow-up clinics for long-term survivors in the USA have predominantly been nurse-run clinics (Hobbie and Hollen, 1993). The nurse practitioner works as part of a multidisciplinary team, including the paediatric oncologist, the radiotherapist, the adult oncologist, the psychologist, the social worker, school liaison and the specially identified physician such as an orthopaedic surgeon or endocrinologist. The nurse practitioner acts as leader/

facilitator, presenting the survivor's case history, and validates the appropriate evaluations and interventions with the other team members.

In developing new roles we must, of course, look to the benefit of such a service to the survivor and family. The advantage of nurse-run clinics as found in the USA would enable the families to have easy access to a specialty care provider, increasing the likelihood of continuity of care.

Long-term survivors are a unique population with high-risk needs. By providing innovative care to a group with common needs, Hobbie and Hollen (1993) suggest that nurse-run clinics 'enhance the service and marketability while reducing costs'. For nurses who wish to specialise in this area there is the opportunity to break new ground in practice in the UK by completing health assessment courses at advanced practitioner/degree level. Although the opportunity, level of education and specialist nursing skills are available, we may need to spend some time convincing our medical colleagues, and indeed our own managers, of the benefits of such a service.

Health education is an individual focused activity, which involves targeting a specific group of individuals who are seen to be 'at risk' of illness, disease or accident due to inherent or environmental risk factors; aiming to promote, maintain or restore health. (Beckman-Murray and Proctor-Zentner, 1989 pp. 25–26). However, by targeting cancer survivors for health education, there is a danger that the individual may fail to perceive the benefit of preventing cancer but may focus on the fact that they have an increased risk of second malignancy or long-term complications. Individuals may have been unaware of the risks of late effects, particularly those children who were too young to remember the experience, and may already indulge in health risk behaviours. Some individuals may find such interest in their future health an undesirable psychological burden. They may feel powerless to alter their current behaviour, or may even have so many other physical, psychological or social problems that such information is too much to cope with. O'Neill, (1975), in his work on the 'psychological aspects of cancer recovery', identifies that patients may have a heightened concern or even a preoccupation with their health, and these individuals need sensitive health education so as not to escalate their fears into an obsession, but still to impart the information they need. It is for this reason that the assessment of individuals must be as sensitive as possible and nurses need to be able to judge when such information would be untimely for the individual.

The concept of risk taking is worth further consideration to help nurses predict individual responsiveness to active health education. Does surviving cancer lead an individual to see cancer as less of a risk because it is survivable, or more of a risk because it may not be as treatable the second time around? Hollen and Hobbie (1996) proposed that survivors may take fewer risks because they have been 'compelled to reprioritise values' due to the illness experience; for example, constant exposure to reducing health risks. However, it is also true that having once beaten cancer, individuals may engage in more risk-taking activity. The experience of having cancer once may invoke feelings of fatalism and inevitability and the individual may not perceive preventative measures to have any real influence on their health. Indeed we have personal experience of an adolescent boy who successfully survived his cancer following bone marrow transplantation and was later tragically killed in an accident in which his family recognise he was taking a huge risk. Indeed since completing his treatment he had particularly enjoyed 'close to the edge' sport and leisure activities. It would be difficult to establish whether the cancer experience had a direct effect on his behaviour or whether he would have enjoyed such experiences anyway, as many adolescent boys do.

Alternatively, 'if people perceive themselves as being susceptible to a serious disease (or late effects), they may be more willing to accept recommendations for prevention and early detection.' McGuire, (1985) and Rose, (1989), suggest that strategies for health promotion should reinforce optimism about the future, encouraging patients to take control, and protect themselves against future problems.

Integrating quality-of-life issues into treatment protocols – promoting a coping model

The final section of this chapter has focused on how we can help survivors adjust to the consequences of their treatment, through effective information giving (understanding the needs of the whole family), facing the ethical dilemma's of cost versus cure with families and survivors from the start of treatment, re-integrating children into school or supporting special needs, reviewing the provision of off-treatment support and developing follow-up support. Addressing all of these issues means moving towards what Chang (1991) calls a 'Coping model' of care. It aims to leave behind the 'Crisis intervention model' that allowed young adults to suddenly discover their infertility years after treatment, as we gave an example of earlier. Chang talks about problem solving and adjusting, advocating a system which 'assists families to cope with the chronicity of the illness and the continuous stress'. Chang talks about cancer survivors needing to be assisted in 'mastering developmental tasks required to cope with the demands of the illness'. However, it is not clear from this one article quite what these developmental tasks are, nor how we can teach people to cope. He suggests that the goal of psychological help should be the promotion of quality of life. Bearing in mind our discussions earlier in the chapter, it can only be assumed that Chang means we should identify for each individual what elements of life constitute quality for them, and employ whatever agencies are needed to teach the individual new skills to achieve more for themselves.

One way to encourage the use of a coping model is to further integrate quality of life issues into treatment protocols. Many protocols and clinical trials available in the 1990s are aiming at modifying treatment to reduce the late effects without compromising survival rates. These modifications however predominantly consider reducing physical late effects. Although this may assist with reducing psychosocial late effects indirectly because of the correlation between the two, it does demonstrate that psychosocial issues may still be secondary considerations.

Eiser and Jenney (1996) make suggestions for raising the priority of quality of life issues in clinical trials. They recognise that little is known about how to 'quantify the impact of treatment' and the actual experience of late effects as opposed to the incidence of late effects. They suggest that measures of impact of treatment should be included in randomised studies.

Once clinical trials and protocols raise awareness of the cost versus cure debate, and long-term sequelae are considered throughout treatment, we will be closer to promoting a coping model of care, where survivors are given the opportunity and support to adjust with the implications of treatment. Indeed through recent discussion with our medical colleagues we can anticipate seeing changes to protocols in the next few years, as quality of life issues increase in profile in the medical profession.

Conclusion

As we move into the twenty-first century, the 'truly cured' child is now an achievable aim for all of us working in the field of paediatric oncology. Given the evidence that is constantly emerging, our whole philosophy of care must encompass a holistic approach. Nurses caring for the childhood cancer survivor must be knowledgeable about chemotherapeutic agents and the potential or actual impact they have on the children's lives, but along with those issues, the more subtle and perhaps more fundamentally challenging to the care of these children are those of a psychosocial nature.

This chapter has attempted to provide the reader with an overview of how children with cancer and their families journey through their survivorship and rehabilitation. The review of the literature and personal experiences enable us to recognise that childhood cancer can bring about many negative experiences for the child and family. However, it can also be related to self improvement and to survivors acquiring values that are likely to change their lives for the better.

An issue that is often raised among survivors, is their need to meet with and talk to other survivors. Lozowski (1993) in her article 'Views of childhood survivors' suggests that:

> Health care providers and administrators should encourage and organize meetings between survivors … Through a national network, survivors with similar experiences can share their concerns, their struggles, and their triumphs.

In the UK there is already a national network of parent support groups. Perhaps they, together with members of the multidisciplinary team, could work together to achieve this level of support for our survivors.

Caring for a child with cancer is always a challenge but, returning to the words of Spinetta (1993), when we care for our children we need to 'hold their hand, walk them through it and teach them how to deal with it'.

References

Barr, R. Furlong, W. & Dawson, S. (1993) An assessment of global health status in survivors of acute lymphoblastic leukaemia in childhood. *American Journal of Acute Lymphoblastic Leukaemia in Childhood*, **15**, 284–290.

Beckman-Murray, R. & Proctor-Zentner, J. (1989) Basic considerations in health and illness *in* Howells, C. *Nursing Concepts for Health Promotion*, 1st adapted edition UK. London: Prentice Hall International (UK).

Blacklay, A.E. (ed.) (1997) (United Kingdom Children's Cancer Study Group late effects group.) *After Cure: Surviving Cancer, what does this mean for you?* Welwyn Garden City, Herts: Serono Laboratories.

Bowlby, J. (1953) *Child Care and the Growth of Love*. London/Tonbridge: Pelican/Whitefriars.

Brouwers, P. & Poplack. D. (1990) Memory and learning sequelae in long-term survivors of acute lymphoblastic leukaemia: association with attention deficits. *American Journal of Pediatric Hematology/Oncology*, **12**, 174–181.

Brown, R. Madan-Swain, A. & Lambert, R. (1992) Chemotherapy for acute lymphocytic leukaemia: cognitive and academic sequelae. *Journal of Pediatrics*, **121**, 885–889.

Burnard, P. & Chapman, C.M. (1992) *Professional and Ethical Issues in Nursing: The Code of Professional Conduct*, 4th edn. Chichester: John Wiley.

Byrne, J., Lewis, S. & Halamek, L. (1989) Childhood cancer survivors' knowledge of their diagnosis and treatment. *Annals of Internal Medicine*, **110**, 400–403.

Cancer Research Campaign (1990) *Childhood Cancer*. Factsheet 153.

Chang, P. (1991) Psychosocial needs of long-term childhood cancer survivors: a review of literature. *Pediatrician*, **18**, 20–24.

Cincotta, N. (1993) Psychosocial issues in the world of children with cancer. *Cancer*, **71**(Suppl.), 3251–3260.

D'Angio, G.M. (1982) The child cured of cancer: a problem for the internist. *Seminars in Oncology*, **9**: 143–149.

Darwin, C. (1859) *The Origin of Species.*

Deasy-Spinetta, P. (1993) School issues and the child with cancer. *Cancer*, **73**, 3261–3264.

Dunstan, G.R. (1986) The doctor as the responsible moral agent *in* Dunstan, G.R. & Shinebourne, E.A. eds. *Doctors decisions; ethical conflicts in medical practice.* Oxford: Oxford University Press.

Eiser, C. & Jenney, M.E.M. (1996) Measuring symptomatic benefit and quality of life in paediatric oncology. *British Journal of Cancer*, **73**, 1313–1316.

Everhart, C. (1991) Overcoming childhood cancer misconceptions among long-term survivors. *Journal of Paediatric Oncology Nursing*, **8**(1), 46–48.

Fitzmaurice, N. (1996) Palliative Care Degree Course, unpublished assignment. University of Central England, Birmingham.

Fraumeni, J.F. (1975) Respiratory carcinogenesis: an epidemiologic appraisal. *Journal of the National Cancer Institute*, **55**, 1039–1046.

Garbett, R. (1996) Did the NHS fail Child B? *Nursing Times*, **92**(36), 33–36.

Gavin, A. (1994) Nurse practitioners; here to stay? *Journal of Community Nursing*, January, 12–14.

Harris, J. (1985) *The Value of Human Life: an introduction to medical ethics.* New York.: Routledge & Kegan Paul.

Hawkins, J.M. (1990) The Hawkins Paediatric Nursing Model for Family Centred Care, unpublished. Oncology Unit, Birmingham Children's Hospital NHS Trust. B16 8ET

Hawkins, J.M. (1994) Ethical Issues in Information Giving about the Late Effects of Cancer

Treatment, unpublished. University of Central England in Birmingham, Diploma in Professional Studies in Nursing Year II.

Hays, D. (1993) Adult survivors of childhood cancer – employment and insurance issues at different age groups. *Cancer* **71** (Suppl.), 3306–3309.

Hobbie, W. & Hollen, P. (1993) Paediatric nurse practitioners specializing with survivors of childhood cancer. *Journal of Paediatric Health Care*, **7**, 24–30.

Hollen, P. & Hobbie, W. (1996) Decision making and risk behaviors of cancer-surviving adolescents and their peers. *Journal of Paediatric Oncology Nursing*, **13**(3), 121–134.

Hoppe-Hirsch, E., Renier, D. & Lelloch-Tubiana, A. (1990) Medulloblastoma in childhood: progressive intellectual deterioration. *Child's Nervous System*, **6**, 60–65.

Hyne, J. & Hully, M. (1993) Using parent held records in an oncology unit. *Pediatric Nursing*, **5**(8), 14–16.

Karon, M. (1973) Problems in the evaluation of long-term results *in* Mathe, G., Pouillart, P. & Schwarzenberg, L. eds. *Recent Results in Cancer Research*, pp. 13–120 New York: Springer-Verlag

Koocher, G. (1985) Psychosocial care of the child cured of cancer. *Pediatric Nursing*, **11**(2), 91–93.

Koocher, G.P. & O'Malley, J.E. (1981) *The Damocles Syndrome.* London: McGraw-Hill.

Kupst, M. (1993) Family coping. Supportive and obstructive factors. *Cancer* **71** (suppl.), 3337–3341.

Lansky, S.B., List, M., Ritter-Sterr, C. *et al.* (1985) *in* Nesbit, M. ed. *Clinics in Oncology: Late effects*

in successfully treated children with cancer, vol. 4, no. 2, pp. 205–221. London: W.B. Saunders.

Levy, M. & Stillman, R. (1991) Reproductive potential in survivors of childhood malignancy. *Pediatrician*, **18**, 61–70.

Lichter, I. (1989) The right to bad news *in* Stall, B. ed. *Ethical Dilemmas in Cancer Care*, pp. 7–16. Basingstoke: Macmillan Press Scientific and Medical.

Lozowski, S. (1993) Views of childhood cancer survivors. Selected perspectives. *Cancer* **71**(suppl.), 3354–3357.

McCaffrey, D. (1991) Surviving cancer. *Nursing Times*, **87**(32), 26–30.

McGuire, D.B. (1985) Preventive health practices and educational needs in families with hereditary melanoma. *Cancer Nurse*, **8**(1): 29–36.

Meadows, A.T. (1989) Second neoplasms in childhood cancer survivors. *Journal of American Pediatric Oncology Nurses*, **6**(1), 7–11.

Medical Ethics Institute Working Group (1986) Report; medical research with children: ethics, law and practice *in* Nicholson, R.H. ed. *Children and the Law*, 1st edn. Chap. 6. Oxford: Oxford University Press.

Moore, I., Glasser, M. & Ablin, A. (1987) The late psychosocial consequences of childhood cancer. *Journal of Paediatric Nursing*, **3**(3), 150–158.

Morris-Jones, P. & Craft, A. (1990) Childhood cancer: cure at what cost? *Archives of Disease in Childhood*, **65**, 638–640.

Mostow, E., Byrne, J. & Connelly, R. (1991) Quality of life in long-term survivors of CNS tumors of childhood and adolescence. *Journal of Clinical Oncology*, **9**, 592–599.

Mulhern, R.K., Horowitz, M.E. Ochs, J. *et al.* (1989) Assessment of quality of life among pediatric patients with cancer. *Journal of Consultant Clinical Psychology*, **1**, 130.

Mullan, F. (1984) Seasons of Survival: reflections of a physician with Cancer. *New England Journal of Medicine*, **313**, 270–273.

Nicholson, H. & Byrne, J. (1993) Fertility and pregnancy after treatment for cancer during childhood or adolescence. *Cancer*, **71**(Suppl.), 3392–3399.

O'Neill, M.P. (1975) Psychological aspects of cancer recovery. *Cancer*, **36**(Suppl.), 271–273.

Rees, G.J.G. & Rees, A.A.D. (1989) Defensive medicine or malpractice suits? *in* Stoll, B. ed. *Ethical Dilemmas in Cancer Care*. Basingstake: Macmillan Press, Scientific Medical.

Robison, L. (1993) Issues in the consideration of intervention strategies in long-term survivors of childhood cancer. *Cancer* **71**(suppl.), 3406–3410.

Rose. M.A. (1989) Health promotion and risk prevention: application for cancer survivors. *Oncology Nursing Forum*, **16**, 335–340.

Ruccione, K. (1985) The role of nurses in late effects evaluation *in* Nesbit, M. ed. *Clinics in Oncology: late effects in successfully treated children with cancer*, vol. 4, no. 2, pp. 205–221. London: W.B. Saunders.

Spinetta, J. (1993) Conference Lecture. Psychological Late Effects: the myths of surviving childhood cancer. Late Effects Conference, Manchester, UK. May 1993. England.

Sposto, R. & Hammond, G. (1985) Survival in childhood cancer *in* Nesbit, M. ed. *Clinics in Oncology: late effects in successfully treated children with*

cancer. vol. 4, no. 2, pp. 195–203. London: W.B. Saunders.

Sullivan. J. (1982) Research on nurse practitioners. Processes behind the outcome. *American Journal of Public Health*, **72**: 8–9.

van Eys. J. (1991) The truly cured child? *Pediatrician*, **18**, 90–95.

Wilde, J. (1989) Caesarean section: whose choice and for whom? *in* Dunstan, G.R. & Shinebourne, E.A. eds. *Doctors Decisions: ethical conflicts in medical practice*, pp. 45–50 Oxford: Oxford University Press.

Woodhouse, S.L. (1997) Winner of Paediatric Oncology Nurses Forum-Best Poster Award. Childhood into the 21st. Century. Joint UKCCSG/ PONF (Paediatric Oncology Nurses Forum) Conference. Birmingham, UK, April 1997.

Zeltzer, L. (1993) Cancer in adolescents and young adults – psychosocial aspects. *Cancer* **71**(Suppl.), 3463–3468.

Further reading

Bisset, D. & Kunkeler, L. (1990) Long-term sequelae of treatment for testicular germ cell tumours. *Cancer*, **62**, 655–659.

Chesler, M. (1993) Introduction to psychosocial issues. *Cancer*, **71** (Suppl.), 3245–3250.

Crooks, G.M., Baron-Hay, G.S. & Byrne, G.C. (1991) Late effects of childhood malignancies seen in Western Australia. *American Journal of Pediatric Hematology/ Oncology*, **13**, 442–449.

Davies, H. (1993) Late problems faced by childhood cancer survivors. *British Journal of Hospital Medicine*, **50**, 137–140.

Dorfman, E. (1996) Observations from a survivor of childhood

cancer. *Journal of Paediatric Oncology Nursing*, **13** (4), 235–236.

Eiser, C. & Lansdown, R. (1977) Retrospective study of intellectual development in children treated for acute lymphoblastic leukaemia. *Archives of Disease in Childhood*, **52**, 525–529.

Feeney, D., Furlong, W. & Barr, R. (1992) A comprehensive multiattribute system for classifying the health status of survivors of childhood cancer. *Journal of Clinical Oncology*, **10**, 923–928.

Frank-Stromborg, M. (1989) Reaction to the diagnosis of cancer questionnaire: development and psychometric evaluation. *Nursing Research*, **38**, 364–369.

Gamis, A. & Nesbit, M. (1991)

Neuropsychologic (cognitive) disabilities in long-term survivors of childhood cancer. *Pediatrician*, **18**(1), 11–19.

Greenberg, H., Kazak, A. & Meadows, A. (1989) Psychologic functioning in 8–16-year-old cancer survivors and their parents. *Journal of Pediatrics*, **114**, 488–493.

Hays, D., Landsverk, J. & Sallen, S. (1992) Educational, occupational, and insurance status of childhood cancer survivors in their fourth and fifth decades of life. *Journal of Clinical Oncology*, **10**, 1397–1406.

Lynam, M. (1987) The parent network in paediatric oncology. Supportive or not.? *Cancer Nursing*, **10**, 207–216.

Noll, R., Bukowski, W. & Davies, W. (1993) Adjustment in the peer system of adolescents with Cancer: a two-year study. *Journal of Pediatric Psychology*, **18**, 351–364.

Pinkerton, R. (1992) Avoiding chemotherapy related late effects in children with curable tumours. *Archives of Disease in Childhood*, **65**, 1116–1119.

Rogers, P. (1992) Late effects in childhood cancer survivors. *Journal of Paediatric Nursing*, **7**, 364–365.

Rosen, D. (1993) Transition to adult health care for adolescents and young adults with cancer. *Cancer*, **71**(suppl.), 3411–3414.

Waber, D., Tarbell, N. & Kahn, C. (1992) The relationship of sex and treatment modality to neuropsychologic outcome in childhood acute lymphoblastic leukaemia. *Journal of Clinical Oncology*, **10**, 810–817.

Waterworth, S. (1992) Long-term effects of cancer on children and their families. *British Journal of Nursing*, **1**, 373–377.

Weekes, D. & Kagan, S. (1994) Adolescents completing cancer therapy: meaning, perception, and coping. *Oncology Nursing Forum*, **21**, 663–670.

Yamamoto, M., Fukunaga, Y. & Tsukimoto, I. (1991) Late effects of childhood acute leukaemia and its treatment. *Acta Paediatrica Japonica – Overseas Edition*, **33**, 573–588.

The dying child   12

SALLY CURNICK AND ANNE HARRIS

Introduction

In the past, the death of a child was not an uncommon event, and it would have been usual for the child to be cared for within the family. The combination of childhood disease and poverty meant that families through the social strata would be at risk of facing the death of a child, therefore death was more commonplace and consequently discussed and coped with in an open manner.

Throughout the second half of the twentieth century as health care became more readily accessible, particularly with the birth of the NHS promising free care for all, medical intervention improved, childhood death through illness became less common and people relied heavily on the props of treatment to prevent or postpone death. When death became inevitable, parents were deskilled, and with demographic changes meaning that people were more mobile and likely to be living away from their extended family, it became more usual for the terminal phase of a child's illness to be managed in hospital. Inevitably death in hospital was managed by medical and nursing staff and was frequently clinical and sanitised (Corr and Doka, 1994). This had the effect of making the death less real to the immediate family, who were often not actively involved in the care of their child. Death became hospital based with little or no involvement on the part of the wider community. As a result the primary health care team did not develop the expertise and confidence required to care for a child dying at home.

As the adult hospice movement developed and raised awareness of the rights and views of dying adults, offering them an alternative to hospital-based death, those involved with the care of children facing death began to explore alternatives.

Throughout the last decade, planned terminal care for children has been increasingly community based. This has required a different focus and the increased involvement of the primary health care team.

Key points
- Planning care
- Symptom control
- Appropriate support
- Siblings
- Bereavement care

Planned and negotiated palliative care

To ensure optimum palliative care, all involved parties need to be working with identical aims and a mutual acceptance of the inevitability of death. Without the mutual understanding and agreement, the family are likely to receive mixed messages about the ultimate outcome. However, professionals working with the family must remember that although they may appreciate that death is inevitable, it is likely that the family will operate at a degree of denial necessary to enable them to cope with everyday living (Case study 12.1). Denial that enables the family functioning is a common response and the professionals should be wary of challenging it:

> It is clear that hope and optimism must be encouraged, but it is vital that parents receive appropriate information and guidance to assist them to make educated decisions about treatment. (Evans, 1987).

Consideration should be given to the person most appropriate to discuss with the child and their family that active curative therapy is no longer appropriate and to start the negotiation of palliative care. As with the initial diagnosis, such information will take time to be absorbed and the discussion may need to be repeated many times. Parents will often need time to assimilate the information before they are able to discuss with their child the altered circumstances: 'Parents also are more willing to be open with their children when given appropriate support' (Bluebond-Laugner, 1992). Information giving is often staggered to go at the child's pace and one at which the family feel comfortable. Parents need to be aware of the information circulating within the community and to set appropriate boundaries to ensure that the child receives relevant information in a manner that they would wish (Case study 12.2).

Case study 12.1

Robyn, a 17-year-old girl in the terminal phase of a disfiguring tumour, was aware that her death was imminent, but after making all the plans that she considered necessary, chose to ignore the fact and carried on with plans for her future. If drawn into discussion about her prognosis, she remained optimistic and denied the possibility of her death until the last few days of her life, when she requested clarification of factual information regarding death. Her parents remained convinced that her optimism prolonged her life and for their part made the terminal phase of her illness more bearable.

> **Case study 12.2**
>
> Laura, a 10-year-old child, returned to a small village for palliative care; at that time she had been told neither her diagnosis or prognosis and her parents did not feel that she would have coped with the knowledge. However, having been home for a few hours, her best friend came to visit and announced 'Mum says you've got a brain tumour and that you are going to die'. This caused Laura to distrust any further information given by her family and led to major difficulties in family functioning.

The Act Charter for Children with Life-Threatening Conditions, highlights the need for children's involvement in planning for their care (Box 1.2). Crompton (1990) states that 'Honesty is the one and only policy'. An important role of the nurse is to help parents reach a stage at which they can be completely honest with their child. It is an understandable parental response to wish to protect one's child from harm or distress, however if the child is to be fully integrated into a partnership of care with both professionals and parents as dictated by the Children Act 1989, then they need to operate from an equal knowledge base.

Open communication is dependent on honesty and trust. To withhold information from children, whatever the motive, merely undermines this trust. However, nurses must remember that honesty can be very painful and must be confident in their ability to convey information sensitively and remain a source of support to the family. Despite explanations of the benefits of a policy of honesty, some parents will maintain their right to withhold the truth from their child. Although this stance can be difficult for the professionals working with the family to accept, parental wishes have to be respected and the professional has no right to over-rule them. In such situations consideration should be given to an agreement being made with the family to the effect that while the decision will be respected, should the child ask a direct question regarding their prognosis, the professional would not lie. Often, however, children are aware of parental reluctance to explore various topics and will rarely raise the subject themselves:

> It is really important to tell people their real condition. If you don't, they'll never trust you. At first my Mom told the Doctor 'We're not telling her' but the Doctor told her they were going to tell me. I knew. There were no secrets between our family, nothing was hidden. Doctor's conferences were held in my room. That made things a lot easier, even if at first it was kind of hard. A dying person usually knows his

condition anyway and can tell if things aren't being told to him. It helps a person accept the truths, the sooner they know the facts. That's the way Doctors and the family can help the patient most. (Spinetta and Deasy-Spinetta, 1981 pp. 15, 72)

Bluebond-Laugner (1992) identifies the idea of mutual presence in which all family members are aware of the truth but collude with each other to avoid meaningful discussion. Children will often adhere to family rules even if it is not comfortable for them.

It is imperative in situations such as that discussed in Case study 12.3 that the professionals involved with the family have an arena in which they can discuss the feelings that are raised by working in an atmosphere of distress. It is important these feelings are acknowledged and worked through to minimise any detrimental effect on the working relationship. Despite differences of opinion, the philosophy of family-led care must remain of paramount importance.

At the time of cessation of active curative therapy, the family should be asked to consider where they would like their child's terminal care to be managed and where they would like their child to die. It should be stressed, however, that they are not required to make a firm unalterable decision at this stage: 'A main feature of the palliative approach is to offer care in a setting of the client's choice' (Farrell and Allen, 1998).

It is not uncommon for parents to opt to return home with a certainty that there would be a bed available should they wish to return to hospital as their child becomes less well.

Young people who are involved in the decision-making process regarding the place of death will often choose to remain at home where they feel they retain some control over their lives, it is also possible to retain a greater degree of normality as regards school attendance, etc. if the child is home based. Adolescents sometimes

Case study 12.3

Gareth, an 18-year-old boy, was dying at home. His family decided that although they were aware of his prognosis, he was not to be informed of his imminent death. His brother found the situation too painful to endure and chose to opt out of family life, his parents continued to make plans for his future and while Gareth entered into these plans, he found it painful and was frequently in tears during these discussions. Despite interventions from the many professionals involved in his care, his mother considered it to be in his best interests for him to remain unaware of his prognosis. An agreement was made with the family, which resulted in no professional being left alone with Gareth to ensure such a discussion would not be possible.

elect to remain in hospital for the terminal phase of their illness, and it is interesting to consider the possible reasons for this:

- The developmental stage of adolescence means that the young person is breaking away from parental control and developing independence; it can be very difficult to readjust to a dependent role within the family and to rely on parental help for the most basic human functions.
- There is often a very strong desire to spare their parents the pain of watching them die while being involved with the day-to-day caregiving.
- Perhaps the adolescent has started to view death in a adult way, that it is something of which our society is ashamed and which should therefore be institutionalised and controlled.
- They are often terrified about their impending death and the process of dying and trust the nursing and medical staff to manage their symptoms more effectively than their parents. Within this there is often a subconscious belief that the staff will prevent death occurring, this is often despite a full understanding of the inevitability of their death.

If the child and family elect to stay in hospital, the agreement should be made that the child is free to come and go as they are able. Within the nursing team, there should be discussion as to how appropriate it is to undertake routine observations and investigations on a child being cared for in the palliative phase of their illness. It should be borne in mind however that if these procedures are abruptly halted, the young person and their family may feel abandoned within the ward setting and feel like intruders who are falsely occupying an acute medical bed.

It is important to consider the effect on the ward staff while caring for a dying child in the ward setting. Nurses' anxieties about their competence can manifest themselves by distancing from the patient and their family. Care should be taken to ensure that adequate support is available to help staff recognise these patterns of behaviour and develop strategies to cope with them: 'Nurses will be able to fulfill their enhanced responsibilities in care of the dying and care of the bereaved most effectively if they are well prepared to do so' (Corr and Doka, 1994).

It is usual for most children and families to return home for at least some of the terminal phase of their illness, therefore it is imperative that direct contact is re-established with the relevant members of the primary health care team. Although throughout the treatment phase of the child's illness the primary health care team should have been kept involved by means of regular dis-charge summaries while planning shared palliative care, it is pre-ferable that a meeting to include hospital- and community-based health staff is arranged. The aim of the meeting is to share information and plan optimum care for the family. The topics for discussions should include:

- the likely progression of disease
- the likely mode of death
- symptom control
- the estimated timescale
- the roles of the involved professionals.

This meeting should also offer an opportunity for professionals to share personal experiences that may make their participation in the care of the family inappropriate – it should always be acknowledged that caring for a dying child is highly stressful and it is vital that all the core members of the care team feel committed to offering ongoing care for as long as necessary without feeling under an unwilling obligation to participate. At the conclusion of the meeting there should be an established programme of care agreed that will ensure the family are adequately supported but not overwhelmed by professionals. There must also be the proviso that the care plan may be subject to unexpected change and professionals must be prepared to remain flexible. It is important that, once established, communication remains open, on a two-way basis with the inclusion of the family.

It is desirable that all professionals involved in the care of the child collaborate to provide seamless care that transfers from hospital to home with minimal disruption to the family. It is vital to ensure that one named professional acts as co-ordinator for the care: 'The named key worker must be acceptable to the family, preferably chosen by them, and used by the family and all involved as the main referral point and channel for discussion and information' (ACT and RCPGP, 1997). It is common for this role to be assumed by the paediatric oncology outreach nurse specialist (POONS). These workers have the advantage of being known to the child and family throughout the treatment process and have access to both community and hospital staff.

Despite the increasing involvement of the primary health care team, it is important that the hospital retains an input with family. This ensures that the family do not feel abandoned by the hospital team once curative therapy has ceased, and also that the primary health care team has easy access to paediatric expertise as necessary.

As has been discussed in previous chapters, it is vital that the general practitioner (GP) has been involved throughout the treatment process. It would be unrealistic of hospital medical staff to expect the primary health care team to re-establish the main care role for a family with whom they have had neither direct nor indirect contact since diagnosis. This difficulty can be heightened if the family perceive that the diagnosis was badly handled by the primary health care team and if this perception has not been addressed by hospital staff during the treatment process.

As has already been mentioned, the child and family will need time to deal with their altered circumstances and the information that they have been given, however it is not uncommon for parents to experience some sense of relief at the cessation of curative therapy. It is acknowledged that families with children with malignant disease experience 'the Damocles syndrome' (Eisenberg, 1981 p. 11), in that they live with continuing uncertainty and the fear of disease recurrence. Once the child has moved to requiring palliative care, the parents' worst fears have been realised and there is some sense of relaxation of anxiety. This can be difficult for parents to manage who experience considerable guilt feeling any sense of relief about their child's inevitable death. It is the first certainty that they will have been given since their child's diagnosis and, although unpleasant, can enable them to move forward.

As the child and family adapt and settle into a new routine at home, the process of information sharing needs to be continued. Again, it needs to be at a pace dictated by the child and family, but needs to include the likely mode of death and assurance that the professional will be honest about any deterioration in the child's condition. Parents are often anxious to be given some idea of timescale, however the professionals should be wary of giving any concrete suggestion of timing which may prove to be incorrect. (Case study 12.4).

It is helpful, if the family are able, that they give thoughts to the arrangements that will be necessary immediately after the death of their child. If possible they need to consider the following issues:

- Which undertaker to employ.
- Whether they would like to keep their child at home until the funeral.

Case study 12.4

A 16-year-old girl with a recurrent relapse of a solid tumour was told her life expectancy was approximately 6 months and that she should plan accordingly. She decided that she would live every day as fully as possible and make no contingency plans for her future. She remained extremely well for 2 years after being given this information, with palliative care being required for a further 6 months. Prior to her death she stated she was very angry she had been given false information, as she viewed it, feeling that she would have behaved differently had she known her life expectancy was longer.

- Whether they wish burial or cremation.
- Type of funeral service.

It is important that any children in the family have an opportunity to express their views and opinions when considering the above.

The involvement of dying children in the making of the above decisions will vary depending on their age, understanding and life experience to date. When attempting to involve children in the decision-making process, an understanding of their awareness of their situation is vital. Lansdown and Benjamin (1985) identified different stages of awareness and understanding that a child with a life-threatening condition goes through:

- I am very sick.
- I have an illness that can kill people.
- I have an illness that can kill children.
- I may not get better.

Most children will know that their illness is serious, even if they do not know that they are going to die, and will plan accordingly (Case study 12.5).

Many young people however will welcome the opportunity to make a formal will. Parents can find this an impossible task to contemplate and children, sensing parental unease, will be reluctant to mention it. Professionals working with the family should be aware that this is a likely scenario (Case study 12.6) and give the young person space to discuss it if they wish.

Case study 12.5

Simon, a 9-year-old boy, was in the terminal phase of his illness, although he had not been included in discussions about his death. However, in the weeks prior to his death he sold all of his toys without making any attempt to replace them. When asked about this he merely stated that he no longer required them.

Case study 12.6

Diana, a 16-year-old girl, made her will and funeral plans in secret as soon as the decision to cease curative therapy was made. She was the only member of her family to have a religious faith and she did not feel that any other family member would carry out her wishes. After her death, her family found written instructions regarding her funeral, will and a headstone, along with letters to each family member.

> **☞** **Case study 12.7**
>
> Darren, a 14-year-old boy, could not discuss his wishes with his family, but insisted that the community nurse brought a typewriter to the home in order to dictate his will and instructions to her. He was clear that his will had to be typed as he was certain that nobody would be able to read her writing!

Another scenario that may arise is described in Case study 12.7. The above two examples highlight the way in which young people will ensure that their wishes are known, while trying to protect their parents. It enables young people to retain control in the situation when they can feel entirely powerless.

Living with dying

While working with children facing death, the underlying philosophy must be to help them live until they die. Once the focus of treatment switches from curative to palliative care, ensuring good quality of life must become of paramount importance:

- maintenance of normality
- optimum symptom control
- minimal medical intervention.

Maintenance of normality

While the concept of maintaining normality can seem out of place when discussing terminal care in childhood, recognition should be given to its importance in coping with these situations.

> The desire for a normal life is palpable, and if achievement of that sense of normalcy means altering the realm of normal to accommodate changes in the patient's condition, so be it. This is not to say that patients and their family members deny what is happening, but rather that they choose to compartmentalize information about the disease and the patient's condition. (Bluebond-Laugner, 1992)

Once the family have adapted to their altered circumstances, in order to maintain family functioning, it is helpful to retain structure to the day. Many children will choose to remain at school for as long as they are able, enjoying the social contact with their peer group and also a break from their home environment:

> The emphasis on securing the child's return to normal

schooling applies equally to children with life-threatening diseases, and dying children, who also have a right to education suited to their age, ability, needs and health at the time. (Department of Health, 1994)

While this choice should be supported and encouraged, it is only fair that contact should be re-established with school. As has been discussed previously, many teachers have considerable anxieties about reintegrating children with cancer back into the class while on treatment. When faced with reintegrating a child known to be dying, many teachers will find the task too daunting to consider.The staff need regular contact with the hospital community team to give them up-to-date information regarding the child's health. They need reassurance that while the child is known to be dying it is not likely that:

- The child will die in school.
- The child will continue to attend school while very sick.

Teachers will often welcome some input as to how to help the rest of the class cope with the altered situation. As previously discussed, prior to entering into discussions of this nature it is vital to establish the wishes of the child and family as regards dissemination of information. Often the family do not want the child's class to be made aware that their classmate is dying, feeling that the child will be ostracised by peers; however at this stage it would be prudent for the teaching staff to remind the class that the child is ill and sometimes may have to miss school.

Some children may be unable to attend full days at school but may wish to attend certain classes or events. With discussion, most schools are willing and able to accommodate this, particularly as the child becomes less well.

The *Guide to Development of Children's Palliative Care Services 1997* (ACT and RCPGP, 1997) highlights the benefits of school attendance in terms of sustaining quality of lifestyle for as long as feasible, but also highlighting the need for adequate information and support.

Some children will be unable to return to school, or will elect not to return to school. For those children it is important that some structure is given to the day. In these circumstances consideration should be given to arranging home tuition for the child. Although it is recognised that educational development is no longer the primary motive, it offers the child some diversion to the day and a break for the carer.

Case study 12.8 an excellent example of the flexibility that can be obtained if hospital and school staff work in co-operation.

For those children who are either pre-school age or unable to

> **☞ Case study 12.8**
>
> Mark, a 14-year-old boy, chose not to return to school when he was told that he was dying. Having not particularly enjoyed school, he viewed this as an excellent excuse not to go, however he missed the company of his peers. After discussion with the school, it was arranged that each week his tutor would visit with a group of his friends for a 'lesson'.

attend school, it can be appropriate to arrange for a play specialist from the hospital to visit at home. As with the provision of home tuition, this provides a structure to the day and also an opportunity for the child to interact with somebody from outside the immediate family group. Parents often welcome regular contact from play specialist staff, as they view it as a link with the hospital. A common fear of families who have elected for home terminal care is that they will be abandoned by the hospital, while they are reassured by contact with liaison nurses, they appreciate the support offered by staff whom they view as safe. The child enjoys having one-to-one attention from somebody with whom they have established a relationship of trust. It is often during these sessions that the child will feel able to discuss their fears and beliefs, particularly while using play as a means of communication. Burton (1974) emphasises the importance of non-verbal communication via toys, favourite clothes, food, etc. to aid verbal communication. It must be recognised that as children will often confide in the play specialist staff, involving them in regular visiting during the palliative phase of the child's care carries a very high stress content. To ensure their professional survival, the play specialist must be offered regular ongoing supervision to enable them to deal with the personal impact of the work. It is also important that the play specialist has the opportunity to discuss with other members of the community team anything they think is relevant to the future planning of the child's care.

Minimal medical intervention

Once the decision to switch from palliative care has been made, then careful consideration should be given prior to undertaking any investigation. Blood counts should no longer be done routinely, only if the child becomes symptomatic. Parents can find the cessation of regular blood counts difficult to accept, feeling that it underlines the significance of the change in the focus of treatment. Reassurance should be given to the family that symptoms will always be treated to ensure a good quality of life with minimal intervention.

This should also be true for children who are hospital based for palliative care, however it must be acknowledged that this can be harder to achieve in the ward situation where the atmosphere is one of acute care. A balance must be achieved between unnecessary medical and nursing procedures and the dying child being left in a bed in the corner of the ward feeling overlooked by staff involved in the more acute aspects of care.

Optimum symptom control

The ultimate aim of good palliative care is to alleviate or prevent any unpleasant symptoms. The symptom the child and the family fear most is unrelieved pain – they need to be reassured that appropriate drugs will be prescribed throughout at a dosage required at that time (see Appendix 12.1).

Adequate symptom control relies on an open two-way communication between the family and professionals – this is particularly important when caring for younger children who may not be able to vocalise their needs but whose behaviour can be interpreted by their parents as to their requirements for analgesia, etc. The drugs and dosages required to keep children symptom free can be quite daunting for families and professionals unused to caring for dying children. However, the enhanced quality of life gained from the use of opiates, etc. quickly becomes apparent, and families usually have little difficulty in increasing the dose to maintain the status quo.

Complementary therapies

A common response to being told that curative treatment is no longer available is for families to search for another option in the many complementary therapies available. Once extended family and friends are made aware of the situation, they will often proffer advice regarding so called 'miracle cures', or the availability of better treatment in other countries. This can be very stressful for families who are having to come to terms with the imminent death of their child. It is a natural parental reaction to wish to do anything to prolong the life of their child, and they will often need the support of professionals to refuse to become involved in following these dreams.

While it is the rule of the professional to actively dissuade parents from anything that would be potentially detrimental to their child, they should support the use of any of the complementary therapies that can be used as an aid to relaxation or to promote well being. Parents will often appreciate actively contributing to their child's well being. If one accepts that parents often experience an overwhelming sense of helplessness, feeling that they have given up on their child and are allowing them to die, then the use of massage, visualisation and aromatherapy can both involve them in active care while giving benefit to both the child and parent.

Spiritual support

Many families will have pre-existing sources of spiritual support which will continue to be valuable throughout the palliative phase of the illness. However it is not uncommon for families with little or no pre-existing religious faith to want to have contact with the relevant spiritual leader appropriate to their culture. There can be issues of faith that families wish to discuss with a neutral person but can be bewildered as to how to begin. Families can be fearful that it will be viewed in a negative light that they are only seeking spiritual support because they are facing the death of their child. However there are often issues around events, such as the baptism of their child, that they may wish to explore. The child facing death may well wish to discuss their own faith and any queries that they have.

It is important in this, as in all other aspects of care, that the child's wishes are respected and acted upon, as shown in Case study 12.9.

It is not an uncommon reaction for families to direct their anger at the situation towards 'God'; often their need to see a spiritual leader is influenced by their wish to vent this anger. They should be reassured that this is a common reaction and that the vicar, or religious leader, will not be threatened or dismayed by it but may help them work through their feelings.

Given the multicultural nature of society, it is important that professionals involved with the family have access to information and advice from differing spiritual leaders. As with all aspects of care, the child and family must be viewed as individuals and time taken to establish individual beliefs and relevant rituals surrounding death.

At times of heightened emotion there can be a danger of imposing one's own views or beliefs: Neuberger (1987) suggests this is rarely out of arrogance, rather out of a lack of understanding.

Case study 12.9

Marie a 13-year-old girl facing death was clear that she wanted to be baptised prior to death. As her parents had no professed religious faith, it was difficult for them to accept, however they arranged for her to meet with a vicar at home and she was baptised 2 weeks prior to her death.

Faith healing

As has been discussed previously, families can find stopping treatment and 'doing nothing' hard to cope with, feeling that they have given up on their child. Embarking on a course of faith healing can often fulfil the need to do something positive while being manageable within the home. Professionals involved with the family should try to ensure that they use a reputable faith healer who will not exploit the family either financially or emotionally.

Professionals can be very disparaging of the use of faith healers, believing that they have no place within palliative care as they have no proven success. However, their beneficial role in terms of the psychology of family functioning should not be underestimated.

Professionals working in this field should be able to set aside their personal views or opinions and support families in the use of any intervention that is not detrimental to the child and facilitates their coping mechanisms.

Terminal care

As the child deteriorates it is likely that there will be increased involvement of professionals.

If the family have elected to care for their child at home, they will require increasing support to enable them to cope. This eventuality should have been discussed at the meeting with the primary health care team and plans made to cover this. The family should have 24-hour access to professional advice and support by telephone, with the knowledge that someone they know will visit as necessary.

It is likely that the family will request daily visits from the community nurses to advise on adequate analgesia and general care. As the child becomes less well, it is usual for them to eat and drink less. This can be a very hard phase for parents to accept – ensuring that your child has adequate nutrition is a fundamental parental role and watching your child fade away has a huge impact on them. The parents need support and reassurance that they are doing the best they can for their child and that they are meeting their needs at that time.

At this time, it is usual for parents to have assumed responsibility for their child's medication and the community team should respect their assessment of their child's requirements on a daily basis. They should also ensure adequate stocks of drugs are readily available should the child have an escalation of pain. It should be remembered that starting opiates can be a difficult step for families, who will often view it as 'the beginning of the end'

– given this, some parents will choose not to be actually involved in its administration.

During this phase there are various practical points that need to be discussed with the family to ensure that they are as well prepared as possible for their child's death. These include:

- The likely mode of death – families are often very fearful about the process of dying. This can be encouraged by the media's portrayal of death.
- How they will recognise that their child has died – it is not uncommon for people never to have seen a dead body and parents can fear that they will miss it.
- Who they need to contact after the death.

Although parents are often reluctant to raise these topics, once the professional has done so they are usually relieved as it can be an issue that has been causing them concern but feel they will be seen as callous discussing their child's death and practical tasks relating to it prior to the event.

It is not unusual for the dying child to have very clear ideas about how they wish their death to be managed, and although these can be uncomfortable discussions for parents to initiate, the professional should encourage them to include the child fully in the decision-making process.

The family should be made aware that, if they want, a member of the community team will go to be with them when their child dies. Some families will request company as they see their child deteriorate, others will not make contact with anyone until after the child has died. It is important that this is led by family wishes, the professional must consider and respect individual family functioning, their role should be supportive and not undermining of parental ability.

After death, parents will often appreciate support while they carry out the practical tasks such as washing or dressing their child. If they elect for their child to be removed by undertakers, they often need support to cope while their child leaves the house. The professional can ease this initial separation by being sensitive to the practicalities necessary. If requested, undertakers will not use body bags for younger children, and will not close the bag if the child is older. It can be advisable to suggest that the family do not watch their child being taken from the house; it can be easier for them to say their initial goodbye and then let the undertaker carry on alone.

Some families will choose to keep their child at home until the funeral. Undertakers can take a coffin to the home, although some undertakers prefer to take the child to their chapel of rest for a few hours prior to returning them to the home. If the family wish to keep their child at home, there are practical considerations that need to be taken into account.

- Where will the family keep the child.
- Will the body be maintained at the correct temperature.
- Does the whole family agree with this decision.

Professionals often express anxieties about the ability of the family to give up their child for burial or cremation if they have not taken the first step of letting the child go to the undertakers. However some families see this decision as an essential first task in the bereavement process.

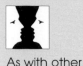

As with other issues, the personal feelings of the professional should not be allowed to sway their interaction with the bereaved family, professionals should be aware of how their experiences may influence their view point.

> It is generally accepted that, given the choice, terminally ill patients prefer to be cared for at home for as long as possible. It would seem that this choice for home care might be even stronger for families of terminally ill children. Farrell and Allen, 1998).

This is not to suggest that adequate terminal care cannot be given in hospital, rather that a switch in nursing emphasis is necessary in the ward situation to ensure that parents continue to feel in control of their child's care.

If the child remains in hospital during the terminal phase of the illness, the family should be given as much responsibility as they wish for their child's care. Difficulties can arise around drug administration, particularly for families who have been at home managing the drug regimen. Parents can find the delay caused by bureaucracy surrounding opiates in hospital difficult to accept and allowances should be made when allocating staff to care for the child.

If the child dies in hospital, the family should be given as much time and privacy as they require to carry out the rituals that they view as important. When possible a member of staff should explain the procedure to parents, including the fact that their child can be returned home if that is their wish.

While the impact of a death on the rest of the ward should not be minimised, the family should not feel under any pressure to leave until they feel ready to do so. If they do not wish their child to return home, they should be told they can return to hospital or the local undertakers to see their child as often as they wish.

The time between death and the funeral is a time of limbo for families. They are busy with the practicalities surrounding death, therefore the start of the grieving process can be delayed until after the funeral. During this time consideration should be given to regular contact with the family, particular if contact leading up to the death has been intense. Abrupt cessation of contact increases the sense of isolation that families experience at a time when familiar routines are important.

Although many families appreciate contact and the attendance of professional staff at the funeral, it should never be assumed that one will be welcome. Some families need to keep this period of their life private as a way of reclaiming their child from the illness experience. While it is acknowledged that staff have a need to complete their contact with the child and say goodbye, the wishes of the family must be paramount and staff may need to find an alternative means of ending contact.

The converse of the scenario is also true in that families often want many hospital staff to attended the funeral and can be very hurt if there is no hospital representative. It should be remembered that families often develop very strong links with each other and exchange experiences – a bereaved family can have problems if they hear of many staff attending one funeral if nobody has attended their child's service.

Although it is recognised that staff will develop different relationships with families, consideration should be given to a ward policy around how to acknowledge the death of a child.

Bereavement care

As with all other aspects of care, it is not possible to suggest a blueprint of bereavement care, it should be tailored to meet the needs of each individual family while accepting that families may not want any further involvement with hospital or community staff. However, it is widely accepted that everybody needs education and information about grief to help them deal with the experience of bereavement. Worden (1991), identified four main tasks for mourning which he states must be completed to resolve one's grief:

- To accept the reality of loss.
- To work through the pain of grief.
- To adjust to an environment in which the deceased is missing.
- To emotionally relocate the deceased and move on with life (the task of resolution).

While remembering that grief is a normal process following death, families can be very fearful of the strong emotions that they may experience and it can be helpful to offer a list of the various support agencies that are available.

Immediately after their child's funeral many families have a need for regular contact with the people who were involved with caring for their child. This transitional phase is necessary to enable them to start letting go of the experience they have gone through and often involves the need to retell their story many times. It can be difficult for close families and friends to cope with hearing the same tale repeatedly at a time when they are also dealing with their grief. This can be an important role for the professional to fulfil – while it is accepted that the professional will also have their feelings of grief, it is to be hoped that the professional boundary will mean that they can step back from the intensity of grief and remain objective. However, it must be remembered that staff need some outlet for their feelings around the death of a child with whom they have developed a close relationship and there is often a possibility of support within the work environment, either through ward meetings arranged specifically to debrief following a death of a child, or through the provision of a work-based counsellor available for one-to-one support. Nevertheless, every individual must take some responsibility for their own support and it is suggested that each professional should ensure they have an external source of support. The effect of working with children facing death should not be minimised and it should be reinforced to each new staff member that without properly arranged support, their professional survival may be compromised. While the benefits of friends and family should not be minimised, it is unfair to rely on them as a sole means of support when dealing with work-related issues.

After the death of a child, the hospital team should try to arrange contact with the primary health care team to evaluate the efficacy of home-based terminal care. This gives an opportunity for professionals to share their feelings and also to make plans to improve their contact/role should a similar situation arise again. Given that GPs often identify a sense of exclusion from the treatment process, if they have been involved in offering palliative care, it is vital that the hospital staff acknowledge their input, without which it is likely that the family would have received suboptimum care. While the hospital input will end with the death of the child, the primary health care team will have an ongoing involvement with the family, and it is therefore important that a working relationship is maintained.

In the period following the death of a child, it is desirable for contact to be made with the child's school. Teaching staff can find it difficult to know how to support other pupils with whom the child was friendly. They can be grateful for advice about how to mark the child's absence in school, perhaps as a memorial assembly or the planting of a tree in the playground. Although the ideas are usually ones with which the staff feel comfortable, they may need reassurance that this is beneficial to everyone in the school environment to give them confidence to pursue the task. Children with whom the child was particularly friendly made need extra support and staff should be given information regarding common manifestations of childhood grief to help them identify those who are having difficulty in coping with their feelings.

Subsequent contact with the bereaved family should be dictated by their requirements, and it is assumed that for the majority of people this will lessen as the months pass. Although the family's grief will not be resolved, they will have developed external coping mechanisms and their need for regular prolonged contact with the hospital staff will decrease. It should be made explicit that this contact can always be re-established as necessary. However hospital-led contact can continue, with cards sent on significant dates to let the family know their child is remembered.

Many units organise an annual memorial service open to all bereaved families as a public acknowledgement of their ongoing grief for their child. This service can involve all family members and gives an opportunity for each to share their emotions. As the time since the death passes, these services gain in significance, offering a legitimate opportunity to remember and grieve for one's child.

Given that grief is individual, it is not possible to offer a service that will meet the needs of every bereaved family. As with families who choose not to retain contact with the hospital following the death of their child, the worker must accept that many families will elect not to attend a memorial service or events arranged by the ward. This does not minimise their grief, merely that they have chosen an alternative means of support. While this can be difficult for staff who would wish to see families again to reassure themselves that they are coping, the decision must be respected and one must remember that in situations such as these it is the family whose needs are of paramount importance.

Complicated grief

As has been discussed, most families will grieve in an entirely appropriate manner. However it is important to identify families who are likely to be at risk of complicated grief. This rarely arises from circumstances around the death alone, rather it is brought about by many factors, but nursing staff should be aware of the two groups most at risk:

- Those bereaved through sudden or unexpected death.
- Those bereaved following a prolonged terminal phase.

Complicated grief can be:

- avoided

- delayed
- excessive
- prolonged.

Staff working with bereaved families need to be aware of the manifestations of complicated grief in order to assess the possible need for referral to further specialist professional help. Although the manifestations of complicated grief are very similar to those grieving normally, i.e. anger, guilt, depression and idealisation, anger and guilt tend to be the most powerful emotions with prolonged anger being directed towards staff involved in caring for their child. If the anger is not given an outlet for expression then it can become internalised, leading to profound depression or suicidal thinking. It is important when embarking on bereavement work with either an individual or family that some though should be given to assessing the risk factors indicating complicated grief. These factors include:

- place of death
- coincidental losses
- successive losses
- nature of the loss
- existing support
- cultural background
- intimacy level of the lost relationship
- grief history of the bereaved person
- emotional complexity of relationship lost
- degree of isolation and capacity to trust others
- ability to express feelings
- ability to tolerate uncomfortable feelings
- desire for change
- preparedness to trust in the counselling relationship.

Given that the whole person needs to be grieved for to ensure that grief is successful, if a number of the above factors are present, consideration should be given to the most appropriate worker to help the bereaved person resolve their grief.

Given that some families will display complicated grief, nursing staff should feel able to refer to specialist bereavement support without feeling that they have failed the family. Staff should remember that their expertise lies in different areas and they may have neither the time nor skill required to offer the necessary depth of support.

Sibling support

As has been discussed in previous chapters, siblings of a child with malignant disease can have a difficult time in dealing with the illness experience. They can have a strong sense of isolation from their parents who are caring for the sick child while they are expected to carry on with their everyday routine with little thought given to their emotions. They can struggle with understanding while their sibling is sick, often fearing that they are in some way responsible. They can be aware that they should treat their sick sibling in a different way while resenting the obligation to alter their behaviour. These feelings can be magnified when it becomes apparent that treatment is not going to be successful and that their sibling will die.

It is desirable for siblings to be kept as involved as they wish during the terminal phase of illness. It is not uncommon for children to elect to stay away for much of the time, finding the situation too painful to bear. In these situations parents should be dissuaded from forcing any involvement which is likely to only increase a sense of resentment felt by the child.

After the death of the child, siblings may experience a wide range of emotions of which, depending on their age, they will have little understanding. It is a time when they need the security of familiar routines, but this can be difficult to maintain given that their parents are grieving.

Fox (1988) describes four tasks for grieving youngsters:

Task I   To understand or begin to make sense out of what has happened or is happening.
Task II   To grieve or express emotional responses to loss.
Task III   To commemorate in some formal or informal manner the life of the person who has died.
Task IV   To learn how to begin to integrate the loss into one's life in order to go on with the everyday activities of living and loving.

The worker should take time to help adults understand the manifestations of childhood grief and different patterns of adult and child grieving. It is important that these are understood to help the adults help their surviving children. Children can appear callous and matter of fact about death and parents who have no knowledge of the patterns of childhood grief can find this difficult to accept.

Remaining children can experience a strong sense of survivor guilt, finding it hard to move on with their lives.

The scenario in Case study 12.10 highlights the need for sibling information and education about the disease process from the outset of the illness and the need to offer healthy children time to deal with their emotions.

Children have a need to complete any unfinished business following a death in order to enable them to move on. This can

Case study 12.10

Dean, a 7-year-old boy, felt responsible for the death of his brother and felt the only way to make amends would be to attempt suicide. He felt that his mother would cope with her pain with less difficulty if she was not faced with a living (but less good) reminder of her loss. He formulated a clear plan which was only aborted when it came to the attention of professionals working with the family. His mother was unable to reassure him of his worth because of her profound grief and previous psychiatric history and, despite the extensive involvement of psychiatric teams, 9 years on his sense of guilt remains undiminished.

be achieved by allowing them time with the person after death to say a final private goodbye, or suggesting that they may like to write a letter to accompany the child in the coffin.

As with adults, complicated grief is exacerbated by the lack of opportunity to say goodbye or by having no permission to mourn the deceased. Children are often encouraged to be 'the strong family member', to help their parents grieve, however this can deny the feelings of sadness that a child has making them believe that their grief is not legitimate.

Siblings' opinions regarding their attendance at the funeral should be sought and listened to. Parents often feel that they will be unable to cope with their other children at a funeral; however if the child wishes to go this should be facilitated by identifying another adult who will care for them. The child who has no opportunity to attend the funeral is likely to develop fantasies about the reality of the situation.

As with adults, grief in children is a normal emotion following death. However they can experience a strong sense of isolation, particularly if they return to school and are expected to carry on with no acknowledgment of their loss. It is important that contact is made with school prior to the child's return and that there is an acknowledgement of their experience.

It can be helpful for children to be invited to join bereavement support groups which help them understand that they are not alone and that there are people who can help them work through their grief. These groups offer a neutral environment of support, but some children will require more intensive one-to-one support to help them move on.

It is important to remember that grief will be long lasting for children and often fuelled by transitional development stages. It is necessary to differentiate between age-appropriate developmental tasks and grief-related behaviour to assess the need for further intervention.

It is not uncommon for bereaved children to feel under pressure to live out the life of the child who has died and to adopt their goals. In these circumstances it becomes increasingly difficult when they overtake their dead sibling in age or experience. However, with support from their parents or professionals, most children will cope with the experience of bereavement and be able to live their own life.

The most important message for a bereaved sibling to receive is that although the death of their sibling is a tragedy, it is alright for them to live their own life and have fun.

Conclusion

The key to good practice when working with a dying child and the child's family should lie in regular ongoing open communication between all key people involved in the care of the child. It is essential that all parties involved in the care are working towards the same goal and have had an opportunity to explore the optimum way to achieve them.

As with all holistic care, the child and family should feel that they are in a position to fully participate in discussions around formulating a plan of care and also feel safe when raising issues that arc causing them concern. However, it must be remembered that in some cases families may find this too difficult and may choose to opt out of much of the planning for care. In these situations it must be remembered that a family who choose not to participate in the formulation of care plans for their child need to be included at all other stages of care.

Optimum palliative care requires professionals to approach the situation with both honesty and commitment, therefore adequate care must be taken of the involved professionals to prevent burnout and the overwhelming stress that can come hand in hand with repeated exposure to families facing the death of their child. Staff support is an element that is often overlooked when planning palliative care, however it should be seen as integral to any workable plan.

While it could be argued that one never gets over the death of a child and it can take years to begin to come to terms with the experience, it should be possible with adequate planning for the family to look back on the experience as one that was well managed and in which they felt they were viewed as equally participative members.

References

ACT & RCPCH (1997) *Guide to Development of Children's Palliative Care Services*. London: ACT/RCPCH.

Bluebond-Laugner, M. (1992) *Children and Death: directions for the 90s*. New Jersey: Princeton University Press.

Burton, L. (1974) *Care of the Child Facing Death*. London: Routledge Kegan Paul.

Corr, C.A. & Doka, K.J. (1994) Current models of death, dying and bereavement. *Critical Care Nursing Clinics of North America*, **6**(3), 545–552.

Crompton, M. (1990) *Attending to Children Direct Work in Social and Health Care*. London: Edward Arnold.

Department of Health (1994) The Education of Sick Children. NHS Executive Circular No 12/94. London: HMSO.

Eisenberg, L. (1981) *in* Koocher, G.P. & Malley, J.E. eds. *The Damocles Syndrome*. New York: McGraw-Hill.

Evans, M. (1987) Learning to lose fear. *Nursing Times*, **83**(17), 55–56.

Farrell, M. & Allen S. (1998) Hospice at home – our first year. *Paediatric Nursing*, **10**(7), 18–20.

Fox, S.S. (1988) *Good Grief: helping groups of children when a friend dies*. The New England Association for the Education of Young Children.

Lansdown, R. & Benjamin, G. (1985) The development of the concept of death in children aged 5–9 years. *Child Care Health and Development*, **11**, 13–20.

Neuberger, J. (1987) *Caring for Dying People of Different Faiths. Lisa Sainsbury Foundation Series*. London: Austin Coluish Publishers.

Spinetta, J.J. & Deasy-Spinetta, P. (1981) *Living with Childhood Cancer*. St Louis, MO: Mosby.

Worden, J.W. (1982) *Grief Counselling and Grief Therapy: a handbook for the neutral health practitioner*. New York: Spiniper.

Appendix 12.1 GUIDELINES FOR DRUGS IN TERMINAL CARE

Dr Joanna Chambers, Bristol Children's Hospital

ANALGESICS

Mild pain

Paracetamol

	Tabs	500 mg (also dispersible)
	Liquid	120 mg/5 ml

Dose

< 1 yr	12 mg/kg	4 hourly
1–5 yr	120–240 mg	4 hourly
6–12 yr	240–500 mg	4 hourly

Moderate pain

Dihydrocodeine

	Tabs	30 mg
		60 mg Continus also available
	Liquid	10 mg/5 ml
	i.v.	50 mg/ml

Dose

	0.5–1 mg/kg	4 hourly

Dose

Maximum dose 60 mg 4 hourly; give after food if possible. NB Can give 1.5 times 4 hourly dose for the last dose at night. For sustained release tablets calculate total daily dose and give as two divided doses.

NSAIDs

- Particularly useful for bone pain
- Care if child thrombocytopenic

Diclofenac

Tabs	25 mg, 50 mg
Dispersible	50 mg
Supp.	100 mg; paediatric 12.5 mg

Dose

> 1 yr	1–3 mg/kg/day in divided doses
> 12 yrs	75–150 mg/day in divided doses

Ibuprofen

Tabs	200 mg, 400 mg
Spansules (m/r)	300 mg (Fenbid)
Tabs m/r	800 mg (Brufen retard)
Syrup	100 mg/5 ml

Dose

Child	20 mg/kg/day in 3 or 4 divided doses
> 12 yr	200 mg t.d.s. to 400 mg t.d.s.
	Give after food

Severe pain

Diamorphine

Oral	Liquid	5–100 mg/ml (water/chloroform water)
	Tabs	10 mg (dispersible)

Doses (starting)

0.1 mg/kg–0.2 mg/kg 4 hourly (usually 0.2 mg/kg if previous dihydrocodeine)

NB: 1000 µg = 1 mg

Parenteral	i.v. or s.c.
i.v./s.c.	4 hourly i.v. push or continuous infusion

Doses

i.v. bolus (slow) half oral dose
i.v. infusion 20–100 µg/kg/h

Tolerance more of a problem with i.v. than oral diamorphine. Intermittent bolus worse than continuous infusion

Morphine

Oral	tabs	10 mg; 20 mg
	liquid	10 mg/5 ml; 100 mg/5 ml

Slow-release tabs – M.S.T.
10, 15, 30, 60, 100, 200 mg tabs
Slow-release suspension
20 mg and 30 mg sachets

Rectal   10 mg, 15 mg, 20 mg and 30 mg suppositories

Dose

Oral

< 1 month	150 µg/kg 4 hourly	
1–12 months	200 micrograms/kg 4 hourly	
> 1 yr	150–300 µg/kg 4 hourly	

usually:

1–5 years	2.5–5 mg	4 hourly
6–12 years	5–10 mg	4 hourly
M.S.T.	6 × 4 hourly dose in 2 doses 12 hours apart	

Assessment prior to each dose.

Guidelines (not rigid) for incremental increases of diamorphine

Doses up to 20 mg 4 hourly	5 mg increment
Doses up to 40 mg 4 hourly	10 mg increment
Doses 40–100 mg 4 hourly	20 mg increment
Doses > 100–150 mg 4 hourly	25–40 mg increment

Alternatively first increase by 50% and then by 25% increments

Table of equivalent doses

10 mg diamorphine orally = 5 mg diamorphine i.v. or subcut.
= 15 mg morphine orally
= 10 mg morphine i.v.
= 30 mg morphine rectally

NB:

- Not all pains are caused by cancer or relieved by morphine. It may be appropriate to use other drugs; e.g. abdominal pain may be caused by constipation, treat with laxatives, or colic, treat with hyoscine butylbromide.
- Neuropathic pain will need coanalgesics such as anticonvulsants or/and antidepressants.
- For the pain of raised intracranial pressure consider high-dose dexamethasone.
- Pain from stretch of liver capsule may also respond to steroids.

LAXATIVES

Start at the same time as dihydrocodeine or diamorphine/morphine. Most patients taking opiates need a softener and a stimulant.

Stimulant laxatives

Bisacodyl
(acts in 10–12 h)

Dose
Oral or rectal
5 mg nocte may be increased to 10–15 mg nocte

Senokot
(acts in 8–10 h)

Dose
age 2–6 yr   syrup (7.5 mg/5 ml)   2.5–5 ml nocte
age > 6 yr   syrup 5–10 ml nocte
               tabs 7.5 mg   1–2 nocte
               also chocolate-flavoured granules (15 mg in 5 ml)

Softeners

Docusate sodium initial doses should be large

Dose
> 6 months 12.5–25 mg t.d.s.
paed – soln (12.5 mg/5 ml).
age > 12 yr 1–2 tab (100 mg tabs) b.d.

Mixed softener and stimulant

Codanthramer
(Danthron 25 mg; Poloxamer 188 200 mg)
Acts within 6–12 hours

Dose
suspension 2.5–5 ml nocte.

Codanthrusate
(Danthron 50 mg; Docusate 60 mg)

Dose
6–12 yr   1 cap. nocte
> 12 yr   1–3 caps nocte

Both may colour urine red and cause skin rash in the incontinent.

Osmotic laxatives

Lactulose
Usually insufficient on its own, takes 2 days to work, give regularly and adjust dose according to requirements.

Dose

　　　　5 ml b.d. (1–5 yr)
　　　　10 ml b.d. (6–12 yr)

Small children frequently refuse all laxatives. Use: intermittent microlette enemas (5 ml) or Dulcolax supp.

ANTIEMETICS

Aim to tailor the antiemetic to the emetic stimulus and site of action.

The main causes of vomiting in advanced cancer are:

1. Chemical

　　　　drugs,　　　　　e.g. narcotics
　　　　biochemical　　　e.g. uraemia, hypercalcaemia
　　　　toxins　　　　　e.g. infection, tumour metabolites

Site of action – chemoreceptor trigger zone.
Neuroreceptor – dopamine D_2 $5HT_3$.
Appropriate group of antiemetics:

　　　　butyrophenones, e.g. haloperidol
　　　　prokinetic agents, e.g. metoclopramide
　　　　phenothiazines

Drug of first choice – haloperidol.

2. Visceral disturbances

　　　　gastric irritation, e.g. drugs intra-abdominal tumours,
　　　　external pressure on stomach, liver stretch,

Site of action – vomiting centre.
Neuroreceptor – histamine H_1, muscarinic cholinergic and $5HT_3$.
Appropriate group of antiemetics:

　　　　antihistamines, e.g. cyclizine,
　　　　belladonna alkaloids, e.g. hyoscine

Drug of first choice – cyclizine

3. Central nervous system disturbance

　　　　pain, fear, psychological factors
　　　　raised intracranial pressure (RIP)
　　　　meningitis – chemical, carcinomatous or infective

Site of action – cerebral cortex.
Neuroreceptor – histamine H_1.
Appropriate group of antiemetics:

　　　　antihistamines, e.g. cyclizine
　　　　steroids for RIP

Drugs of first choice – cyclizine, dexamethasone

4. *Vestibular disturbances*

> local tumours −1° or 2°
> bone meets at base of skull
> motion sickness, labyrinthitis

Site of action – vestibular nucleus.
Neuroreceptor – muscarinic cholinergic, histamine H_1.
Appropriate group of antiemetics:

> belladonna alkaloids, e.g. hyoscine
> antihistamines, e.g. cyclizine

Drugs of first choice – cyclizine or hyoscine.

5. *Gastric stasis*

> narcotics
> gastric outlet obstruction

Site of action – periphery.
Use prokinetic agents, e.g. metoclopramide or domperidone.

Drugs and their doses

Cyclizine

Dose

> Oral and i.v. doses equivalent   > 10 yr 50 mg t.d.s.
> 1–10 yr 25 mg t.d.s.
>
> or
> 50–150 mg in 24 hours as 24 hours infusion with opiate

Haloperidol

Tabs/caps	0.5 mg, 1.5 mg, 5 mg, 10 mg
Liquid	1 mg/ml, 2 mg/ml, 10 mg/ml
Injection	5 mg/ml, 10 mg/ml

Dose

> oral or subcut
> 25–50 µg/kg/24 hours as b.d. dose
> can consider single night-time dose

Hyoscine hydrobromide

Dose

> 10 µg/kg s.c. may be given 6–8 hourly
> > 12 yr 600 µg/dose
> can be given as 24 hour infusion with diamorphine s.c. or i.v.

Scopoderm patches (transdermal hyoscine hydrobromide each patch releases 500 µg/72 hours)
1 patch behind the ear each 72 hours (only licenced for motion sickness in children age > 10 yr, but we have found it useful – takes 6 hours to work

Metoclopramide

(NB: dystonic reactions)

Dose

up to 1 yr (10 kg)	1 mg b.d.
1–3 yr (10–14 kg)	1 mg b.d. – t.d.s.
3–5 yr (15–19 kg)	2 mg b.d. – t.d.s.
5–9 yr (20–29 kg)	2.5 mg t.d.s.
9–12 yr (> 30 kg)	5 mg t.d.s.
> 12 yr	10 mg t.d.s.

Treat dystonic reactions with procyclidine i.m. or slow i.v. single dose may be repeated after 20 min if necessary

<2 yr 500 µg-2 mg

2–1 yr 2–5 mg

> 10 yr 5–10 mg

Domperidone

tabs	10 mg
susp.	5 mg/5 ml
supp.	30 mg

Dose

oral	child	200–400 µg/kg every 4–8 hours
	> 12 yrs	10–20 mg t.d.s.
rectal	3 times oral dose	

Prochlorperazine – oral, rectal and i.v.

Dose

250 µg/kg 8 hourly

often 5 mg 8 hourly but can increase frequency for greater effect – warning parents of possible dystonic reaction and hypotension with i.v. route

Rectal	1–4 yr	2.5 mg t.d.s.
	> 5 yr	5 mg t.d.s.
Buccal	3 mg tabs available (Buccastem)	

OTHER USEFUL DRUGS

Diazepam rectal solution

Stesolid   2 mg/ml – 2.5 ml tube i.e. 5 mg

4 mg/ml – 2.5 ml tube i.e. 10 mg

Dose

1–3 yr 5 mg

> 3 yrs 10 mg

Sodium valproate
When oral anticonvulsant not possible

Dose
i.v. (over 3–5 min) 20 mg/kg daily – see data sheet

Tranexamic acid
25 mg/kg 8 hourly orally for bleeding in the absence of haematuria.

Temazepam
Occassonally required for night sedation.

Chlorpheniramine

Dose

1–2 yr	1 mg twice daily
2–5 yr	1 mg 4–6 hourly max. 6 mg/24 h
6–12 yr	2 mg 4–6 hourly max. 12 mg/24 h

Useful for itching that occurs in some children on opiates.

Midazolam
Terminal sedation may occassionally be necessary in children; it may also be useful as an anticonvulsant by s.c. or i.v. infusion.

Injection   2 mg/ml;   5 mg/ml

Dose

50–400 µg/kg/h

Spironolactone
For malignant ascites

Dose

Child	3 mg/kg daily in divided doses
> 12 yr	100–200 mg daily increased to 400 mg if needed

Abbreviations

s.c. = subcutaneous	i.v. = intravenous
t.d.s. = three times daily	b.d. = twice daily
caps = capsules	tabs = tablets
NSAID = non-steroidal antiinflammatory drugs	soln = solution

Conclusion – the challenge for the future

HELEN LANGTON

Ending a book on paediatric oncology with a chapter on death and dying, whilst logical, does not fit with the fact that long-term survival rates for many childhood cancers are steadily improving.

While death will continue to be an outcome for some children, this book has focused on the fact that, as physical quantity of life has been extended through treatment, the psychosocial aspects which determine the quality of life through treatment and either into survivorship or death have become equally as important when caring for the child and family with cancer.

The understanding of the lived experience of the cancer journey is necessary if health care professionals are to continue to improve care and enhance partnership in care.

This understanding has been dominated by the necessary empirical view of the experience, in order to extend quantity of life. However, it is now possible to look at other perspectives in this experience such as a social science view or a phenomenological approach. These allow the nurse to develop an understanding of the interaction between the person with cancer, their culture and environment, throughout different stages of the disease process. Furthermore, by encouraging the expression of the meaning of illness through narrative, the patient's perspective comes to the forefront, encouraging insight into the fact that the patient's complaint is more extensive than the patient's symptoms.

Whilst this insight can lead to more complexity, it must be remembered that an ill person does not exist in isolation, and a cancer experience affects many others as well as the individual with the disease. Stages of illness such as these described by Mathiesan and Stam (1995) in Box 13.1 need to be explored through listening to children and their families if the nurse is to be able to offer an holistic approach to partnership in the care of the child.

As advocated in the Calman–Hine report (Department of Health, 1995), the involvement of users of the service to take the service forward is paramount. In order to foster this approach there needs to be some clarity as to the role of users. We would suggest that

---

Box 13.1   Stages of illness (adapted from Mathiesan and Stam, 1995)

- Uncertainty – symptoms detected; attempt to make sense of this
- Disruption of fit – illness real; help sought; crisis, loss of identity and control
- Striving – to regain self; self preservation; making sense of illness; prediction of the future
- Regaining wellness – regain former relationships; regain control; adaption

---

part of their role is to tell their story. This would enable nurses to identify gaps in the service and develop initiatives to diminish these gaps.

This book, by adopting a psychosocial approach to the care of the child with cancer and their family, has attempted to provoke the reader into thinking and learning more about this experience. The use of a partnership model throughout has enabled a consistency of approach, helping an exploration of the role of the child, the family and the nurse in all aspects of care.

It is hoped that this text will enable an in-depth exploration of the effect of cancer on the child, family and nurse from a psychosocial perspective. The use of reflection, action points and case studies is aimed to stimulate application of theory to practice and provide the reader with scope for further inquiry. The quality of life for children and families experiencing cancer is vitally important. This book encourages oncology nurses to listen to them and learn from them if a true partnership in care is to be achieved.

References

Department of Health (1995) *A Policy Framework for Commissioning Carer Services.* London: Department of Health.

Mathiesan, C.M. & Stam, H.J. (1995) Renegotiating identity: cancer narratives. *Sociology of Health and Illness*, **17**, 283–306.

Index

Numbers in **bold** refer to tables or illustrations